A School of Struggle

A School of Struggle

Durban's medical school and the education
of black doctors in South Africa

Vanessa Noble

UNIVERSITY OF KwaZulu-Natal Press

Published in 2013 by University of KwaZulu-Natal Press
Private Bag X01
Scottsville, 3209
South Africa
Email: books@ukzn.ac.za
Website: www.ukznpress.co.za

ISBN: 978-1-86914-252-0

Managing editor: Louis Gaigher
Editor: Jane Argall
Typesetter: Patricia Comrie
Proofreader: Lisa Compton
Indexer: Ethné Clarke
Cover design: Nicolene van Loggerenberg, Ideaexchange

Printed by Paarl Media Paarl

Contents

Acknowledgements

The writing of this book, which has taken more than a decade to complete, and has travelled with me in my journeys across a number of continents, could not have been accomplished without the kindness and generosity of many people. In its first incarnation as a dissertation at the University of Michigan, I am indebted to numerous individuals who were instrumental in its inception and development. My dissertation committee, which included David William Cohen, Carol Boyd, Nancy Rose Hunt and Catherine Burns, provided the most rigorous and astute critical readings, helped sharpen my arguments, and led me to countless sources. Two people need special mention. In his own quiet and unassuming way, David guided my thinking and writing in innumerable ways. Still waters run deep for this gentle man, upon whose incredible insights I owe so much. Catherine, too, has been an invaluable supporter in this book's journey. A special person with a warm and giving heart, enormous enthusiasm, and a fierce defender of her students, I will be forever grateful to her for her intellectual generosity and emotional support.

Over the years, many other people at the University of Michigan, particularly Frederick Cooper, Mamadou Diouf, and Elisha Renne, provided important insights and guidance in discussions with them. I also had the privilege of learning from many of my graduate student peers, primarily Caroline Jeannerat, Vukile Khumalo, Katherine Luongo, Monica Patterson, and Bhavani Raman. I thank them for their friendship too, which made a long and difficult academic journey easier. Two South Africans, Stephen Sparks and Nafisa Essop Sheik, who fortuitously started their studies at the University of Michigan when I was in my final year, provided much needed distraction and light-hearted humour. Their friendship and support was a treasure. Mention should also be made of the kindness shown to me by David's partner, Gretchen Elsner-Sommer. The caring support she showed me in the final stages of my dissertation will not be forgotten. Financial support provided over many years by the University of Michigan, is gratefully acknowledged too.

In South Africa, I would like to extend my thanks to a number of people in History at the University of KwaZulu-Natal (formerly the University of Natal), where I began my academic studies and returned to work after I completed my PhD. The Howard College campus in Durban, which I used as my research base during my visits from the USA, provided much intellectual nourishment. In later years, my colleagues on the Pietermaritzburg campus did much to give me the space to revise my manuscript. For all of their assistance, first as my mentors, but also later as my co-workers, I would like to express my deep gratitude to Keith Breckenridge, Catherine Burns, Marijke du Toit, Mandy Goedhals, Jeff Guy, Kalpana Hiralal, Vukile Khumalo, Julie Parle, Jabulani Sithole, Goolam Vahed and Thembisa Waetjen. A valued colleague, but more importantly, a dear friend, I would like to mention Julie Parle's influence on my thinking and writing. Julie provided immense encouragement and invaluable advice, especially during the process of revising my dissertation into a book, which I am so thankful for. From the title, which she helped brainstorm, to guidance on the structure and content, her influence is interwoven everywhere in the fabric of this work. I am also grateful to a number of other colleagues, graduate students and seminar participants, who read various chapters, made suggestions for references, and gave other practical advice, particularly, Peter Alegi, Prinisha Badassy, Fiona Bell, Julian Brown, Suryakanthie Chetty, Scott Cooper, Nafisa Essop Sheik, Janet Giddy, Mike Mahoney, Gerry Maré, Mandisa Mbali, Steve Reid, Gail Robinson, Paul Rouillard, Stephen Sparks and Sandi Thomson.

In Switzerland, I would like to recognise the support received from Patrick Harries and three of his graduate students, particularly Marcel Dreier (for our wonderful Swiss and South African adventures!), but also Lukas Meier and Pascal Schmid, all based at the University of Basel. I was introduced to this special group of Africanist historians through my research on another UKZN project with Catherine Burns and Julie Parle, and through UCT-based medical historian Howard Phillips. Between 2008 and 2011, I was privileged to participate in several workshops and conferences on various aspects of medical history in Africa. Moreover, they introduced me to a wide network of international medical historians who read and commented on my work. In addition to the names mentioned above, I would especially like to thank Harriet Deacon, Anne Digby, Simonne Horwitz, Shula Marks,

Glen Ncube and Helen Sweet. At one of these Basel conferences in 2011, I was also fortunate enough to cross paths again with Nancy Rose Hunt. She provided me with invaluable references and supportive advice at a crucial stage of my revisions. Her astute intellectual presence throughout the research and writing stages of this work, made this a better book, and I owe her immeasurably for that.

There are many others on whose expertise and support I leaned at various times. I owe a huge debt of gratitude to many archivists. I would like to record my special thanks to a number of people in KwaZulu-Natal, where I did most of my research. At the Campbell Collections in Durban, I would like to mention Stacey Gibson, Bobby Eldridge and Nellie Somers; at the Durban medical school's library, Norma Russell, Rani Moodley and Gail Robinson; and at the University of KwaZulu-Natal Archives in Pieter-maritzburg, Bronwyn Jenkins, Carol Jacobs and Mirenda Selepe. I am also grateful to many archivists around the country. In particular, I would like to thank those working at the National Archives Repository in Pretoria; University of the Witwatersrand staff at the Faculty of Health Science Registry Archives and Central Records Office Archives; staff at the South African History Archive in Johannesburg; those working at the Faculty of Health Sciences Registry Archives and Manuscripts and Administration Archives at the University of Cape Town; at the Medical University of Southern Africa Archives in Limpopo; at the University of Fort Hare's Archives in the Eastern Cape; and at the University of the Western Cape Mayibuye Archives Centre. I am indebted as well, to a number of deans at the time, who gave me permission to use their medical schools' archives, particularly, M. Barry Kistnasamy, Max Price and Nicky Padayachee. Helga Holst, the recently retired CEO of McCord Hospital in Durban, must also be acknowledged for making this hospital's archival documents available for research.

The research for this book also depended much on the generosity of my interview participants. I would like to record my sincere thanks and admiration for all those who willingly participated in this study. The information they provided me with, as well as the time they invested – sometimes in more than one sitting to accommodate their busy schedules – was very much appreciated. The memories of these informants' student days at the medical school in Durban provide an invaluable part of the complex history I have tried to capture in this book.

The team at University of KwaZulu-Natal Press, especially my managing editor, Louis Gaigher, must be thanked for their interest in this book and for all their hard work getting it ready for publication. It has been a great pleasure working with University of KwaZulu-Natal Press and copy-editor, Jane Argall. I am also grateful to the anonymous reviewers who gave generous advice on my manuscript.

Finally, I wish to thank my friends and family for their emotional support. Janet Duncan has been a wonderful friend and been there for me from the beginning of this process. In addition to reading parts of my work and occasionally taking notes for me in seminars, she also provided fun-filled distractions and much needed encouragement at key moments. Michelle Powell-Rees, whose friendship also extends over many years, must also be acknowledged for her unfailing support. My deepest thanks go to my mom, Heather, who was my emotional rock through the years it took to bring this book to fruition. In addition to her steadfast encouragement, she has also been a valued travel companion and occasional research assistant on a number of archival trips around South Africa. I would also like to thank my dad, Norman, my step mom, Maureen, my sister, Lauren, my gran, and my extended family. My family's love and constant support made everything possible. I could not have started this long journey, nor completed it, without them.

Abbreviations

ABM	American Board of Foreign Missions
ANC	African National Congress
ATR	Alan Taylor Residence
BCM	Black Consciousness Movement
BCP	Black Community Programmes
BPC	Black People's Convention
CHW	Community Health Worker
COPC	Community-Oriented Primary Health Care
HHMI	Howard Hughes Medical Institute
IFCH	Institute of Family and Community Health
IFP	Inkatha Freedom Party
K-RITH	KwaZulu-Natal Research Institute for Tuberculosis and HIV
MASA	Medical Association of South Africa
MB ChB	Bachelor of Medicine and Surgery
MEDUNSA	Medical University of Southern Africa
MSRC	Medical Students' Representative Council
NAMDA	National Medical and Dental Association
NHSC	National Health Services Commission
NP	National Party
NPA	Natal Provincial Administration
NUC	Natal University College
NUSAS	National Union of South African Students
PAC	Pan Africanist Congress
SAMDC	South African Medical and Dental Council
SASO	South African Students' Organisation
SCF	Student Christian Fellowship
SPFM	Social, Preventive and Family Medicine
SRC	Students' Representative Council

UCT	University of Cape Town
UDF	United Democratic Front
UDW	University of Durban-Westville
UKZN	University of KwaZulu-Natal
UN	University of Natal
UNB	University of Natal Black Section
UP	United Party
UNISA	University of South Africa
UNNE	University of Natal Non-European Section
UWC	University of the Western Cape
WITS	University of the Witwatersrand

Introduction

When in 1950 the apartheid government created a 'black faculty' in a 'white institution' it shaped an environment ordained to nurture a commonality of purpose that would far exceed its expectations. For not only was the Medical School of the University of Natal destined to produce doctors of international quality, it was also to provide the anvil on which the tools to fight its creator would be fashioned . . . [Its students] came from disparate backgrounds, but they were united in adversity . . . The corridors of the University's Faculty of Medicine became a hub of political activity, and the Alan Taylor Residence at Wentworth, the target of many raids by the security police, provided an uneasy setting for the planning of subversive actions against the state. As a result, the Medical School quickly became synonymous with the struggle against apartheid . . .

— 'History's hand in the shaping of the medical school',
*University of Natal Nelson R. Mandela School of Medicine:
50 Years of Achievement in Teaching, Service and Research*

These words, recorded in an early twenty-first-century University of KwaZulu-Natal[1] (UKZN) Medical School brochure to mark the school's 50th anniversary, highlight a number of pertinent issues that this book seeks to explore. During the apartheid years the medical school was known variously as the University of Natal Faculty of Medicine, the University of Natal Non-European Section, the University of Natal Black Section, the Durban Medical School, or more simply as 'Wentworth' after the school's segregated residence. Today, it is named the Nelson R. Mandela School of Medicine, in honour of the country's first democratically elected president. It is widely celebrated by alumni as a progressive institution, both educationally and politically, and remembered as a place where students and staff alike 'struggled' against many hardships, stood 'united in adversity' and

1

survived to tell a triumphant tale of their achievements. These sentiments have been captured in numerous university publications since the early 1990s.[2]

However, the constructions of partial, public memory narratives, such as those quoted above, are also one-sided and hide a much more complicated history of this medical school. A bleaker view of many tensions and contradictions which played out within and around this institution was also central to the existence of this place and the people who worked and studied there. In fact, like any institution with a changing mix of students and staff over many decades, the medical school's history is one that could claim significant advances or successes in a number of areas, but also deep disappointments, ambiguities, tensions and divisions. This institution and the many people who walked its corridors over many decades and occupied its lecture and laboratory rooms and clinical learning spaces, not to mention its dormitories, *both* reflected and opposed apartheid influences in complex ways. Taking seriously the various sides of this institution's historical development during the apartheid years, not just the publicly celebrated versions, are vital to understand more fully the school's fascinating history.

Opened in 1951, this institution was not the first to train black students in South Africa. It was the first of its kind, however, to make the training of black – 'African', 'Indian' and 'coloured' – students as medical doctors its mandate or its main focus or concern.[3] Unlike earlier aborted medical-training schemes that were attempted, the medical degree it offered was recognised on a par with those provided by the country's established white medical schools and allowed its graduates to register with the South African Medical and Dental Council, the body responsible for regulating the practice of medicine in South Africa. This Durban Medical School gave black students the rare opportunity to enter one of the most prestigious and highly paid professions in the country at the time. Funded largely by the Afrikaner-led National Party state, inevitably apartheid policies would influence its operation in decisive ways.

From the late 1950s rigid, racial segregation legislation restricted access to even the token numbers of black students, particularly African students, who were granted permission to study at the universities of the Witwatersrand (Wits) and Cape Town (UCT) from the 1940s right up until the late 1970s when the Medical University of Southern Africa (MEDUNSA) was opened. This meant that for many years Durban's medical school was *the only* place of its kind to train African students. Between 1957, when its first students graduated, until the 1994 political transition to democracy, the University of Natal produced 2 413 medical graduates, increasing in number per year from about 25 graduates in the 1960s to about 65 during the 1970s, and to about 100 during the 1980s and early 1990s. While, therefore, this book appears at first glance to be an account of the history of one particular province's medical school, it is an account which has a national resonance. The University of Natal's medical school was in many ways a national institution: for many years it was the only institution willing to train African students and by 1994 it had produced the largest number of black doctors in South Africa. These graduates went on to play a vital role in the provision of biomedical health-care services for various communities in South Africa's racially divided health-care system.

This is evident even in recent years. Today the school is often in the news for its many achievements. As a thriving institution with over 2 000 students, it is considered one of UKZN's greatest assets. It boasts amongst its staff some of the most prestigious names in South African medical science, and it has an excellent reputation for its research and teaching innovations which have attracted generous international sponsorships for research projects and centres.[4] These include, for example, the world-renowned Doris Duke Medical Research Institute which, since its inception in 2003, has focused on researching diseases affecting the poor and vulnerable in sub-Saharan Africa, especially those affected by HIV and AIDS, tuberculosis and malaria.[5] Another multimillion-dollar research centre, the KwaZulu-Natal Research Institute for Tuberculosis and HIV (K-RITH), has recently been opened in partnership with the Howard Hughes Medical Institute (HHMI). To date, this is the largest infrastructural investment made by the HHMI outside the United States.[6]

The medical school is also well known today for some of its alumni who, in the post-apartheid period, have become recognised business people. Dr Mamphela Ramphele, for example, former vice-chancellor of the University of Cape Town and managing director at the World Bank and Standard Bank, was also, until recently, the chairperson of the mining company Gold Fields until she resigned to play a greater role in politics. Distinguished academics and medical researchers – such as Professor Hoosen ('Jerry') Coovadia, who has contributed much on child health and HIV/AIDS research – are also former graduates of the medical school.[7] Some have become important politicians in high-profile government positions and have guided and influenced South Africa in many ways. These include, for example, the current national minister of health, Dr Aaron Motsoaledi; the premier of KwaZulu-Natal, chancellor of UKZN, and treasurer-general of the African National Congress, Dr Zweli Mkhize; the MEC for health in KwaZulu-Natal, Dr Sibongiseni Dhlomo; the current vice-chancellor of UKZN, and internationally recognised molecular immunologist and HIV/AIDS researcher, Professor Malegapuru Makgoba; Dr Nkosazana Dlamini Zuma (formerly minister of health, foreign affairs and home affairs, and now the chairperson of the African Union); the now retired Professor Ronald Green Thompson, the longest-serving superintendent-general of the province of KwaZulu-Natal's Department of Health between 1995 and 2005; and former provincial premiers of health in KZN, such as Dr Frank Mdlalose and Dr Ben Ngubane (who was also national minister of arts, culture, science and technology, and is currently chairperson of the board of directors of the South African Broadcasting Corporation) – to mention but a few.[8] Some of these very people, and many others, learnt to become political activists as students on the Durban medical campus.

During the apartheid era, the government's attempts to manipulate and control black students at racially segregated, tertiary institutions proved enormously contradictory as they became fertile breeding grounds for widespread anti-apartheid sentiment and action. Opened just three years after the National Party government came to power in 1948 and reliant on substantial financial backing from the state, the Durban Medical School's development occurred in complex ways, sometimes in line with, but at other times in opposition to, the state's desired policies. Created as an institution whose students were technically part of but geographically separated from the main University of Natal's white campus in Durban, the school's anomalous set-up offered aspiring black students the rare opportunity to improve their socio-economic life chances and professional standing in the country by studying to become doctors. However, it also forced them to suffer myriad hardships and subjected them to humiliating racial discriminations in their clinical training and residential arrangements. Yet, in unanticipated ways, the medical school environment helped bring students from culturally diverse backgrounds to live and study together, creating opportunities for interracial socialisation not commonly available elsewhere in South Africa. At times, this created a strong spirit of unity in adversity.

The experience of inequality angered and frustrated the school's students and politicised many. Some turned to direct involvement in anti-apartheid political activities as a way to address their grievances. Others, such as Steve Biko, who was a medical student in Durban between 1966 and 1972, became active leaders in the fight to end apartheid in South Africa. The politicisation process saw the emergence of a confident and defiant black consciousness student politics on the Durban medical campus in the late 1960s and through the 1970s – a consciousness that worked actively to transcend apartheid-created racial divisions and to stress pride and a celebration of 'blackness'. This made the school a fulcrum of student politics, especially during the 1970s and 1980s, posing a serious challenge to the state and also, at times, the university itself. Often, anti-apartheid political initiatives led by medical students were in the news. This put the school in the firing line for political interference and police harassment during the latter apartheid years, with harsh consequences for student leaders and other student supporters, as well as for innocent bystanders who were merely associated with them. Some activists, like Biko, paid dearly for their activism. Biko was expelled from his studies after repeated course failures at the school which resulted from his political activities; he was arrested and detained, experienced first-hand the violent nature of police brutality and eventually paid the ultimate price for his activities with his life.[9]

While these many educational and political accomplishments will be recounted, there is also a messier and more complex story to tell. The history captured in this book will certainly show that apartheid-state policies were contested and challenged by many medical students in Durban. The challenges these students faced were serious enough to warrant constant state surveillance and frequent police interventions, and ultimately did produce a defiant anti-apartheid politics that fuelled the broader liberation struggle leading to the collapse of the apartheid state in the early 1990s. But the story will also show the ruinous successes of apartheid on the medical school and health-care system in South Africa more generally. While the anomalous arrangement to provide medical training to state-designated 'non-European' students in Durban produced at key historical moments a sense of political unity amongst black students who stood up to contest apartheid, it also resulted in deep divisions amongst its student body over the years.

Together with other medical schools in operation in South Africa during the apartheid period, the University of Natal Medical School played a pivotal role in buttressing a racially divided and inherently unequal medical profession whose legacies still haunt this country today. This is evident in a floundering present-day health-care system that continues to provide inadequate facilities, massive disparities in resource allocations and insufficient numbers of adequately trained health-care personnel, many of whom are emigrating to seek greener pastures elsewhere.[10] In other words, the formation and operation of this school was critical to *both* the struggle against apartheid and the construction of a racially segmented medical profession, the unequal health-care effects of which are still very much a part of the post-apartheid democratic South Africa.

Medicine, methodology and memory

A number of books have been written about the contributions of some of the oldest and most esteemed historically white medical schools in the country.[11] However, there has been no comprehensive, book-length published study done on the history of South Africa's first successful black medical school. In 1966 Edgar Brookes published a history of the University of Natal, providing an important summary of the medical school's history in one of his chapters. Its institutional focus, however, does not consider the students' experiences and perspectives, and does not cover the school's tumultuous latter decades leading up to the country's political transition.[12] And, although the University of Natal has published numerous glossy booklets on the medical school's history, these publications are celebratory and commemorative types of productions to mark main anniversary occasions.[13] A warts-and-all, critical approach covering its development and operation is absent. The narratives in these glossy publications conceal as much as they reveal.

This book will attempt to fill this lacuna by telling the complex history of the Durban Medical School from the years leading up to its formation in the early 1950s to the years following the transition to democracy in 1994. It must be stated up front, however, that although this book is a history of Durban's medical school, it does not claim to be a definitive one, covering all aspects of its history or the persons who worked or studied there. That is an impossible feat. Hopefully, in the years to come, graduates as well staff members will write about their individual experiences and make them available to the general public. This will add to the historical account I produce here. Conducting the research for this book was a multifaceted endeavour that required searches in archives across South Africa. During the early 2000s I found little archival material on the medical school's institutional history on the school's premises itself. This was no surprise on a campus where there have been enduring problems with the availability of space as well as human and financial resources for the preservation of historical documents. With the help of the head librarian at the time, I was able to find a few drawers in filing cabinets – in the head librarian's office and hidden away behind the old journal stacks in the medical school's library – containing a mixture of documents, photographs and newspaper clippings. Although it provided a beginning, the material collected in these filing cabinets seemed random and disorganised, and missing documents appeared to have been either lost or destroyed over the years.[14] Many of these documents also tended to highlight the triumphs of the school's achievements, including those of its many celebrated alumni. The research process had to recognise that there could and probably would be biases and gaps in the archival sources.[15] To look for these gaps, I have used a variety of archives and sources to flesh out as much as I could about the Durban Medical School's history.

The University of KwaZulu-Natal's main archive located in Pietermaritz-burg provided useful official documents on the establishment and financing of the school, as well as a complete collection of the Faculty of Medicine's handbooks, useful faculty biography files, newsletters, minutes,[16] and commemorative brochures from the university's public-relations office.[17] The university's Campbell Collections, located in Durban, was pivotal too. Donated private collections, such as the Mabel Palmer Collection, the E.G. Malherbe Collection and the Gordon Papers, held valuable documents that helped uncover the motivations and experiences of individuals who worked at or were personally associated with the medical school's formation and operations. Through research on another project, I have also had access to archival materials related to the McCord Hospital which are presently being prepared for donation to the Campbell Collections.[18] They provided crucial material on the school's early formation, particularly the central role that Christian missionary doctors played in its establishment. Following this, research at the National Archives Repository in Pretoria produced useful material on the state's policies and perspectives on black medical education and training. This expanded the focus beyond the specific history of the Durban Medical School. To bolster this broader perspective, additional materials were found at a variety of other South African universities. Documents in archives at UCT, Wits and MEDUNSA recording staff discussions of what was going on in Durban, as well as their own difficulties around training black medical students, provided important comparisons. Furthermore, materials found on students' involvement in anti-apartheid activities at archives at these institutions, but also at other universities, such as collections at the University of the Western Cape's Mayibuye Archives Centre, were helpful in reconstructing the educational *and* political history of the Durban Medical School.

Part of the medical school's history can be told through official or institutional records – government and university reports, minutes of meetings, letters, statistics, memoranda – held in diverse archives across the country. Newspaper clippings from the apartheid period, too, have much to say about how the medical school was viewed by the media. The aim of the research for this book was to provide much more than a bland institutional or publicly recorded history of the medical school. People's lived experiences and personal perspectives were imperative too. These were drawn in part from student publications housed at an array of different universities as well as personal narratives, including autobiographies and biographies written by alumni of the school.[19] Significantly, a number of oral interviews were conducted to get to grips with the variety of people's personal experiences at the medical school – educational, social and political – and what motivated those individuals who worked, studied and shaped the school over the years.

This book draws therefore on about 30 qualitative, in-depth, oral interviews which I conducted in the late 1990s and early 2000s, some of which required follow-up interviews to complete. Although this sample is in no way representative of the many hundreds of employees and thousands of students who worked and studied at the school during the years covered by this book, I purposefully chose a variety of people from different cohorts, who came from different 'race' or ethnic groups and whose collective involvement with the school spanned the apartheid years.[20] Those interviewed included both men and women, though I interviewed more men in line with their historically greater demographic numbers in the medical profession.[21] Some people's perspectives were particularly interesting as they had been both students and staff at some point in their lives. Ultimately, however, those chosen for interviews also boiled down to the individual's interest, availability and working schedule. Other time constraints and geographical distance also played a limiting role.[22] In addition, while I did try to contact doctors engaged in various types of work, including private practice and government service after they graduated, there can be little doubt that my sample is biased towards those who ended up in academic medicine, having spent a great deal (if not all) of their working lives at a medical school, and still feeling a strong connection with the Durban Medical School.

This book also draws on a number of transcribed interviews conducted by other researchers with black doctors who trained in South Africa during the apartheid period. Interviewed during the late 1970s and through the 1980s for other research projects, many of these doctors were politically active and living in exile at the time.[23] These interviews are available for use as part of the Karis-Gerhart Collection in the South African History Archives at Wits in Johannesburg. Some of Padraig O'Malley's political interviews, which are hosted by the Nelson Mandela Centre of Memory and Dialogue and record the perspectives of prominent political role-players in South Africa during the apartheid and post-apartheid periods, were also useful.[24] Finally, use of written and transcribed oral-interview documents collected by the faculties of medicine at Wits, UCT and the University of Natal as part of their submissions to the Truth and Reconciliation Commission hearings in 1997 and 1998 proved extremely valuable in portraying some of the diverse experiences and perspectives of black students and doctors who studied and worked in South Africa during apartheid.[25]

While a wide range of archival and oral sources have much to offer a social and institutional history of the Durban Medical School, it is essential to keep in mind the issue of memory and its 'constructed' nature when writing any history.[26] It is vital to keep this idea in mind when reading this book. An individual alumnus's oral and written memory narratives certainly give us valuable information about a particular event, or a person's life story, or a particular historical moment that cannot be gleaned by analysing official sources alone. But these cannot be treated naively as transparent or authentic historical 'facts' that have simply been 'recovered' for use by the historian. Just like written sources, oral sources should be problematised as they are not objective but rather 'constructed' accounts. Memories produced long after the events can be distorted by physical deterioration of the informant's memory over time, or hindsight, when an informant's later-life experiences can cause them to revise their earlier stories. One also has to take into account the issue of nostalgia in old age, personal bias, selectiveness and silences, but also distortion of facts, as well as exaggeration, which influences the knowledge that is ultimately produced.[27] Interviewees are not simply subjects, but 'constructors of knowledge'.[28] Moreover, interviewers are co-creators of stories, and the types of questions they ask, and the anticipated audience that both interviewees and interviewers expect will hear their words, also influence the process of remembering done by interviewees.[29]

It is also essential to emphasise that remembering is not merely a process located in the individual mind, but is a social phenomenon too that has relational dimensions. Our memories are rooted in social environments and are thus constructed in dialogue with other people. Moreover, they are 'collective' in the sense that individuals try to locate their own individual memories in a wider social framework, placing their memories in the perspective of a group when they remember, to help them make meaning of their lives.[30] As one oral historian has asserted, 'The act of remembering goes on inside our heads but not independently of the social relations of which we are a part. What we remember and what we forget is to a greater or lesser extent shaped by the social environment in which we are embedded.'[31] In addition, oral historians have discovered how whole communities have 'rearranged their recollections collectively' to make them more 'relevant to the present . . .'.[32]

Thus, when interpreting memory narratives, we need to understand the societies that informants live in, as well as how individuals link their own lives to broader historical events and currents of their times, including political agendas. The past is not simply some given 'fact'. Rather, aspects of the past are actively remembered in the light of factors related to the present. African oral literature specialist Isabel Hofmeyr captured this notable feature of memory aptly when she wrote: 'Not only do historical narratives refer to the past and mediate an understanding of the past through their form; the stories and their tellers also pass through time and are shaped by its often precipitously changing circumstances. Stories, then, comment on the passing of time and times past.'[33] Recognising that memory narratives, like all other sources, are constructed, and that they are also affected by the passing of time and the politics of the present, including political agendas and personal interests, forces researchers to approach these sources critically. It also helps us to understand that studying people's memories tells us as much about the present as it does about the past.[34] The past and present are closely intertwined in shaping how, when and why people remember their pasts.

Many of the alumni's memories used in this book were written down or recorded as oral interviews in the post-1994 period in South Africa. Thus, it is imperative to consider the dynamics of the post-apartheid transformation process on what they remember.[35] The immediate post-1994 years were concerned with building a new, more unified nation and promoting reconciliation for South Africans just emerging from the apartheid era. President Nelson Mandela's first democratic government worked hard to promote an overarching or 'master' nationalist narrative of a multicultural 'rainbow nation' that incorporated everyone and tried to undermine the many decades of apartheid that had divided South Africa's population by race. This narrative, which simplified complicated and untidy pasts in the interests of promoting social cohesion, also actively worked to celebrate and commemorate anti-apartheid heroes.[36]

Influenced by this broader context, many medical graduates recalled their past experiences in ways that were shaped by nostalgia, perhaps even through a romanticising lens.[37] They focused on promoting the idea – evident in university commemorative publications and newspapers, and even in interviews – of the school as a significant 'barometer' or 'hub of political activity', that it had a student body that stood firmly together, 'united in adversity' against their apartheid enemies, and that it produced leaders 'who were in the forefront of the struggle for political freedom in South Africa'.[38] These public stories highlighted how living and studying in Durban was a harmonious and unifying experience, and one immune to political or ethnic tensions, class antagonisms or gender divisions. In addition to reflecting a changed historical and political reality, these celebratory narratives by alumni were also influenced by the desire to gain social acceptance and public affirmation for their achievements, as well as served to legitimate their role as contributors in an emerging new social order.

It took the school's 50th anniversary celebrations in 2000, in a changed, less euphoric, historical context with some distance from the immediate post-1994 period, and probing questions asked during interview sessions for alumni to reflect more critically on their time spent at this institution. Some alumni were invited to be speakers at the prestigious July 2000 banquet, which included guest dignitaries such as the former president Nelson R. Mandela, then deputy president Jacob Zuma, Zulu king Goodwill Zwelithini, Dr Nkosazana Dlamini Zuma, Dr Zweli Mkhize and Dr Ben Ngubane. Some used the occasion to raise a number of controversial memories about studying and working at their alma mater, about which, until then, they had kept publicly silent. One of the big issues highlighted was the deeply rooted racial divisions and tensions, particularly between African and Indian students, that had caused disharmony over the years amongst the school's student body.[39] The anomalous set-up at the school's Alan Taylor Residence (ATR) allowed black students from diverse racial backgrounds to live and work together for the first time. It laid the foundations for special friendships to develop, but it also produced tensions. These tensions played themselves out in educational, social and political ways, as this book will show.

Of course, these less than 'politically correct' alternative memories were not merely contentious factual windows into some distant apartheid past. They burst into public discourse in recent years because they were very much alive in a school desperately struggling to transform itself in the post-apartheid period. Many years after their studies, there was still much unhappiness about unequal opportunities that some Africans believed some Indian alumni received during the apartheid era, including what they regarded as favoured treatment by certain staff members, enabling them to advance as undergraduate and postgraduate students, and in employment and promotion opportunities at the school.[40] One such alumnus, Dr Kgotsi Letslape, made an impassioned speech at the July 2000 banquet, saying: 'We plead for the systematic persecution of our people in the institution to stop.' He raised these issues for discussion to promote strategies for change. Until Letslape's public statement in July 2000, only a handful of Africans had been appointed to head departments at the medical school and, while being a historically black medical school, it had not yet had an African appointed as dean. Although improvements have been made, including student admissions that are now representative of wider demographic trends, and greater numbers of black South Africans appointed to faculty positions, some black doctors continue to live in a world in which many aspects of the racially defined past remain stubbornly in place.

Certainly, close friendships were forged at the medical school, and some graduates experienced a genuine sense of political unity in, what they regarded as, the common fight to end apartheid. This book affirms these positive examples as part of the multifaceted story of this institution and its diverse student body. However, not all students experienced their time at the medical school in the same way; nor did they suffer or struggle in the same way. During the apartheid years, student interactions were not all rosy, despite being viewed in recent years through a more romanticised lens. Relationships were often complicated by race, class, ethnic and gender differences and many other things. Simply focusing on the dominant triumphalist and celebratory narratives, which dovetail so well with the grand narratives of South Africa's struggle history, hides the enormous complexity and messiness of this school's history. It also blinds us to the diverse types of interactions that occurred amongst its students who lived through a very difficult historical period.

This book will focus on both the positive successes and achievements that occurred, despite the enormous odds stacked against the school's staff and students, but also on the ambiguities, contradictions, tensions and frustrations. Taking seriously what is remembered but also actively silenced, and thus considering both common and dissenting, or alternative, memory narratives, will be essential to get at the different sides of this medical school's fascinating story. Spanning over a half-century, segregated medical education in apartheid South Africa developed as a site of great struggle and a setting of deep contradictions, at times reproducing apartheid conditions, but also unlocking the essential failure of an apartheid ideology, fulfilling some objectives of policies of separate development, but also contributing to the apartheid state's demise.

A School of Struggle addresses the histories of medical education, professionalisation and student politics in South Africa during the apartheid period. It opens with an analysis of some of the early twentieth-century debates, initiatives and difficulties in providing medical education for black students in South Africa. Medical education for black students in the pre-apartheid years was unequal and was geared towards producing inferior categories of health personnel that would serve 'their own communities' in a racially segregated health service. Early in the twentieth century Christian missionaries made efforts to train 'medical assistants', and in the late 1930s the government of the day started a 'Medical Aid' training scheme for

Africans at the South African Native College of Fort Hare. Some of these early medical-training initiatives for black South Africans were hard fought for by people with the very best of intentions, such as doctors McCord and Taylor at the McCord mission hospital in Durban, but had compromised outcomes because of the racially unequal context in which they were developed. Ultimately this led to their failure. They were followed by efforts to train small numbers of black students at the established white medical schools of the universities of Cape Town and the Witwatersrand during the Second World War.

The establishment of the University of Natal Medical School in Durban forms the subject of chapter 2. Funded largely by the National Party government, whose apartheid racial policies came to influence the school's formation and operation in essential ways, the school provided the main training facility for black medical students in South Africa from the early 1950s through to the early 1990s. Focusing on the institutional history of the school, this chapter discusses some of the contradictions that arose around its creation and operation. During its early years, the school became a significant showpiece of apartheid; however, it also became a complex anomaly that worked to undermine apartheid-state directives and policies in numerous ways.

Chapter 3 moves away from the institutional perspective to consider the difficult personal journeys black students made to get to the Durban Medical School. Most black students in the apartheid years faced racial, financial and gender obstacles that made advancement through secondary school a challenging and unlikely possibility. Aspects of the personal and educational backgrounds of medical students could work to hinder or advance their progress. Only a tiny and determined few successfully struggled to make the journey to the tertiary level and gained admittance into the University of Natal's medical school, which had very limited spaces available for each year of training. This chapter looks at what motivated these students to get there.

For the few who did make it and who travelled across the country to settle in Durban, many further hardships awaited them. Chapters 4 and 5 dwell on some of the positive and negative social and educational experiences of students who gained admission to the school. Its irregular establishment as a black faculty within the historically white University of Natal forced its students to suffer many painful and humiliating racial inequalities academically, and in its segregated clinical teaching arrangements. The school's segregated residence – ATR – which allowed African, Indian and coloured students to live and study together, also produced contradictory outcomes. While this arrangement enabled some students to bond at a level rarely seen in apartheid South Africa, motivating and inspiring some, it also produced difficulties. In addition to the physical hardships that students had to endure at this grossly inferior residence, this chapter will discuss some of the tensions and divisions that emerged amongst the students living there.

Chapters 6 and 7 expand the analysis of Durban medical students' experiences to the political realm. Recognising, as in the previous chapters, the racial, class and gender schisms that plagued the student body, they discuss some of the complicated responses that emerged amongst black students to the many forms of discrimination students encountered while studying in Durban. While some students tried to remain apolitical to get on with their medical studies, hoping for social and professional rewards once they had graduated, others became involved in extracurricular political activities to try to address their many grievances. Starting with an analysis of some of the reasons for the lower level of medical student political involvement in the 1950s and the early 1960s, chapter 6 ends with a consideration of what mobilised a growing number of students to get involved in anti-apartheid politics from the late 1960s. In 1969, the early leadership and headquarters of a defiant, black consciousness, student politics developed at ATR. The South African Students' Organisation, or SASO, provided a broad political education that helped to conscientise its members and encouraged some to stand up in opposition to their apartheid oppressors.

By the 1970s, the state's provision of discriminatory facilities and its attempts to rigidly control the activities of black students at racially segregated tertiary institutions proved enormously contradictory, as they provided opportunities for the growth of anti-apartheid sentiment and action. Chapter 7 focuses on those black medical students who actively involved themselves in politics, particularly in the activities of SASO in the 1970s and the African National Congress-aligned United Democratic Front in the 1980s. It will consider a number of examples of the issues and types of political activities students got involved in, as well as staff responses to these activities. Students protested against the discrimination and inequality they encountered at the hands of both the apartheid state and the University of Natal. This chapter looks at some of the varied and serious consequences of their political activism. During the 1970s and 1980s, the Durban Medical School became an important seat of anti-apartheid political activity, which brought harsh state responses to silence activists, but also helped reinvigorate the wider, nationalist anti-apartheid opposition.

Chapter 8 brings the material covered in the book into the post-apartheid era and focuses on some of the legacies of apartheid-era, medical educational and political struggles. It highlights changes that have occurred, but also points to some remarkable continuities. Finally, it considers medical educational developments in the post-1994 years. The short concluding chapter ends the book with a few reflections.

Notes

1. This university has gone through a number of name changes over the years. Before 1949, it was known as the Natal University College. In 1949, when it received full university status, it was renamed the University of Natal. In 2004, after a number of tertiary education institutions in KwaZulu-Natal were merged under its control, it was renamed the University of KwaZulu-Natal (UKZN).
2. See the University Publications section in the bibliography for examples of these commemorative publications.
3. Terminology in South Africa has a contested history. Under apartheid, all South Africans were classified into one of four 'race' groups. In this book terms such as 'African', 'Indian', 'coloured' and 'white' will be used to denote specific racial groupings of people, while the terms 'non-white' or 'non-European', which were used by the state during this period, as well as 'black', which is commonly used today, will be used to refer to African, Indian and coloured people as a collective group. An additional difficulty with using generalised categories such as these is their tendency to hide further schisms within population groups – for example, in ethnicity, language, religion, class, gender, and so on. Furthermore, sometimes these overarching categories of identity have been actively claimed by people who over time promoted them, while others have vehemently rejected them. While I recognise that racial classifications are contentious social constructions and hide a great deal, their usage had very real socio-economic and political effects before 1994 and still has resonance today. Use of these terms as descriptive and analytical categories is a necessary part of trying to understand any history dealing with the apartheid period. For more on this complicated subject of classifying and naming based on race and ethnicity, see, for example, Gerry Maré, *Ethnicity and Politics in South Africa* (London and Atlantic Highlands, NJ: Zed Books, 1993); and Goolam Vahed, 'The making of "Indianness": Indian politics in South Africa during the 1930s and 1940s', *Journal of Natal and Zulu History* 17 (1997).

4. UKZNA MF3/1/1-8, Patrick Leeman, 'From humble beginnings to an institution of excellence', *MedNews: Faculty of Medicine Newsletter* 1 (January–May 2000), 3.

5. 'R40 mln research facility opened at Durban Medical School', *Natal Witness* (20 July 2003); Dasarath Chetty and Smita Maharaj, eds, *Doris Duke Medical Research Institute* brochure, UKZN Public Affairs and Corporate Communications (2007). The institute houses a number of research initiatives such as CAPRISA (the Centre for the AIDS Programme of Research in South Africa), HPP (HIV Pathogenesis Programme), ECI (Enhancing Care Initiative) and the Women's Health Unit.

6. 'UKZN's Nelson R. Mandela School of Medicine celebrates its 60th anniversary', *Mercury* (27 May 2010). Also see Chris Ndaliso, 'HIV and TB: US medical institute, UKZN in joint research programme', *Witness* (12 May 2011); and Lunga Memela, 'Groundbreaking ceremony of major tuberculosis and HIV research institute', *Mercury* (26 July 2011).

7. 'UKZN academic named as one of the top 50 most influential individuals in HIV/ AIDS in the world', *College of Health Sciences Newsletter* 5, no. 1 (May 2009).

8. For a list of other illustrious graduates, see Melanie Peter, 'Hallowed halls of medicine: Fifty years old with an illustrious list of university graduates', *Independent on Saturday* (29 July 2000). Also see UKZN EGML Patrick Leeman, 'Calling back the past', *NU Focus* 11, no. 2 (2000); and C.C. 'Noddy' Jinabhai, 'Medical school: The other struggle', *NU Focus* 11, no. 2 (2000); as well as 'UKZN's Nelson R. Mandela School of Medicine celebrates its 60th anniversary', *Mercury* (27 May 2010).

9. UKZNA MF3/1/1-8, 'From Biko we have much to learn – Brenda Gourley', *MedNews: Faculty of Medicine Newsletter* 1 (January–May 2000), 6.

10. 'Alarming lack of doctors', *Star*, 8 July 2008; Lucas Ntyintyana, 'How can we stop the rot?' *Sunday Times* (31 May 2009); Nathaniel Lee, 'Government must act fast on health and education', *Star* (7 June 2010).

11. For UCT, see, for example, J.H. Louw, *In the Shadow of Table Mountain: A History of the University of Cape Town Medical School* (Cape Town: Struik, 1969); R. Kirsch and C. Knox, eds, *UCT Medical School at 75* (Cape Town: UCT Department of Medicine, 1987); and Anne Digby, Howard Phillips, Harriet Deacon and Kirsten Thomson, *At the Heart of Healing: Groote Schuur Hospital, 1938–2008* (Auckland Park: Jacana Media, 2008). For Wits, see, for example, Bruce K. Murray, *Wits the Early Years: A History of the University of the Witwatersrand Johannesburg and its Precursors, 1896–1939* (Johannesburg: Witwatersrand University Press, 1982); and *Wits the 'Open' Years: A History of the University of the Witwatersrand, Johannesburg, 1939–59* (Johannesburg: Witwatersrand University Press, 1997).

12. Edgar Brookes, *A History of the University of Natal* (Pietermaritzburg: University of Natal Press, 1966). See also B.T. Naidoo, 'A history of the Durban Medical School', *South African Medical Journal* 50, no. 41 (25 September 1976).

13. See, for example, *1951–1976: 25 Years of the Faculty of Medicine at the University of Natal*, University of Natal: Communication and Publicity (1977); *The University of Natal Medical School 1951–1991: Meeting the Challenge of Change*, University of Natal: Communication and Publicity (1991); and Jack Moodley and Smita Maharaj,

eds, *University of Natal Nelson R. Mandela School of Medicine: 50 Years of Achievement in Teaching, Service and Research*, University of Natal Nelson R. Mandela School of Medicine: Communications Office (2001). Unpublished university-commissioned reports as well as unpublished theses were also drawn upon to write this book. See the bibliography for a list of these works.

14. Fortunately, priorities have changed since the late 1990s and through the early 2000s when I conducted my research. In 2011, a researcher, Gail Robinson, was employed by the medical school to gather together archival material on the school's history and to sort and catalogue this material into a formal archive. This archive was opened in late 2011 as part of the school's library.

15. Michel-Rolph Trouillot, *Silencing the Past: Power and the Production of History* (Boston: Beacon Press, 1995); Carolyn Hamilton, Verne Harris, Jane Taylor, Michele Pickover, Graeme Reid and Razia Saleh, eds, *Refiguring the Archive* (Cape Town: David Philip, 2002); and Antoinette Burton, ed., *Archive Stories: Facts, Fictions and the Writing of History* (Durham and London: Duke University Press, 2005).

16. Although the council and senate minutes were available at the University of KwaZulu-Natal archives, the minutes of the board of the Faculty of Medicine were not. These were housed in the administration section of the medical school.

17. Many of these brochures were also available for use at the Special Collections Section (lower ground floor) of the E.G. Malherbe Library on the Howard College campus in Durban and at the medical school's library.

18. Together with medical historians Catherine Burns and Julie Parle, as well as a team of other researchers, during the last few years I have been researching and writing the history of McCord Hospital, an important mission hospital based in Durban, which celebrated its centenary in 2009.

19. James B. McCord, *My Patients were Zulus* (New York and Toronto: Rinehart and Co., 1951); Mamphela Ramphele, *Across Boundaries: The Journey of a South African Woman Leader* (New York: Feminist Press, 1995); Malegapuru W. Makgoba, *Mokoko: The Makgoba Affair: A Reflection on Transformation* (Florida Hills, RSA: Vivlia Publishers, 1997). Also see Adam Starz, *Between Laughter and Tears* (Ladysmith, RSA: Sinclair Publishing, 1986) for a fictionalised account of life as a black medical student and doctor in apartheid South Africa.

20. It should also be noted that because there were fewer doctors trained in the 1950s and early 1960s, and a larger number from this cohort are now deceased, my interview sample is also skewed towards people who trained and worked at the medical school from the 1970s onwards. In addition, I interviewed a few white doctors who had studied with black students, trained at the medical school's King Edward VIII teaching hospital or taught black medical students.

21. See the Interviews section of the bibliography for more on this. Ten women doctors were interviewed in total, with five having completed their undergraduate degrees at the Durban Medical School. The other women interviewed had either completed their internship training at King Edward VIII Hospital, had done their postgraduate studies at this institution or had worked for some years at the medical school.

22. Most interviews were conducted in South Africa. I also sent out questionnaires to people who were not available for interviews. However, very few responded to these questionnaires.

23. See Thomas G. Karis and Gail M. Gerhart, *From Protest to Challenge: A Documentary History of African Politics in South Africa, 1882–1990* (Pretoria: UNISA Press, 1997).

24. See Padraig O'Malley Political Interviews, http://www.nelsonmandela.org/omalley/index.php/site/q/03lv02424/04lv02730.htm. Padraig O'Malley's interviews, captured between 1989 and 1999, have been archived as written transcriptions and on audio tapes at the University of the Western Cape's Mayibuye Archives.

25. Wits FHSR M3/40 Internal Reconciliation Commission, 1998; UCT Faculty of Health Sciences, 'Truth and Reconciliation: A Process of Transformation at UCT Health Sciences Faculty'; University of Natal Medical School's submission to the TRC Commission, 23 June 1997.

26. Much scholarly work has been done on the complex issue of orality, memory and narrative construction in the writing of history in the last 30 years. Useful starting points are to be found in general readers, such as Robert Perks and Alistair Thomson, eds, *The Oral History Reader*, 2nd ed. (London and New York: Routledge, 2006); and more recently, Donald A. Ritchie, ed., *The Oxford Handbook of Oral History* (Oxford and New York: Oxford University Press, 2011).

27. For more on the issue of the dialectic between remembering and forgetting, see, for example, David William Cohen, *The Combing of History* (Chicago and London: University of Chicago Press, 1994); Trouillot, *Silencing the Past*.

28. D.A. Ritchie, 'Introduction: The evolution of oral history', in *The Oxford Handbook of Oral History*, ed. Donald A. Ritchie (Oxford and New York: Oxford University Press, 2011), 13.

29. Alessandro Portelli, 'What makes oral history different', in *The Oral History Reader*, 2nd ed., eds Robert Perks and Alistair Thomson (London and New York: Routledge, 2006), 39–40; and Sean Field, 'Turning up the volume: Dialogues about memory create oral histories', *South African Historical Journal* 60, no. 2 (2008), 182.

30. See, for example, Paul Connerton, *How Societies Remember* (Cambridge: Cambridge University Press, 1989); Lewis A. Coser, ed., *Maurice Halbwachs: On Collective Memory* (Chicago and London: University of Chicago Press, 1992); Elizabeth Tonkin, *Narrating our Pasts: The Social Construction of Oral History* (Cambridge: Cambridge University Press, 1992); Susan A. Crane, 'AHR Forum: Writing the individual back into collective memory', *American Historical Review* (December 1997), 1376; and Alistair Thomson, 'Memory and remembering in oral history', in *The Oxford Handbook of Oral History*, ed. Donald A. Ritchie (Oxford and New York: Oxford University Press, 2001), 87.

31. Brian Conway, 'Active remembering, selective forgetting, and collective identity: The case of Bloody Sunday', in *Identity: An International Journal of Theory and Research* 3, no. 4 (2003), 311.

32. Ritchie, 'Introduction: The evolution of oral history', 13.

33. Isabel Hofmeyr, 'We Spend our Years as a Tale that is Told': Oral Historical Narrative in a South African Chiefdom (Portsmouth, NH: Heinemann; Johannesburg: Witwatersrand University Press; and London: James Currey, 1993), xi.

34. Susannah Radstone and Bill Schwarz, 'Introduction: Mapping memory', in Memory: Histories, Theories, Debates, eds Susannah Radstone and Bill Schwarz (New York: Fordham University Press, 2010), 3.

35. Field, 'Turning up the volume', 188. Also see Sarah Nuttall and Carli Coetzee, eds, Negotiating the Past: The Making of Memory in South Africa (Oxford and New York: Oxford University Press, 2002); and Cheryl McEwan, 'Building a postcolonial archive? Gender, collective memory and citizenship in post-apartheid South Africa', Journal of Southern African Studies 29, no. 3 (September 2003).

36. See, for example, Nuttall and Coetzee, eds, Negotiating the Past; Annie E. Coombes, Visual Culture and Public Memory in a Democratic South Africa (Durham and London: Duke University Press, 2003); Gary Baines, 'The master narrative of South Africa's liberation struggle: Remembering and forgetting June 16, 1976', International Journal of African Historical Studies 40, no. 2 (2007).

37. For a fascinating discussion on nostalgia, see Jacob Dlamini, Native Nostalgia (Auckland Park: Jacana, 2009).

38. See 'Message from Dr U.G. Lalloo, President, Medical Graduates Association', in The University of Natal Medical School 1951–1991: Meeting the Challenge of Change, brochure to mark the fortieth anniversary of the Faculty of Medicine of the University of Natal, (University of Natal: Communication and Publicity, 1991); 'Reflections on life at the medical school by Dr M.M.R. Belle', in University of Natal Medical School Reconciliation Graduation Booklet 1995 (Durban: Indicator Press, December 1995), 13. See later commemorative publications for similar themes: for example, Moodley and Maharaj, eds, University of Natal Nelson R. Mandela School of Medicine: 50 Years of Achievement in Teaching, Service and Research, 9; UKZNA MF3/1/1-8, 'Reminiscence of Dr Theven "BT" Naidoo, Mednews: Faculty of Medicine Newsletter 1, no. 2 (June–December 2000), 14; and newspaper articles such as Melanie Peters, 'Hallowed halls of medicine: Fifty years old with an illustrious list of university graduates', The Independent on Saturday (29 July 2000).

39. University of Natal, Nelson R. Mandela School of Medicine, Fiftieth Anniversary Banquet, (University of Natal, Durban: Audio-Visual Centre, 29 July 2000); Patrick Leeman, 'University's medical school criticised', Mercury (31 July 2000); and 'Day of shame for NU medical school', Mercury (11 August 2000).

40. Ali Modiba, 'MSRC, Racism Report presented to the faculty and students of the University of Natal, Nelson R. Mandela School of Medicine' (26 September 2004); and Reena Budree and Pitika Ntuli, 'UKZN report change strategy workshops, Nelson R. Mandela School of Medicine' (12 April 2006).

CHAPTER 1

Black medical education in South Africa, 1910–45

Early in the twentieth century South Africa's public health-care services and medical-education provisions were directly influenced by the state's policies of racial segregation that discriminated against people designated as 'non-European'.[1] In this context a wide range of political considerations and economic disparities mediated and shaped competing claims to health care and medical training for different population groups in the country. Politically oppressive laws, economically exploitative labour policies, social dislocations, poverty and poor municipal service delivery in separately created African, Indian and coloured rural 'reserves' or urban 'township' areas helped create environments in which diseases proliferated in subordinate 'non-white' communities. The regions or provinces which formed the country of South Africa at Union in 1910, and in the decades that followed, were ill served outside of the main 'European' urban centres by any organised, centralised form of public health-care service. Responsibility for health provision was divided amongst central government departments, provincial administrations and local authorities. Indeed, until the early 1940s, when the National Health Services Commission was instituted to investigate and improve health-care services in the country, those services provided for black South Africans were found to be disorganised, underfunded and in a state of general neglect.[2] As a 1940s *South African Medical Journal* editorial lamented about South Africa's public health-care services: '... it is all patchwork, a patch here and a patch there and no planning'.[3] In addition to being racially segregated, public health-care services also tended to focus on treating already established diseases, while health educational and preventive approaches were largely ignored. Thus, many preventable infectious diseases were rampant in many black rural and urban areas.

This public health-care situation was aggravated by the lack of medical-training facilities for black students in South Africa as well as the state's attempts to criminalise – through its passage of the 1928 Medical, Dental and Pharmacy Act – what it considered as 'harmful' and 'backward' indigenous healing practices.[4] Although two medical schools – one at the University of Cape Town (UCT) and the other at the University of the Witwatersrand in Johannesburg (Wits) – were opened in South Africa in the 1910s and 1920s to train white male and female medical students in the country for the first time, black students were prevented from studying at these medical establishments.[5] The country had a long history of exclusion of black students from admission into its historically white medical schools, which were the official gatekeepers to the country's prestigious medical profession. Reasons used to exclude black students from South Africa's early medical schools included the rampant prevalence of scientific racism in the medical profession, which led to concerns over the mental capacity of blacks to master a difficult subject like medicine; anxieties that their admission into the profession would lower medical standards; and that these medical schools lacked clinical training facilities for black trainees.[6] In addition, fears were expressed that social and academic fraternisation might lead to racial mixing at these schools, not to mention the potential economic threat black doctors would pose to white doctors once in practice. Furthermore, the South African Native College of Fort Hare, which had opened in 1916 to train black students in professional subjects, did not offer a medical degree.

Consequently, in the early decades of the twentieth century, black students living in South Africa who wanted to enter the medical profession had two options. First, as had been the case for white students before UCT and Wits medical schools were opened, African, Indian and coloured students wanting to obtain a full medical qualification were required to go overseas to study. Although a lucky few won university scholarships, were sponsored by overseas organisations (such as missionary bodies) or had wealthy families who could afford to support them through their long medical studies programmes, the numbers of those venturing overseas to study – primarily to Great Britain, the Republic of Ireland, the United States or Canada – rarely exceeded more than a handful every year. The great distances and huge costs involved proved strong deterrents. But a few did succeed. For example, Steven Gish documented the story of Alfred B. Xuma's extraordinary journey to qualify as a doctor at Northwestern University in

Chicago during the 1920s, while K. Goonam wrote of her own experiences as an Indian South African woman receiving her medical training in Edinburgh during the late 1920s and early 1930s.[7]

The lack of medical schools to choose from in African countries also proved a deterrent. It is imperative to note that the provision of a full medical training for Africans came late to most of the continent. By the time of the opening of South Africa's black medical school in Durban in 1951, there were fewer than ten African medical-training institutions available north of the Limpopo River to serve the whole of sub-Saharan Africa, and most did not provide a full medical training. Many had opened during the interwar years and included, for example, schools in Dakar in Senegal, Ayos in the Cameroon, Abidjan in Côte d'Ivoire, in the Congo, Yaba Medical Training College just outside Lagos in Nigeria, Khartoum in the Sudan and Makerere in Uganda. As Adell Patton and John Iliffe highlight in their accomplished books on the medical training of Africans in West and East Africa respectively, most of these medical schools actually focused on producing African medical 'assistants' who were ranked professionally below physicians and were trained to work with, and usually under the supervision of, European doctors in the colonies.[8] By the 1960s, Patton argued, most African countries had not founded their own medical schools. In fact,

> [t]he Dakar Medical School served the vast region of Francophone Africa, Khartoum served the Sudan, and Makerere served East Africa. Ghana, Sierra Leone, and Gambia relied solely on the Ibadan facility [which opened in Nigeria in the 1950s] to meet their needs for medical personnel. Ethiopia, Tanzania, and Kenya were only in the initial stages of developing their own training facilities. Liberia had certified only 2 doctors by 1955 . . . In Central Africa, Salisbury University of Rhodesia . . . was still only in the planning stages. The Congo, with only 12 university graduates at the time of independence in 1960 out of a population of 13.5 million, had not graduated a single physician by that same time. Similar to Dakar and Yaba, the Congo first produced only medical assistants until the 1960s.[9]

The lack of local and international training opportunities seriously hindered the chances of black South African students studying medicine, and resulted in an acute shortage of black doctors available to work in the country's segregated public health-care services. By the period of the Second World War, over 95 per cent of doctors registered to practise in South Africa were white.[10]

The second and more readily used option was that black students wanting to enter the health field trained as nurses, as Shula Marks's comprehensive book *Divided Sisterhood* has demonstrated,[11] though this was usually a field reserved for women in South Africa.[12] Furthermore, potential applicants could lower their professional aspirations and train as auxiliary health personnel, such as medical assistants, who would aid white doctors in their public or private practices.[13] During the early twentieth century, Christian missionaries were some of the first people in South Africa to train black medical assistants for their hospitals and clinics. During this period, medical education for black South Africans developed in a way that was unequal, and was geared towards producing subordinate categories of health personnel who would serve 'their own communities' in a racially segregated service. Although this was not the intended outcome of most liberal-minded Christian missionaries, even these early compromised training schemes had to be hard fought for.

Christian missionaries and early black medical assistants in South Africa

Until the early 1930s, the South African state left most health-care services for the majority of the country's rural and predominantly African population to faith-driven and philanthropic-inspired European doctors and nurses from various missionary bodies. Many of these doctors and nurses had come to the country in the late nineteenth or early twentieth centuries as part of foreign missions from Britain, Europe or the United States, to work amongst and convert local peoples to their Christian faith. Scholars such as Michael Gelfand have written valuable surveys about their work and contributions.[14] Scattered about in largely remote rural areas, with little in the way of funds, and facing many personal hardships, these health pioneers set up early churches and schools, as well as rudimentary clinics and later hospitals. These doctors and nurses viewed biomedicine and Christianity as a 'team effort' to heal patients, to facilitate religious conversions and to undermine what they perceived as the 'dangerous' and 'backward' indigenous healing beliefs and practices which had been in existence in the country for centuries before their arrival.[15] In many places, their biomedical health-care services were often the first that black communities encountered, and although resistance was experienced initially in some places, over time Christian missionary doctors and nurses played a pivotal role in winning converts to Western forms of religion, education and health care.

In an environment where only small numbers of white doctors and nurses were available to help large numbers of underserved black populations, and with philanthropic intentions to advance the welfare of their black patients, Christian medical missionaries were also at the forefront of training black South Africans as nurses and medical assistants and providing them with work opportunities in their clinics and hospitals.[16] Anne Digby's book *Diversity and Division in Medicine* discusses early missionary initiatives in the wider Cape region, such as the efforts by the Victoria Hospital to recruit prominent Lovedale Mission School African students to train as hospital orderlies and medical assistants.[17] In the Natal region, the province where the first black medical school in the country would later be opened, James B. McCord from the American Board of Foreign Missions (ABM) was one of the first medical missionaries to train and employ black medical assistants and nurses.[18] They provided him with vital assistance at his first clinic on a mission station in Amanzimtoti, just south of Durban, in the late nineteenth century, and at his second clinic located in a more central area in the bustling city of Durban in the early decades of the twentieth century. Moreover, from 1909, when he opened his first hospital (which in time became known as McCord Zulu Hospital and then McCord Hospital) on the Berea in Durban, until his retirement in 1940, James McCord relied heavily on the help of his black male and female medical assistants.[19]

Since no medical schools were available to train blacks in South Africa in these decades, early missionary medical assistants were trained 'on the job' in basic first-aid work. They were also taught how to mix drugs, sterilise the clinics and the doctors' surgical instruments, and provide health education to patients sitting in the clinics' waiting areas. Furthermore, they served as vital interpreters between the missionary doctors and nurses and their African patients in consultation rooms. McCord, like other missionary doctors at the time, recruited many of his early assistants from amongst his former patients. One African male assistant, Umqibelo, who worked for McCord for many years, was recruited in this way. This was highlighted by

Katie Makanya, another of McCord's assistants, whose words were captured by his daughter in oral interviews just before Makanya's death in the mid-1950s:

> [B]orn in Zululand . . . as a child he had suffered much from ear infections but somehow he had heard about the Doctor, and while still very young he had walked more than a hundred miles to the dispensary. The Doctor had operated on his ears three times in the old cottage hospital, and in-between operations put him to work washing bottles and running errands.[20]

A significant criterion for these early recruits was that they were Christian. This was essential for medical missionaries because they were also charged with spreading the Christian faith to their patients. The provision of religious sermons to patients awaiting medical examination was a duty that many medical assistants performed.[21] McCord and his missionary contemporaries worked hard to dislodge what they regarded as the 'superstitious' healing beliefs and practices of the ubiquitous 'witch-doctor' healers.[22] They believed that religious conversions and the training of Africans in 'rational', scientific medicine approaches would eventually suppress and ultimately replace them. Although some recruits were converted while convalescing from illness or when working for missionaries, others were acquired from better-educated, literate, Christian communities.[23] For example, Katie Makanya, a medical assistant who worked for McCord for almost 40 years, had parents and grandparents who were Christian and literate; she herself had attended mission school, had reached the level of Standard 6 (Grade 8) and could speak six different languages.[24] Edward Jali, another mission-educated African medical assistant, who had come to work for McCord in Durban during the early twentieth century, wrote a letter in 1940 that captured something of these assistants' deeply intertwined biomedical and Christian healing convictions:

> My duty is not [only] to examine patients and prescribe some wonderful drug but to teach people better ways to live. It is the kind of work a Christian should do, the work Christ did when here on earth. He wandered from place to place teaching the people. Now and again He healed the sick and raised the dead.[25]

These early Christian auxiliaries also played important intermediary roles helping to bridge the cultural divide between European missionary doctors and nurses and their African patients. As cultural brokers they operated in contexts where western (or biomedical) and African healing beliefs and practices stood in opposition, a phenomenon that has been well researched in the last fifteen years.[26] They worked to overcome their patients' scepticism about western forms of medicine, helped to translate religious and medical concepts into languages and idioms understandable to their patients, and assisted European doctors and nurses to better appreciate their patients' needs. Some medical assistants were well regarded amongst their own communities for the healing services they provided, and were highly valued as medical assistants by mission doctors who relied heavily on their services. Although Christian missionaries and their assistants were not able to dislodge the work of indigenous healers, nor convince their patients that western medicine was the only or best option, since through the years Africans remained eclectic consumers who drew upon a wide range of healing paradigms, they ultimately helped facilitate the spread of western medicine as a more popular healing choice for Africans. However, despite the many contributions they made, they earned lower wages than white doctors and nurses, and remained subordinate in South Africa's racial hierarchy, as well as within the South African medical profession.

McCord Hospital's early efforts to train African doctors in Durban

In addition to training medical assistants, James McCord also broke new ground in his efforts to train African doctors in South Africa by building, equipping and staffing his own small and private school. After his hospital was opened in 1909, McCord was an early proponent of the training of 'dozens of our most intelligent Zulu youths in modern medicine'.[27] A great believer in the value that locally trained, Christian, African doctors could bring to South Africa's segregated society, especially to 'combat the evils associated with witch doctors and witchcraft', McCord took every opportunity to inform and mobilise locals and international 'friends' about the importance of 'the education of the Native along medical lines'.[28] During the early twentieth century, he wrote many letters to people of influence on the inadequacy of biomedical services available for Africans. He gave speeches to various associations, such as the Native Affairs Reform Association, on this subject; 'pleaded with the Durban Medical Society for a government commission to be appointed to investigate the health conditions prevailing among Africans'; and wrote papers to enlighten the public on these matters.[29]

However, while McCord believed that Africans were capable of achieving the highest medical-training standards and trusted that there would 'come a time when a medical class of natives will become possible, with a medical examination and full medical qualifications . . .', he was also a pragmatist.[30] Facing opposition from white medical professionals who feared that admission of blacks would lower the profession's standards, as well as the economic competition that black doctors would bring, McCord promoted a cost-effective and less threatening interim measure. He advocated for a five-year, shortened course of study in medicine (with the Junior Examination Certificate as the minimum qualification for entrance) to produce graduates who would practise medicine only amongst black communities under the direct supervision of white doctors.[31] Although few in South Africa were prepared to listen to his proposals in 1914 and 1916, McCord was undeterred and took his efforts to raise support for his shortened medical-training scheme overseas.

In 1918, McCord returned to the United States on furlough so that he could join the United States Army as a medical officer during the First World War. He hoped that this opportunity would enable him to raise the necessary funds for 'opening a school . . . in training young Zulus in medicine'.[32] He also wanted to use this furlough period to find a missionary doctor to accompany him back to Durban to assist him with these efforts. In October 1918, after being discharged from his army duties at the end of the war, McCord wrote to Reverend Enoch F. Bell, the foreign secretary of the ABM, expressing his determination to raise funds in the United States to open a medical school for Africans in Durban:

> The medical education of the Zulus looms up so big in relative importance that the work I have been doing seems of small account. I am henceforth a man of one idea and that idea is the medical education of the Zulu. I have about twenty more years of active work in the field. I want that twenty years to be put into the medical education of the Zulu. I should like to practice medicine also, in fact that is necessary to get clinical material for my students, but that is going to take a secondary place hereafter.[33]

The following year, McCord travelled to various parts of the USA to 'exhaust . . . every possibility' for cash and pledged donations from various church congregations, philanthropic organisations and interested individuals.[34] In December 1919, he insisted that he would only leave the USA with the 'understanding and belief that the project of medical education is going to be a "going concern" . . . Nothing else will be considered or contemplated.'[35]

In 1921, having returned to South Africa with a strong determination, McCord, together with Alan B. Taylor, the young American doctor he had recruited to assist him with his hospital work and with the teaching of medical students, began to work towards bringing his medical-education dream to fruition. During this period, McCord made it clear that he wanted to provide African students on his McCord Hospital premises with a five-year medical training – 'practically equal to that of the white medical men' – entitling them once they graduated 'to practice only among the native people', and without government recognition because they lacked the necessary British medical degree to properly register in South Africa.[36] This inferior qualification, he hoped, would also prevent 'the native medical men leaving their own people for more lucrative service among the whites', and prevent the threat of competition with white doctors in practice.

While the medical school buildings were being erected, McCord, in preparation for the opening of this school, sponsored 'six bright-eyed, alert' young African men, who each had two or three years of high school education, but 'who spoke English fluently and were eager to study medicine', to be taught a number of premedical chemistry, biology, zoology, botany, anatomy and physiology subjects over a period of two years at the Amanzimtoti Institute at Adams Mission Station.[37] In a letter addressed to friends in the USA in early 1923, McCord wrote enthusiastically about the near completion of the medical school building, named 'Piedmont Hall' in honour of the Piedmont Church in Worcester, Massachusetts, which supplied most of the donations needed to build the school.[38] In this letter he told his audience how this new school was built using every cost-cutting measure possible, including the labour of 'my medical students [who helped to] erect . . . their own medical school', and that, when completed, it would provide both dormitories and classrooms for the first class of five medical students who had by then successfully passed their preliminary science courses at Adams Mission.

Although McCord did not know where the money was to come from to pay for the running expenses of 'the first South African native medical school' once it opened – many of the pledges that had been promised to him in the USA were never paid – he was so certain about its significance that he was prepared to run the school 'on a financial shoestring' until such time as it won over local sceptics.[39] During 1923, he optimistically maintained his faith that the 'good Lord' would provide the financial means for his medical school project, and was confident that his pioneering medical students would excel in any examination they might have to face.[40] McCord also felt hopeful that once he had 'gone ahead and blazed the trail', demonstrating 'the Zulu's ability to master the subject of medicine . . . and at a moderate expense', then the South African government would help pay for at least some of the school's annual running costs.[41]

However, even before their clinical training of students could properly begin in the latter half of 1923, strong opposition from South Africa's white medical authorities – who were responsible for registering and managing the quality of medical services in South Africa – forced McCord and Taylor to abandon their medical-training efforts. In 1955, Taylor, then the medical superintendent at McCord Hospital, remembered how the secretary of health at the time had been particularly opposed to their school. The authorities refused to recognise or tolerate any inferior qualification to that ordinarily required for the registration of medical practitioners in the country, which they argued threatened to undermine the white medical profession's standards.[42]

What also undermined their private medical school training scheme was the news learnt from McCord's friend, C.T. Loram (an influential Natal educationalist, long-standing member of the Native Affairs Commission and liberal politician who was a founder member of the Institute of Race Relations), that a better training programme had just been started at the South African Native College of Fort Hare.[43] Alexander Kerr, the Scottish principal of Fort Hare at the time, who publicly argued against McCord and Taylor's private scheme to produce 'half-baked doctors', had started offering matriculated African students the chance to study preclinical medical subjects. In his estimation, the Fort Hare scheme was a better option as it would lead to a full medical qualification once the students had completed their final clinical years overseas.

By 1930, ten students had passed their preclinical subjects at Fort Hare and gone on, with the aid of scholarships, to complete their medical studies in Britain or the USA.[44] In time, it was hoped, the whole medical course would be given at Fort Hare. Although McCord raised concerns about the possibility of foreign degrees alienating these African students 'from [their] people' by training overseas, he also saw the merit in sponsoring his five medical students to complete their matriculation qualifications at Fort Hare. It offered them a real chance of qualifying, registering with the South African Medical and Dental Council (SAMDC) and then practising as fully trained doctors in South Africa. Unfortunately, only one of his five students passed the difficult matriculation examinations, which their inadequate primary and secondary schooling had ill-prepared them for, and even this student failed to complete his first-year medical training at Fort Hare. In *My Patients were Zulus,* McCord wrote despairingly:

[M]y medical students were scattered, with the exception of Edward Jali [the same person who had been trained by McCord as a medical assistant in earlier years], who came to work for me in the dispensary. The funds with which I'd hoped to train them were gone, either in buildings or in paying their tuition and board at Fort Hare. With the coming of the depression to America, pledges of support for my school were no longer being paid, making it unlikely that I could revive my own plan.[45]

We should not write off McCord's early medical assistant and then medical school training schemes for Africans as simply the efforts of a prejudiced or narrow-minded person. Believing early on that social and medical opinion would eventually shift in support of the provision of a full medical training of Africans, who formed the majority population in South Africa, McCord was also a realist in a racially discriminatory and segregationist context, where the medical profession stood 'bitterly opposed to the local training of natives in medicine'.[46] In view of the urgent medical needs of Africans in South Africa's deteriorating rural reserves that he had witnessed as a medical missionary, this sincere but paternalistic doctor was determined to make at least some movement forward on the issue of medical training for Africans, even if this meant providing lower qualifications for his recruits until such time as full qualifications could be provided. We should see his efforts as a strategic, provisional measure, and a classic manoeuvre made by white liberals in South Africa at the time, to attempt to move developments for Africans gradually forward without challenging too vigorously the white ruling establishment's status quo.[47]

McCord, while advocating some of the most progressive medical educational efforts for Africans in the country at the time, was also a man of his time, and was thus caught up in, influenced by and ultimately helped to sustain the hegemonic, racial segregation ideology of white South Africa. The concept of training blacks to 'serve their own people' in a racially segregated service was both an acknowledgement that blacks had the potential to become skilled medical professionals *and* an upholding of the separateness of white-controlled medical knowledge and practice as the norm or standard by which blacks continued to remain a racial, and professional, inferior 'other'. The fact that men were chosen to study for this five-year medical diploma and not women demonstrates, too, the wider perspective about unequal gender capabilities and social roles in operation in missionary, medical and wider societal thinking at this time.

Although McCord's black medical-training scheme was in shambles by the end of 1923, he never gave up on the possibility of achieving his medical school dream. Though disheartened, he asserted that he was 'determined to keep working for some form of native medical training', and from then onwards he and Taylor made it 'our mission, whenever we were with other white doctors, to win additional converts to this idea'.[48]

These early Christian missionary medical-training efforts, though premature in the early twentieth century, succeeded in drawing attention to the need for the provision of medical education for Africans in South Africa. Their black health-care work and public advocacy efforts to win support for their black medical-training schemes also challenged the complacency of the state, which during the 1930s increasingly came to view these tasks as its responsibility.

The interwar years and the state's 'Medical Aid' training scheme

By the late 1920s, a number of factors encouraged the South African government to consider providing better health services and a medical education for Africans. Mounting evidence of poor health in South Africa's congested and impoverished African rural reserve areas was a growing concern. So too were the potential disease threats that increasing African urbanisation posed to white urban areas, as well as the economic productivity of African labourers on the mines and industries.[49] During the 1920s, even the gold-mining industry had started providing better health services for its African workers on the mines when they realised that African worker illnesses endangered the productivity of their cheap labour supplies.[50]

In 1928, a government commission, headed by C.T. Loram, after several years of investigation, met to discuss and report back on its inquiry into 'The Training of Natives in Medicine and Public Health'.[51] It recognised the severe shortage of black public health-care services in the country, particularly the services of doctors in 'Native territories',[52] and recommended that equal medical qualifications be provided for black South Africans but on a segregated basis. To cut costs and to build on established experience, the commission looked to the two existing white medical schools to provide such facilities, but only Wits in Johannesburg was willing to consider providing 'a Medical School for Natives segregated from the existing Medical School of the University of the Witwatersrand but under its control'.[53] About this time, one of America's famous philanthropic organisations, the Rockefeller Foundation, also offered Wits $300 000 towards the building costs for such a school.[54] However, severe funding shortages between 1929 and 1932 – the Great Depression years – and 'the bitter hostility' of many members of the medical profession to these plans were essential factors leading to the shelving of these suggestions. So, too, was minister of native affairs E.G. Jansen's public assertion in June 1931 that '[w]e do not think that the time has yet arrived when an institution should be established for the training of natives in medicine'.[55] As a result, no positive actions were taken based on the Loram Committee's recommendations.

Although no momentum was achieved at this point on the issue of providing black students with a medical education, many heated debates raged during the late 1920s and early 1930s in government and medical circles. Analysis of these debates reveals that opinions were largely split between those arguing for the provision of a full medical qualification for Africans, and those arguing for a 'second-rate' medical-training scheme where subordinate categories of African auxiliaries would be restricted to working amongst 'their own communities' in a racially segregated medical service. Overseas-trained black doctors also weighed in on this debate. For instance, A.B. Xuma voiced strong opposition to the provision of inferior medical qualifications for black students in South Africa, using his ability to obtain his medical degree from a prestigious American university as a prime example of what Africans could achieve when given the chance to do so.[56]

Essentially, what was at stake was how much medicine to teach Africans and where best to locate them in the medical hierarchy in order to protect white social, economic and professional control. What most white stakeholders did agree on, however, was their opposition to black students going overseas to complete their medical studies. Concern was raised by individuals on both sides of the debate about a number of issues. Firstly, much unease stemmed from the exposure these students would likely gain to more liberal social and political ideas and conditions overseas. Linked to this, secondly, was the concern that overseas students were allowed to work with white patients and cadavers, which were tabooed practices in South Africa at the time. Thirdly, these stakeholders were anxious that these candidates, having been exposed to more open and democratic societies overseas, would then forget their 'proper' place as political and economic subordinates in South Africa's social hierarchy when they returned to practise.[57] However, because no progress was made on the issue of supplying black students with a full medical-training opportunity in the country at this time, those students who sought to become doctors were compelled to continue applying to overseas universities for their training.

A few years later, once the hardships of the Depression years had eased and growing ill health in the congested black reserves became a state priority once again, those who argued for an inferior medical-training scheme won favour. Such schemes were growing in popularity in other European colonies in Africa as part of their post-war 'development' and social welfare programmes, and in South Africa too, following the introduction of increasingly discriminatory racial legislation by the interwar governments.[58] In 1933, under the leadership of Edward Thornton (then secretary of public health for the Union), an interdepartmental government committee on 'Native Medical Education' came up with a plan that would address the gaps in health provision while keeping healing and economic power in white hands. It suggested the establishment of a scheme similar to one operating successfully in French West Africa at the time, which would train Africans not as doctors but as medical auxiliaries or assistants in a shortened medical course. They would receive diplomas entitling them to practise under the supervision of white medical officers in needy 'Native areas', and work as salaried employees in government service.[59]

Far less progressive than the Loram Committee's recommendations, Thornton's committee did not view the full training of black doctors as 'practical politics' at the time; nor did it consider that there were sufficient numbers of suitably qualified black candidates to warrant the expense of creating a separate medical school.[60] Furthermore, it felt that a shorter-length course would lower the training costs borne by the state, enable the quicker production of black medical assistants and aid the development of a completely separate 'Native Health and Medical Service', jointly administered by the Department of Public Health and Department of Native Administration. This scheme would also appease the white medical fraternity by providing better health-care services for black South Africans while reducing the potential threat that competition posed to white doctors in practice.[61]

Thus, in a changed historical context from the time when McCord attempted his earlier medical-training scheme, a five-year 'Medical Aid' (also sometimes spelt 'Aide') training course was started in 1935. The Chamber of Mines, interested in improving the health of potential labour supplies in the reserves, put up a donation of £75 000 (or $300 000) to help provide classroom facilities and bursaries for students.[62] Reflecting a similar gender bias as McCord's 1920s scheme, 'Native males' with at least a Junior Certificate were targeted for this training programme, but preference was given to applicants who had passed their matriculation (Standard 10 or Grade 12 high school qualification) examinations. The first three years of the course was provided at the Native College of Fort Hare in the Eastern Cape, where students studied botany, zoology, chemistry and physics during their first year; anatomy and physiology in their second year; and, finally, pathology, bacteriology, public health work and laboratory procedures in their third year. This was followed by a fourth year of study in medicine, (minor) surgery and midwifery at the Victoria Hospital in Lovedale, also in the Eastern Cape. Involvement by James McCord, whose continued interest in the provision of medical education for Africans saw him become a key member of the initiating committee of this training course, persuaded the committee to send all final fifth-year students to complete their practical training at the McCord Hospital in Durban.[63]

As a result, and fittingly, the large square building that had been erected on the McCord Hospital property in 1923 for McCord and Taylor's failed private medical school became used by Medical Aids doing their clinical training between 1939 and 1943 while the scheme lasted.[64] So enthusiastic was McCord's support for this training scheme that he recommended and helped sponsor Edward Jali, one of his most trusted and valued African medical assistants, to train as one of the country's first Medical Aids, which he successfully completed in 1939.[65] McCord wrote that Medical Aids were given a thorough curative and preventive training at the busy McCord Hospital, where they

> took case histories, helped with major operations and performed minor surgery themselves, watched and attended confinements, accompanied Durban health officers on their rounds of the city, or travelled over the country with Government health officers to study malarial, sanitation or other conditions. In addition to all this, they attended surgical-clinical lectures given by Dr Taylor and other doctors, worked with microscopes and various laboratory equipment, and carried out much of the examination routine necessary in a hospital. The training of student aides particularly emphasised midwifery and gynaecology, practical minor surgery, the administration of medicines in various ailments, eye work, dentistry, and the treatment of venereal diseases.[66]

Jali was, however, one of only a few to graduate from this course. Although it was anticipated that ten students would graduate annually, only twelve of the expected 30 candidates graduated at the end of the first three years of the course, and during all the years of this course's operation, just 35 students graduated.[67] As a 'near-medical' training that turned out to be only one year short of the standard, six-year medical degree provided for white students at the time, it produced anger and frustration amongst its students, who found themselves ambiguously placed between white doctors and black nurses. As noted in a 1942 government report on the issue, their duties were 'in the main restricted to those of male nurse and orderly', which produced high levels of dissatisfaction 'as they had been trained to do very much more, and had been led '[to] expect that they would be given independent posts where they would practice virtually as doctors'.[68] As graduates soon found out, their 'pseudo-medical' training limited their status and work opportunities, which were essentially restricted to low-paying, state public-service work in black rural areas under the supervision of white district surgeons.[69]

It also resulted in strong opposition from the SAMDC, the legislative body responsible for regulating the standards of medical training and practice in South Africa, which had not been consulted in the development of the course.[70] The course gave instruction in curative procedures reserved for medical practitioners only, and produced 'pseudo-doctors' with inferior medical degrees in contravention of the 1928 Medical, Dental and Pharmacy Act. Once again, another medical-training initiative was halted by the South African medical authorities, who refused to recognise any inferior qualifications.

McCord was aware of the inequalities and restrictions the course produced for its black graduates. He had adopted a gradualist and reformist approach, shared with many other white liberals on the founding committee. For him the exercise was a

> chastening experience . . . [it] . . . had taught us that it was wiser to move slowly than to arouse the antagonism of the *back-veld* [rural] doctors and make no progress at all. The best we could hope for was that the medical aides might soon win a firm place for themselves. Then it would be possible to take the final step toward a full medical course and medical recognition for non-Europeans.[71]

For these liberals, who were hopeful that a full medical training would be provided for black students some day in the future, it was better to produce an inferior type of black biomedical practitioner than none at all. Ultimately, however, as a result of the many objections, the Medical Aid training scheme was abandoned at Fort Hare at the end of 1942, which instead opted to develop a BSc Hygiene course emphasising public health work, and McCord Hospital ended the clinical training for these students in 1943.[72] However, this did not occur before the training of black doctors had officially commenced in South Africa at the Wits and UCT medical schools. During the early 1940s, some trained Medical Aids resigned from their state public-health service appointments and opted to start their medical studies again to obtain a recognisable degree that would enable them to practise as fully qualified doctors in South Africa.[73]

The Second World War and the training of black doctors at Wits and UCT

During the early 1940s, once again, altered historical circumstances shifted the debate about the standard of medical education for black students in South Africa. This time, however, the debate swung in favour of providing a full biomedical training for African, Indian and coloured students. There were four main reasons for this. Firstly, the existence of a more reformist and liberal political climate during the Second World War was pivotal. The atrocities committed by the Nazis revitalised egalitarian politics across the world and led a number of influential white South Africans to question the racist foundations of their society. This era saw the temporary suspension by the United Party government of what had been growing legislative moves towards institutionalised racial segregation and discrimination in the country. This period provided a rare window of opportunity for social welfare improvements, including reforms in the health sector, such as was clearly evident in the Pentz Commission on free hospitalisation in 1943, and the Gluckman Report of 1944, which sought to reorganise and improve South Africa's health-care services.[74] Secondly, the state needed to address the growing number of black patients seeking treatment at urban public health facilities, which had been inundated during the war years.[75] For example, between 1936 and 1946, the population census recorded an average increase of Africans in South Africa's major industrial centres by nearly 60 per cent.[76] While the availability of more effective biomedical treatments, including antibiotic therapies, helps explain this increase, so does the growing number of Africans migrating from deteriorating rural areas to get jobs in the cities, and finding themselves often in even worse informal urban settlements.

Thirdly, the war years witnessed the emergence of a more radical and mass-based black nationalist opposition politics under organisations such as the African National Congress and worker trade unions. The influx of black South Africans into what were considered white urban areas, together with growing political solidarity and stronger calls for improvements in available services and wages, promoted greater urgency and demand on the state to improve the available public health-care services for the country's majority.[77] Finally, the submarine war prevented black students from travelling by ship to study medicine overseas, increasing the pressure on schools within South Africa to accept black applicants. The fact that many white English-speaking students left South Africa to fight as soldiers also opened up spaces at medical schools like Wits and UCT for black candidates during the war years.[78]

As a result, from the early 1940s, small numbers of Indian and coloured students were admitted to complete their full medical training at Wits and UCT, and a small number of African students were also admitted to the

Wits Medical School.[79] The first black doctors began graduating from these schools from the end of 1945.[80] This admission policy was maintained until 1959, when more restrictive apartheid-government legislation closed the doors of these universities to black student applicants, unless they first obtained ministerial permission. It is interesting to note that before the passage of the 1959 Extension of University Education Act, which gave the state power to influence South African universities' admissions policies, it was university authorities, not the state, who determined which students were accepted or excluded.[81] For example, African students remained excluded from UCT during this period and were denied placements right up until the late 1980s, ostensibly because of insufficient clinical material for teaching purposes at its Groote Schuur teaching hospital, and to fall in line with the apartheid state's separate-development policies after 1948.[82] This university's dependence on government funding and its desire to maintain good relations with the public meant that administrators and lecturers were desperate not to offend white South African social mores.

Medical historian Howard Phillips argues that during these early years, despite the official position of these white medical schools, the policy was one of 'grudging tolerance' of their black students, and educational opportunities were riddled with racial quotas and reservations.[83] Between the early 1940s to late 1950s, black students rarely exceeded 6 per cent of the total student bodies of these universities, enabling these universities to remain de facto white institutions.[84] In addition, black doctors who graduated from Wits in the 1950s spoke of feeling insecure as students as there were only 'seven or eight of us in a class of over a hundred white students', and perceived their white colleagues' attitudes as 'patronising us at every opportunity'.[85] The scarcity of places reserved for black students at these institutions also meant that competition was fierce, requiring black matriculants, already disadvantaged in coming from poor families and with inferior secondary school instruction in science and mathematics, to work much harder than their white counterparts to be accepted into the same universities.

The segregation and later apartheid context of South Africa greatly influenced Wits's and UCT's unequal admissions policies, as well as black and white student relationships on these campuses. Although black and white medical students were taught in the same classes at these universities, racially mixed classes were considered anathema to many whites in South

Africa at the time, as they feared the miscegenation outcomes of fraternisation amongst university students, as well as professional competition.[86] As a result, Wits university's authorities, concerned about alienating public opinion in the prevailing social order, petitioned the state for funding on numerous occasions during this period, to help it establish a separate medical college for black students to reduce racial tensions.[87] This funding was not provided, however.

As a result, historian Bruce Murray, who has done extensive research on Wits during the 1940s and 1950s era, argues that Wits adopted a policy of 'academic non-segregation and social segregation', where a colour bar limited 'racial mixing' to purely academic, not social, activities.[88] This social segregation policy applied at UCT too, as was captured in a letter between the Students' Representative Council president and the university registrar in 1959: '[I]n non-academic or social matters such as pertains to dances, it is most desirable and in the best interest of the University that the University abide by the customs and conventions of the community in which it exists.'[89] This segregation policy applied to student participation in sporting events and other recreational and social functions. Careful monitoring of social interaction across the colour line was observed, with harsh punishments meted out for even petty 'offences'. As one black student who attended UCT argued, 'We had our own social life, our own social circles, and only went there for the purposes of attaining our academic qualifications.'[90] Although there were exceptions of close friendships that did develop, as well as examples of multiracial cooperation in student organisations on these campuses, such as students who participated as members of the National Union of South African Students (NUSAS),[91] most white students accepted these universities' segregation policies and there was little socialisation with black students. As one UCT medical graduate explained: '. . . [we] didn't get to know them that well; you didn't know what their issues were. I think we lived in a bit of a white bubble most of the time in terms of the realities of fellow students' lives.'[92]

Black students were not allowed to live in university residences, which were located in Group Areas Act-designated white residential areas. This produced greater hardships for many as they found it difficult to find suitable accommodation close to their university campuses.[93] During the late 1990s, following the 1997 Truth and Reconciliation Commission health-sector hearings, as part of their process of transformation in the post-apartheid era, the universities of Cape Town and the Witwatersrand undertook their own internal reconciliation hearings in an attempt to acknowledge the racial discriminations they perpetuated. Many graduates recounted in submissions their discriminatory educational experiences at these universities. Common issues discussed included the cramped, noisy and candle-lit housing conditions that many were forced to endure whilst living in the townships, as well as the expense and wasted time involved in travelling long distances between their university and township homes on inadequate public transport.[94] As Shan Naidoo, a Wits graduate, noted in a written questionnaire, 'I hated studying at Wits. Travelling was a nightmare. It took us an average of one hour in peak traffic one way from our "black townships" to Wits.'[95]

Moreover, although Wits and UCT officially portrayed their institutions as providing academic training for blacks on an equal, non-segregated basis, there were many humiliating academic restrictions that black students were forced to endure on a daily basis, which ultimately undermined the quality of their academic training. For example, while it is true that black students did attend the same classes as white students, they were forced to leave when white patients or cadavers were demonstrated on, and could not examine white patients in clinical rounds in their teaching hospitals or wards. They were only allowed to treat black patients in 'non-European' teaching hospitals, such as at Baragwanath in Soweto, just outside Johannesburg, and were restricted to the black wards of their teaching hospitals, such as Groote Schuur, UCT's main teaching hospital.[96] At UCT, black students even had to sign documents accepting these policies upon entering medical school, and if they disobeyed, they faced immediate expulsion.[97]

Ralph Hendrickse, one of the first coloured doctors to graduate from UCT, in 1948, and who then went on to do his internship at McCord Hospital, recalled the deep embarrassment he felt at being forced to leave when white patients or cadavers were demonstrated on by his professors:

> In the medical school, non-white medical students were prohibited from entering the white wards of Groote Schuur Hospital, and in outpatients, where the consultants saw both white and Coloured patients, we were constrained to perform a jack-in-the-box act by popping outside when a white patient entered the clinic and popping in again when a Coloured patient entered ... We were also not allowed to be present when case

presentations to our class involved white patients, whether alive or dead. Yes, even autopsies were segregated and white bodies were not defiled by the eyes of non-white medical students . . .[98]

In contrast, white students were encouraged to learn from and examine both black and white patients and cadavers, and were allowed to rotate through black and white teaching hospitals or wards. Therefore, black students were ultimately denied access to learning about the full spectrum of diseases in South Africa's diverse population.

Black graduates also felt that they had less access to their white professors and senior lecturers. Over the years it was noted that senior members of the teaching staff often restricted their clinical rounds of instruction to white hospitals and clinics located near to their universities, to accommodate their busy schedules.[99] As a result, many black graduates argued that they did not get the same level of clinical supervision compared to their white colleagues, and were sometimes not taught by specialists in certain areas.[100] Moreover, many black students often had to travel great distances to receive their clinical instruction, when there were insufficient black clinical facilities to accommodate them at Wits or UCT. Some students even travelled as far away as McCord Hospital in Durban to do their obstetrics and gynaecology rotations.[101]

In addition, the hospitals or wards that black students were allowed to rotate through had inferior facilities and equipment. Most were vastly overcrowded and short-staffed compared to white clinical facilities. This inevitably compromised the quality of instruction given to black students. Groote Schuur Hospital often operated with a 100 per cent occupancy rate in its black wards and less than 70 per cent in its white wards.[102] Baragwanath Hospital, which was opened in 1948, had about 2 500 beds to serve an estimated population of over one million people. At these overcrowded black hospital facilities, many patients were often forced to sleep on floor beds, were discharged early or were turned away if they were not considered emergency cases.[103] Furthermore, the requirement that black students and doctors use separate toilets, dining rooms and change-room facilities in public hospitals were petty and hurtful practices they endured on a daily basis.[104]

Many black students reported feeling academic isolation and social alienation on their mostly white university campuses, and received no additional educational assistance, despite coming from racially disadvantaged educational backgrounds.[105] Some black graduates, recalling their training experiences, have expressed deep resentment towards their training institutions for making them feel like outsiders in a hostile environment. Joe Veriava, a medical graduate from Wits, makes this clear: 'When I completed my medical studies . . . I, like many other black students before me, was left with a feeling of resentment towards an institution which trained me but never made me feel a part of it.'[106] Powerful memories of 'being humiliated', being 'cheated', of having 'missed out' or being 'ignored', and treated as 'second-class citizens' came up often in post-apartheid internal reconciliation hearings and written submissions.[107] Many black graduates, still to this day, abstain from participating in their alma mater's alumni activities, as Hugh Philpott, a medical graduate who attended UCT during the late 1940s and early 1950s, recalled: '. . . some of them [black students] felt so bitter about it that they didn't come to the reunion . . . because of what [they] suffered 50 years ago . . . It hurt them in a way we will never understand.'[108]

Thus, while the authorities at Wits and UCT maintained that the training they gave to black students was exactly the same as their white students received, in fact, it perpetuated an educational system that prevented black students from obtaining equality in their university training. Ideologies and practices of exclusion and racial discrimination were encountered and experienced by black students on a daily basis in both their social and academic lives. Most students quietly accepted these conditions because they had little alternative. However, this situation of training token numbers of black students at the country's two white medical schools was less than ideal. As the 1940s continued, the provision of a completely separate black medical school facility was increasingly mooted as the best way forward if the country was to continue providing a full medical qualification for black students.

Notes

1. See, for example, Anne Digby, *Diversity and Division in Medicine: Health Care in South Africa from the 1800s* (Oxford: Peter Lang, 2006); and Randall M. Packard, *White Plague, Black Labor: Tuberculosis and the Political Economy of Health and Disease in South Africa* (Berkeley and Los Angeles: University of California Press, 1989).

2. *Report of the National Health Services Commission on the Provision of an Organised National Health Service for all Sections of the People of the Union of South Africa, 1942–4* (Pretoria: Government Printer, 1944).

3. 'The National Health Service', *South African Medical Journal* 19, no. 2 (27 January 1945), 19.

4. Catherine Burns, 'Louisa Mvemve: A woman's advice to the public on the cure of various diseases', *Kronos: Journal of Cape History* (23 November 1996); and Karen Flint, *Healing Traditions: African Medicine, Cultural Exchange, and Competition in South Africa, 1820–1948* (Athens: Ohio University Press; Pietermaritzburg: University of KwaZulu-Natal Press, 2008).

5. Bruce K. Murray, *Wits the Early Years: A History of the University of the Witwatersrand Johannesburg and its Precursors, 1896–1939* (Johannesburg: Witwatersrand University Press, 1982); and Anne Digby and Howard Phillips with Harriet Deacon and Kirsten Thomson, *At the Heart of Healing: Groote Schuur Hospital, 1938–2008* (Auckland Park: Jacana, 2008).

6. Murray, *Wits the Early Years*, 35–6 and 300–2; Saul Dubow, *Scientific Racism in Modern South Africa* (Cambridge: Cambridge University Press, 1995); Anne Digby, 'Early black doctors in South Africa', *Journal of African History* 46, no. 3 (November 2005); and Phillip V. Tobias, 'Apartheid and medical education: The training of black doctors in South Africa', *The Leech* 60, no. 1 (March 1991).

7. Steven Gish, *Alfred B. Xuma: African, American, South African* (London: Macmillan Press, 2000); K. Goonam, *Coolie Doctor: An Autobiography* (Durban: Madiba Publications, 1991). Also see Adam Cassimjee, '"A good training ground": The lives of four South African Indian doctors who graduated in the Republic of Ireland during the 1960s and 1970s' (Honours thesis, University of KwaZulu-Natal, 2011).

8. G.W. Gale, 'Medical schools in Africa: A short historical and contemporary survey', *Journal of Medical Education* 34, no. 8 (August 1959); Adell Patton, *Physicians, Colonial Racism, and Diaspora in West Africa* (Gainesville: University of Florida Press, 1996), 24, 32–7; and John Iliffe, *East African Doctors: A History of the Modern Profession* (Cambridge: Cambridge University Press, 1998). For a similar situation in central Africa, see Willy de Craemer and Renee C. Fox, *The Emerging Physician: A Sociological Approach to the Development of a Congolese Medical Profession* (Stanford, CA: The Hoover Institution, 1968).

9. Patton, *Physicians, Colonial Racism, and Diaspora in West Africa*, 34–5. For more on other medical-training facilities opened in Africa in the twentieth century, see Marion Wallace, *Health, Power and Politics in Windhoek, Namibia, 1914–1945* (Basel: P. Schlettwein Publishing, 2002); and Claire L. Wendland, *A Heart for the Work: Journeys through an African Medical School* (Chicago and London: University of Chicago Press, 2010).

10. Bruce K. Murray, *Wits the 'Open' Years: A History of the University of the Witwatersrand, Johannesburg, 1939–1959* (Johannesburg: Witwatersrand University Press, 1997), 173. Also see Tobias, 'Apartheid and medical education' for further statistics.

11. For more on the well-researched history of nursing in South Africa, see Shula Marks, *Divided Sisterhood: Race, Class and Gender in the South African Nursing Profession* (Johannesburg: Witwatersrand University Press, 1994). Also see T.G. Mashaba, *Rising to the Challenge of Change: A History of Black Nursing in South Africa* (Cape Town: Juta, 1995); and Mazo Sybil T. MaDlamini Buthelezi, *African Nurse Pioneers in KwaZulu-Natal, 1920–2000* (Canada, USA, UK: Trafford Publishing, 2004).

12. For more on the gendered aspect of nursing, see Catherine Burns, 'A man is a clumsy thing who does not know how to handle a sick person: Aspects of the history of masculinity and race in the shaping of male nursing in South Africa, 1900–50', *Journal of Southern African Studies* 24, no. 4 (December 1998).

13. Karin A. Shapiro, 'Doctors or Medical Aids: The debate over the training of black medical personnel for the rural black population in South Africa in the 1920s and 1930s', *Journal of Southern African Studies* 13, no. 2 (January 1987).

14. Michael Gelfand, *Christian Doctor and Nurse: The History of Medical Missions in South Africa* (Sandton: Mariannhill Mission Press, 1984).

15. By the early twentieth century, western forms of medicine increasingly moved away from using supernatural explanations and instead used science, particularly 'germ theory', to explain the causes of diseases. See Digby, *Diversity and Division in Medicine*, chapter 7, for a useful summary of the main differences between these approaches.

16. See, for example, Gelfand, *Christian Doctor and Nurse*; and Marks, *Divided Sisterhood*.

17. Digby, *Diversity and Division in Medicine*, especially chapters 2, 3 and 5.

18. James B. McCord, *My Patients were Zulus* (New York and Toronto: Rinehart, 1951).

19. Also see Vanessa Noble, 'Health is much too important a subject to be left to doctors: African assistant health workers in Natal during the early twentieth century', *Journal of Natal and Zulu History* 24 and 25 (2006–7).

20. These oral interviews were used to write a book. See Margaret McCord, *The Calling of Katie Makanya* (Cape Town and Johannesburg: David Philip, 1995), 198. For more on Umqibelo, see McCord, *My Patients were Zulus*, 107 and 117.

21. McCord, *My Patients were Zulus*, 59.

22. See above, 88, 196, 223, 231; and James B. McCord, 'The Zulu witch doctor and medicine man', *South African Medical Record* xvi, no. 4 (April 1918).

23. One such school included Inanda Seminary for girls in Natal. See Meghan Healy-Clancy, *A World of their Own: A History of South African Women's Education* (Pietermaritzburg: University of KwaZulu-Natal Press, 2013).

24. McCord, *The Calling of Katie Makanya*, 178; and McCord, *My Patients were Zulus*, 60.

25. McCord, *My Patients were Zulus*, 273.

26. For more on the issue of cultural brokers and situations of medical pluralism in African contexts, see, for example, Burns, 'Louisa Mvemve'; Nancy Rose Hunt, *A*

Colonial Lexicon: Of Birth Ritual, Medicalisation, and Mobility in the Congo (Durham and London: Duke University Press, 1999); Anne Digby and Helen Sweet, 'Nurses as culture brokers in twentieth-century South Africa', in *Plural Medicine, Tradition and Modernity, 1800–2000,* ed. Waltraud Ernst (London and New York: Routledge, 2001); Digby, *Diversity and Division in Medicine*, especially chapters 8 and 9; Julie Parle, *States of Mind: Searching for Mental Health in Natal and Zululand, 1868–1918* (Pietermaritzburg: University of KwaZulu-Natal Press, 2007); and Flint, *Healing Traditions.*

27. CC MH Houghton Library, Boston (HLB), Papers of the American Board of Commissioners of Foreign Missions (ABCFM), ABC 15: Letters from Missionaries to Africa, 1834–1919, Vol. 29, No. 170, Reel 203 and 204, Report of the Medical Department of the American Zulu Mission for 1916.

28. CC MH HLB ABCFM, Vol. 29, No. 186, Reel 203, Newspaper article 'Natal Native Affairs, Annual Meeting and Report of Reform Association, Dr McCord on the "medicine man": Brutality and ignorance of native doctors', [1917?].

29. CC MH HLB ABCFM, Vol. 29, No. 186, Reel 203, Newspaper article J.B. McCord, 'The Zulu witch doctor and medicine man'.

30. CC MH HLB ABCFM, Vol. 29, No. 116, Reel 203, Report of the Medical Department for 1913–14, 31 July 1914 [26 June 1914].

31. CC MH HLB ABCFM, Vol. 29, No. 170, Reel 204, Report of Medical Department of the American Zulu Mission for 1916; as well as McCord, *My Patients were Zulus*, 223–4. The Junior Certificate was equivalent to Standard 8 or Grade 10 of a high school qualification.

32. McCord, *My Patients were Zulus*, 224.

33. CC MH HLB ABCFM, Vol. 31, Reel 207, McCord Letter 141, James B. McCord, Oberlin, to Reverend E. Bell, Boston, 29 October 1918.

34. McCord, *My Patients were Zulus*, 228.

35. CC MH HLB ABCFM, Vol. 31, Reel 207, McCord Letter 163, McCord, Granville Illinois, to Rev E F Bell, Boston, 31 December 1919.

36. CC MH HLB ABCFM, Vol. 48, Reel 211, Zulu Mission 1909–29, Documents Letters [Supplementary], James B. McCord, 'Medical work among the Zulus', n/d [1936?]; McCord, *My Patients were Zulus*, 231.

37. CC MH HLB ABCFM, Vol. 48, Reel 211, Zulu Mission 1909–29, Documents Letters [Supplementary], Letter from James B. McCord to 'My dear friends', 5 April 1923; and McCord, *My Patients were Zulus*, 231, 234.

38. CC MH HLB ABCFM, Vol. 48, No. 292, Reel 211, Zulu Mission 1909–29, Documents Letters [Supplementary], Letter from J.B. McCord to 'My dear friends', 5 April 1923; and Vol. 48, No. 291, Reel 211, Letter from J.B. McCord to Rev. Enoch F. Bell (Boston, Mass), 8 May 1923; and McCord, *My Patients were Zulus*, 234.

39. McCord, *My Patients were Zulus*, 228–30.

40. CC MH HLB ABCFM, Vol. 48, No. 292, Reel 211, Letter from J.B. McCord to 'My dear friends', 5 April 1923.

41. CC MH HLB ABCFM, Vol. 29, No. 130, Reel 203, 'Medical work among the Zulus' signed by James B. McCord, [1918?].
42. CC MH Pretoria Disk 2 Doc 65, Annual Report of the Medical Superintendent of McCord Hospital 1955, 16.
43. McCord, *My Patients were Zulus*, 230–8.
44. Shapiro, 'Doctors or Medical Aids', 247.
45. McCord, *My Patients were Zulus*, 239–40.
46. CC MH HLB ABCFM, ABC 15: Letters from Missionaries to Africa, 1834–1919, Vol. 29 Reel 204, No. 170, 'Report of Medical Department of the A.Z.M. for 1916', not signed, stamped rec'd 10 Sept 1917, 3.
47. For more on liberals, see Paul Rich's books, *White Power and the Liberal Conscience: Racial Segregation and South African Liberalism, 1921–60* (Manchester: Manchester University Press, 1984) and *Hope and Despair: English-Speaking Intellectuals and South African Politics, 1896–1976* (London: British Academic Press, 1993).
48. McCord, *My Patients were Zulus*, 239–40.
49. 'Report of the Department of Public Health for year ending 30 June 1925', *Medical Journal of South Africa* 21, no. 9 (April 1926), 259–62; and James B. McCord, 'A native medical service in South Africa', *Journal of the Medical Association of South Africa* 14 (September 1930), 511.
50. See, for example, A.P. Cartwright, *Doctors on the Mines: A History of the Mine Medical Doctors Association of South Africa* (Cape Town: Purnell, 1971); and Jock McCulloch, *Asbestos Blues: Labour, Capital, Physicians and the State in South Africa* (Oxford: James Currey; Bloomington and Indianapolis: Indiana University Press, 2002).
51. *Report of the Committee Appointed to Inquire into the Training of Natives in Medicine and Public Health*, or the 'Loram Committee Report' (Pretoria: Government Printer, 1928).
52. In 1937, the proportion of medical practitioners to the black population in South Africa was 1 : 3 829. This average conceals the degree of imbalance in African rural reserve areas. In Zululand, for example, at this time, the ratio of doctors to the African population was 1 : 21 319. See Shapiro, 'Doctors or Medical Aids', 239.
53. UKZN MSA, Prof. Isidor Gordon, 'The Durban Medical School 1951–197_', 1.
54. CC MH HLB ABCFM, ABC 15: Letters from Missionaries to Africa, 1834–1919, Unit 2 Reel 211, Southern Africa Vol. 48, Zulu Mission 1909–29, Documents Letters [Supplementary], James B. McCord, 'Medical work among the Zulus', n/d [1936?], 3–4.
55. CC MH HLB ABCFM, Vol. 48, Reel 211, Zulu Mission 1909–29, Documents Letters [Supplementary], James B. McCord, 'Medical work among the Zulus', n/d [1936?], 4; and Shapiro, 'Doctors or Medical Aids', 249.
56. A.B. Xuma, 'The training of natives in medicine: Notes on a native medical service in rural areas', *Journal of the Medical Association of South Africa* (24 January 1931).
57. I. Seboko Monamodi, 'Medical doctors under segregation and apartheid: A sociological analysis of professionalization among doctors in South Africa, 1900–80' (PhD diss., Indiana University, 1996), 273–4.

58. See, for example, Maryinez Lyons, 'The power to heal: African medical auxiliaries in colonial Belgian Congo and Uganda', in *Contesting Colonial Hegemony: State and Society in Africa and India*, eds Dagmar Engels and Shula Marks (London and New York: British Academic Press, 1994); Patton, *Physicians, Colonial Racism, and Diaspora in West Africa*; Iliffe, *East African Doctors*; and Hunt, *A Colonial Lexicon*.

59. NAR GES 2271, 61/38B, Native Medical School Training of Native Doctors and Health Inspectors, 1933–39, E.H. Cluver (Union Health Dept), 'Native Medical Aids', 10 March 1936.

60. Shapiro, 'Doctors or Medical Aids', 251.

61. Edward Thornton, 'A medical and nursing service for natives in South Africa', *Journal of the Medical Association of South Africa* 5 (13 September 1930), 509; and H.S. Gear, 'The South African native health and medical service', *South African Medical Journal* xvii, no. 11 (12 June 1943), 168.

62. CC MH HLB ABCFM, ABC 15: Letters from Missionaries to Africa, 1834–1919, Unit 2 Reel 211, Southern Africa Vol. 48, Zulu Mission 1909–29, Documents Letters [Supplementary], James B. McCord, 'Medical work among the Zulus', n/d [1936?], 4–6; and NAR GES 2271, 61/38B, Cluver, 'Native Medical Aids', 10 March 1936.

63. McCord, *My Patients were Zulus*, 267–8.

64. Gelfand, *Christian Doctor and Nurse*, 190; CC MH, PDF Scans 1, 'Golden Jubilee, 1909–59: A Report on McCord Zulu Hospital', 1959, 8.

65. McCord, *My Patients were Zulus*, 269–72.

66. McCord, *My Patients were Zulus*, 270.

67. Shapiro, 'Doctors or Medical Aids', 253.

68. NAR GES 2957, PN 5, Native Medical Aids, 'Report of the committee of enquiry on the medical training of natives to the Minister of Public Health', 15 June 1942, 5.

69. McCord, *My Patients were Zulus*, 268–9.

70. NAR GES 2957, PN 5, Native Medical Aids, 'Report of the committee of enquiry on the medical training of natives', 15 June 1942, 9; and Letter from G.W. Gale, Dean of the Medical School, to Dr Le Roux, Secretary for Health, 19 May 1952.

71. McCord, *My Patients were Zulus*, 268. Other important liberals on the initiating committee included Principal Kerr from Fort Hare, several faculty members of the Lovedale Native College, Dr Neil MacVicar of the Victoria Native Hospital at Lovedale and Dr Eustace Cluver, who was later to become secretary of health for the Union – all men who had devoted most of their lives to improving the welfare of Africans in South Africa. See Monamodi, 'Medical doctors under segregation and apartheid', 259.

72. See NAR GES 2957, PN 5, Native Medical Aids, 'Report to the Governing Council, South African Native College, Fort Hare from Prof. W. Norman Taylor, Department of Hygiene concerning course of instruction for B.Sc. (Hygiene), with suggestions for future development', March 1952; NAR NTS 2862, 7/303 Part 4,

Dr McCord's Mission Nursing Home 1942–45. Medical superintendent's report for McCord Hospital in the year ending December 1942.

73. For example, Aaron Lebona went on to complete his medical training at Wits in 1948. See Digby, *Diversity and Division in Medicine*, 191–8.

74. Shula Marks and Neil Andersson, 'Industrialisation, rural health and the 1944 National Health Services Commission in South Africa', in *The Social Basis of Health and Healing in Africa*, eds Steven Feierman and John M. Janzen (Berkeley and Los Angeles: University of California Press, 1992); Derek Yach and Steve M. Tollman, 'Public health initiatives in South Africa in the 1940s and 1950s: Lessons for a post-apartheid era', *American Journal of Public Health* 83, no. 7 (1993).

75. For example, between 1946 and 1959 the number of black patients treated in urban public hospitals in the city of Johannesburg more than doubled. See Murray, *Wits the 'Open' Years*, 174.

76. Deborah Posel, *The Making of Apartheid 1948–61: Conflict and Compromise* (Oxford: Clarendon Press, 1991), 23–4.

77. William Beinart, *Twentieth-Century South Africa* (Oxford and New York: Oxford University Press, 1994), especially chapter 5, 'The settler state in Depression and War, 1930–1948'; and Tom Lodge, *Black Politics in South Africa since 1945* (London and New York: Longman, 1983), especially chapter 5, 'Black protest before 1950'.

78. Merle Naomi Mindel, 'The construction of medical education in an unequal society: A study of the University of Cape Town Medical School, 1904–97' (PhD diss., Institute of Education, University of London, 2003), 94.

79. Wits CRO 570 Medical School by Department, 'Medical school: Bantu students welcome', *Wits Views* (18 March 1941); UCT AA Med/7 Medicine: General, 1953–8, Thos B. Davie, 'Admission of non-European students to medical faculty', 11 May 1995.

80. '50 years ago in *The Leader*: First "crop" of locally qualified medics lauded', *The Leader* (8 December 1945).

81. See Monamadi, 'Medical doctors under segregation and apartheid', 276–85.

82. Howard Phillips, 'White coats and stethoscopes: Doctors and medical students at GSH', in *At the Heart of Healing: Groote Schuur Hospital, 1938–2008*, Anne Digby and Howard Phillips with Harriet Deacon and Kirsten Thomson (Auckland Park: Jacana, 2008), 194.

83. Howard Phillips, *The University of Cape Town 1918–48: The Formative Years* (Cape Town: University of Cape Town Press, 1993), 192–3.

84. Bruce K. Murray, 'Wits as an "open" university 1939–59: Black admissions to the university of the Witwatersrand', *Journal of Southern African Studies* 16, no. 4 (December 1990), 674; and Digby, *Diversity and Division in Medicine*, 206.

85. See Digby, 'Early black doctors in South Africa', 438.

86. Murray, *Wits the Early Years*, 35–6, 300–2.

87. Murray, *Wits the 'Open' Years*, 28, 37–45. Also see Wits CRO Box No. Reg. 00885, File no. 3, B19/2, Blacks – Training of Black Medical and Dental Students, June

1944 – July 1962, 'Memorandum: Medical education for non-Europeans in the Union, 1944', 4; and NAR UOD 1546, U3/40/4, Natal University College for Establishment of Medical School for Natives, 1945–48, 'University of the Witwatersrand, Johannesburg. Memorandum on non-European medical education', signed H.R. Raikes (Principal of Wits), 1947.

88. Murray, *Wits the 'Open' Years*, 28.

89. UCT AA F2/1 Non-Europeans, Vol. II, Letter from David Clain (SRC President) to Mr Benfield (UCT Registrar), 11 August 1959; and Mindel, 'The construction of medical education in an unequal society', especially chapters 3 and 4.

90. Quoted in Anne Digby, 'From racial segregation towards transformation', in *At the Heart of Healing: Groote Schuur Hospital, 1938–2008*, Anne Digby and Howard Phillips with Harriet Deacon and Kirsten Thomson (Auckland Park: Jacana, 2008), 118.

91. For more on the history of NUSAS, see Wits SAHA South African Political Materials 1964–1990s, The Karis-Gerhart Collection, Part III: Political Documents, NUSAS, Folder 575: Martin Legassick, 'The National Union of South African Students: Ethnic cleavage and ethnic integration in the universities' (University of California, L.A.: Occasional Paper No. 4, 1967); and Graeme C. Moodie, 'The state and the liberal universities in South Africa: 1948–90', *Higher Education 27* (1994).

92. Interview with Janet Giddy, Hillcrest, 24 May 2003.

93. Wits CRO Box No. Reg. 00885, File no. 3, B19/2, Blacks – Training of Black Medical and Dental Students, June 1944 – July 1962, 'Admission of non-European students: The special case of medical education', 11 March 1954.

94. Wits FHSR M3/40 Internal Reconciliation Commission, 1998, Jules Browde, Patrick Mokhoba and Essop Jassat, 'University of the Witwatersrand Faculty of Health Sciences Internal Reconciliation Commission Report' (November 1998); and *Truth and Reconciliation: A Process of Transformation at the UCT Health Sciences Faculty* (Cape Town: UCT Faculty of Health Science, 2002).

95. Shan Naidoo, Questionnaire, 2003.

96. For Wits, see Murray, *Wits the 'Open' Years*, 35–6, 52; and Simonne J. Horwitz, '"A phoenix rising": A social history of Baragwanath Hospital, Soweto, South Africa, 1942–90' (DPhil diss., Oxford University, 2006). For UCT, see UCT M&A, 'Academic segregation: Non-white students barred from attending post-mortems on white bodies', *Varsity 20*, no. 5 (7 April 1961); Phillips, 'White coats and stethoscopes', 118; and Phyllis Naidoo, *Footprints in Grey Street* (Durban: Far Ocean Jetty Publishing, 2002), 186. This last book has a section on the experiences of 'Dr Suleman Ismail', an Indian doctor who graduated from UCT in 1955.

97. Mindel, 'The construction of medical education in an unequal society', 132–5.

98. UCT M&A, 'Coming home: A son of South Africa returns for recognition and remembrance', *UCT News 25*, no. 1 (December 1998), 48.

99. Browde, Mokhoba and Jassat, 'University of the Witwatersrand Faculty of Health Sciences Internal Reconciliation Commission Report', 16; and Wits FHSR M12/

1/17/2 Black Students – Clinical Facilities, August 1980 – August 1984, Letter from Prof. Phillip V. Tobias (Dean of Wits Faculty of Medicine) to Prof. John Gear (Dept of Community Medicine) re 'Difficulties of black students', n/d.

100. Wits FHSR M12/1/17/2 Black Students – Clinical Facilities, August 1980 – August 1984, Letter from Prof. Phillip V. Tobias (Dean of Wits Faculty of Medicine) to Prof. John Gear (Dept of Community Medicine) re 'Difficulties of black students'.

101. NAR NTS 2862, 7/303 Part 5 Dr McCord's Mission Nursing Home 1944–49, Letter from Dr Alan B. Taylor to the Secretary for Native Affairs, Pretoria, 5 October 1946 re 'Additions to the McCord Zulu Hospital' and Correspondence from McCord Zulu Hospital, 26 September 1948.

102. For more on the discriminations experienced by black medical students at UCT and its teaching hospitals, see Mindel, 'The construction of medical education in an unequal society'.

103. Horwitz, '"A phoenix rising"'; Aziza Seedat, *Crippling a Nation: Health in Apartheid South Africa* (London: International Defence and Aid Fund for Southern Africa, 1984), 64–5; and Wits CRO Box No. Reg. 00550, File no. 4, S6/5, Senate: Faculty of Medicine Documents, 1984, Yousouf (Joe) Veriava, 'Medical school and apartheid medicine', February 1984, 2–3.

104. Browde, Mokhoba and Jassat, 'University of the Witwatersrand Faculty of Health Sciences Internal Reconciliation Commission Report', 13–4; and *Truth and Reconciliation: A Process of Transformation at the UCT Health Sciences Faculty*.

105. Esline Nozipho Shuenyane, 'Black medical students' perceptions of medical school and the medical course' (MEd diss., University of the Witwatersrand, 1991), 45.

106. Wits FHSR M3/40 Internal Reconciliation Commission, 1998, Yousouf (Joe) Veriava, 'Submission to the Wits Internal Reconciliation Commission' (17 June 1998), 104.

107. See Browde, Mokhoba and Jassat, 'University of the Witwatersrand Faculty of Health Sciences Internal Reconciliation Commission Report'; and *Truth and Reconciliation: A Process of Transformation at the UCT Health Sciences Faculty*.

108. Interview with Hugh Philpott, Kloof, 14 July 2003.

CHAPTER 2

The establishment of the University of Natal Medical School

'There were many Hills and Valleys, Road Blocks and Detours in the Road . . .'
— Dr Alan B. Taylor in a letter to 'Our Friends in America', 1958

In 1951, another medical school was officially opened in the province of Natal to augment and ultimately supplant the training of token numbers of black students at Wits and UCT. It was thus a second attempt to open a training institute for black students in Durban. Fortunately, it would have greater staying power than its predecessor. The Durban Medical School was developed as a separate faculty under the auspices of the historically white University of Natal – not for whites, but to train African, Indian and coloured medical students. It was officially opened less than three years after the Afrikaner-led National Party assumed power in South Africa – on an apartheid platform of the segregation of the races – and was funded mostly by the apartheid state, whose racial policies came to influence its operations in decisive ways.

From the late 1950s, when Wits and UCT were forced to close their doors to black students without ministerial permission, through to the late 1970s, when MEDUNSA, a second, apartheid-funded, African medical-training institution was opened to help meet the growing shortage of black doctors in the country, Durban's medical school was really the only institution available for aspiring black doctors, especially Africans. And, in time, it would come to play a pivotal role in the provision of medical education for black doctors in South Africa. Its founders struggled many long years to bring this institution into existence, and once it was opened, it would be plagued by ambiguities and contradictions. In some ways it became a significant showpiece of apartheid policy; however, in other ways it became a complex and prickly anomaly for the state. Even during this school's early teething years, it did not develop in the exact manner that the Afrikaner-led state hoped it would, and on occasions even produced ideologies and practices that threatened to undermine apartheid-state directives and policies.

'Durban would be the most suitable centre': Growing support for a black medical school in Natal

Support for a separate black medical school gained momentum in the years just before the Second World War. Ten years after the Loram Committee had recommended the establishment of a segregated, black medical school, another government committee – the Botha Committee (1938) – was appointed to investigate and report upon the state of medical training in South Africa.[1] Committee members included Professor M.C. Botha (the secretary for education), Sir Edward Thornton, Dr S.M. de Kock (the president of the South African Medical and Dental Council), Dr Karl Bremer (who later became minister of health), and Mr P.J. du Toit (later president of the Council for Scientific and Industrial Research). The secretary appointed to this committee was Dr E.G. Malherbe, who would later become the principal of the Natal University College, the university under whose aegis the future black medical school would be established. Noting the many problems affecting the inferior Medical Aid training scheme, as well as the insufficient numbers of doctors to treat the growing numbers of black patients seeking care in biomedical facilities, the Botha Committee repeated the Loram Committee's earlier recommendations to provide a full medical training for black students in South Africa. Taking the argument one step further, the committee was also the first to recommend the city of Durban as 'the most suitable centre' for the 'the establishment of a separate medical school for non-Europeans'.[2] The committee's recommendations were delayed with the outbreak of the Second World War, however. It suggested that the existing white medical schools accept token numbers of black students as a cheaper and temporary expedient in the interim.

A few years later, in 1942, two central developments reinforced state thinking towards establishing a 'non-European' medical school in Durban. Firstly, in the more liberal wartime political climate, and in the need to address the growing health demands of a swelling urban and rural African population, the National Health Services Commission (NHSC) was set up by the Jan Smuts United Party (UP) government. The commission was led by forward-thinking individuals, among them, Henry Gluckman, and charged with investigating the disastrous state of public health-care services in South Africa.[3] As chairman, Gluckman, a medical graduate himself, had the task of reorganising the country's inefficient and poorly organised public health-care services, and establishing an effective, more centrally controlled national health services system to be rolled out after the war. He was also charged with providing segregated but improved health-care services for all South Africans, which included a mandate to improve the medical-education situation too. In 1944, when the commission had completed its investigations, including weighing up the claims of Durban against those of Johannesburg, Gluckman concurred with the Botha Committee's findings, and in his report recommended Durban over Johannesburg 'as a site of a medical school primarily for non-Europeans, but also for those whose object is to serve non-Europeans'.[4]

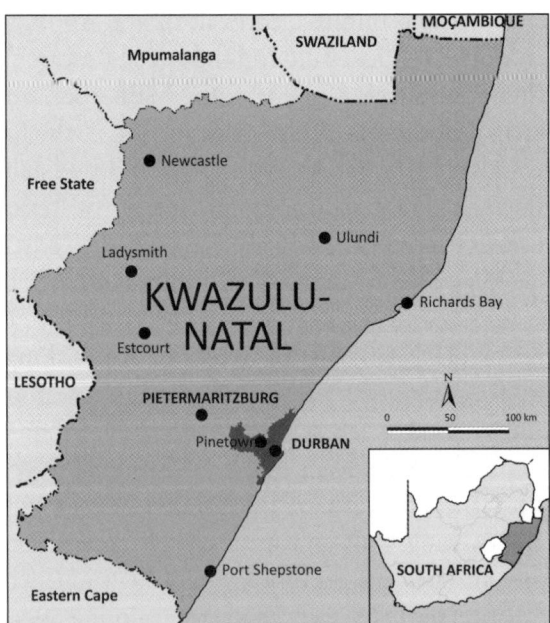

Map 2.1   Map showing Durban, the site of the 'non-European' medical school. Durban is a large city within the province of KwaZulu-Natal on the east coast of South Africa.

Interestingly, of the ten people who made up this commission, only one came from Natal, and none from Durban. Despite this, Gluckman and his team foresaw the significance that a medical school would have for the medical practice and research standards of the province of Natal, which did not have its own medical school.[5] He felt that the city of Durban would provide an advantageous location for a new medical school. It offered much in the way of clinical material for training in various established black hospitals, such as King Edward VIII Hospital (a large state-funded, public hospital), McCord Hospital, King George V Tuberculosis Hospital and Addington Hospital (one of the oldest white, public hospitals in the province, but which had a segregated section designated for 'coloured' patients), as well as various smaller government health centres and clinics.[6] And, because coastal Natal was 'near-tropical' in climate, he felt that 'there were many diseases there which could be studied more fully than elsewhere in the Union', and stressed also its 'proximity to great African tribal areas as well as to the major portion of the Indian population'.[7]

Despite having loyalties to Wits (as an alumnus), Gluckman did not favour extending Wits's or UCT's existing racially mixed training arrangement, which produced overcrowded conditions and racial tensions. Furthermore, this set-up offered limited clinical training opportunities for black students, some of whom were forced to travel to other provinces to get experience.[8] The fact that Wits and UCT could train only a small number of black students per year was also vastly insufficient to meet the country's segregated medical needs, where one-fifth of the population's needs were met by three white medical schools (a third, exclusively white, Afrikaans-medium school was opened in Pretoria in 1948), while four-fifths of the population, the African majority, had no such facilities.[9] Gluckman became the national minister of health in the UP government in 1945, and was placed in charge of implementing the NHSC report's recommendations by the Department of Health. This also helped propel Durban to the fore as the site for a future black medical school.

Secondly, during the 1940s, Alan B. Taylor, a long-time advocate of black medical education, did all he could to generate support in the province for the choice of Durban for the new school.[10] Although James McCord's early 1920s private medical school initiatives had been shattered, Taylor, who succeeded him as superintendent of McCord Hospital after his retirement, continued his fight for black medical education. Soromini

Kallichurum, who was to become one of the first Indian graduates of the school and later the first woman dean of the University of Natal's Faculty of Medicine, spoke of the major influence of medical missionaries on the school's formation:

> [During the 1940s] . . . the whole thing was led by Dr Taylor from McCord's. And you see the beginnings of this medical school . . . lay with the missionary, not the academic or the [medical] profession. And I think working at McCord's, he saw the neglect, you know, of black patients, and so he just fought for a medical school in Natal that would take black students.[11]

Between 1943 and 1945 Taylor, who had been in Durban for over twenty years by this time, chaired a number of meetings in Durban that drew together many of his large network of personal and professional contacts, which extended to 'friends' on the Federal Council of the Medical Association of South Africa (MASA), the Natal Coastal Branch of MASA, the Durban Rotary Club and others.[12] In his book *A History of the University of Natal*, Edgar Brookes, who was a noteworthy educationist, author and liberal leader, and knew Taylor personally, noted that he was a force to be reckoned with.[13] He was a man who 'combined a forcefulness and good humour' with a huge 'capacity for work', and moreover was 'a good "mixer"', a quality which stood him in good stead in his long struggle for African medical education'.[14] Confronted with a burgeoning hospital workload on a daily basis, Taylor wanted desperately to meet the needs of a growing number of black patients living and working in the city of Durban. He was also concerned that the Witwatersrand might have prior claim, since medical education for black students had already been started there, and strong calls were being made by powerful mine owners to build a school to train more black doctors to help keep their labour force healthy.[15] As president of the Natal branch of MASA between 1945 and 1946, Taylor was, however, determined that Durban should not be overlooked in the deliberations.

At these meetings, representatives from the Natal Coastal Branch and Federal Council of MASA, the Natal University College (NUC), which since 1928 had included the establishment of a medical school in its development plans, the Natal Provincial Administration (NPA) as the government body which controlled provincial hospital services in Natal, the local Durban City Council and other influential Natal-based persons discussed ways to promote the opening of a medical school in Durban.[16] At a July 1945 meeting, the motion was passed unanimously: '. . . that immediate steps be taken towards the establishment of a medical school in Durban . . . to be designed primarily for the medical education of the Bantu, with this proviso, that no person be excluded from attending on the grounds of race or colour'.[17] It was felt that white students from Natal, especially those who expressed an interest in working amongst black patients, should not be excluded should this school be opened.

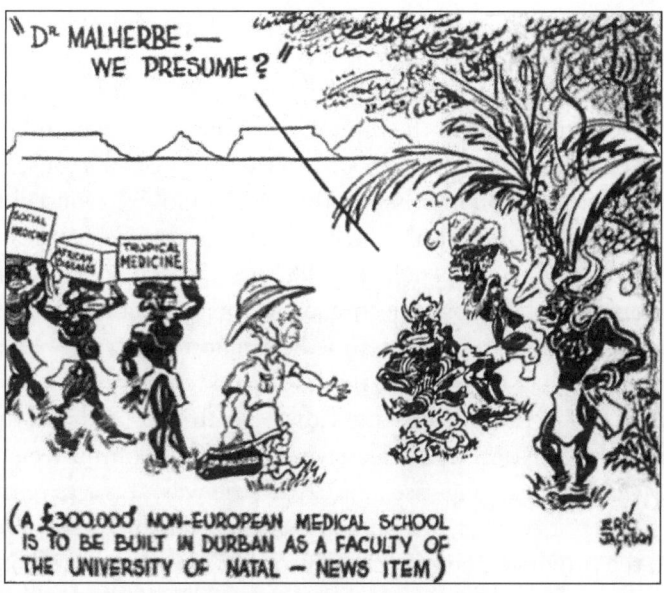

Figure 2.1   A cartoon that appeared in the *Sunday Post* on
19 September 1948, highlighted the pioneering, but
also, contentious nature of the formation of Durban's
medical school.

Later that year, in November 1945, Jan H. Hofmeyr, the minister of education (and ex-chancellor of Wits), came to Durban and met a deputation of about 50 representatives of 'prominent citizens of Natal' under the chairmanship of Taylor. Although attendance was overwhelmingly white, this meeting listed at least one 'non-European' professional – 'a Dr Naiker' – as a key speaker.[18] Following this meeting with an ambivalent Hofmeyr, and to keep the momentum going, Taylor was elected as the chairman of a Durban Medical School 'Joint Action Committee'.[19] This was a strong lobby group that was formed to raise public support for their cause. It consisted of representatives of the NUC Council (including Dr G.G. Campbell, Dr L. Sormany, Mr Humphrey Jones, and the principal, Dr E.G. Malherbe); of the Medical Association (including drs Alan B. Taylor, J.A. Macfadyen, A. Broomberg and H. Grant-Whyte); of the Department of Health (Dr D. Landau, followed after his untimely death in 1948 by Dr Sidney Kark, who would become an important early faculty member of the Durban school); and of the Natal Provincial Hospital services (Dr R.E. Stevenson). In this position, Taylor then led a number of delegations to Pretoria between 1946 and 1947, including a pivotal one made up of himself, E.G. Malherbe and Dr S.F. Oosthuizen (representing the Medical Research Section of the Council for Scientific and Industrial Research), to persuade various ministers in the capital, including Hofmeyr and Gluckman (who had by then become minister of health), of Durban's cause.[20]

Like the Gluckman Commission, this Durban lobby group did much to highlight the wealth of clinical material available for medical teaching and research in the province of Natal. In a 1964 presidential address at a medical-education conference, Taylor, reflecting on factors motivating the government to consider Durban as the site of a medical school, asserted: 'The fact that 2.5 million whites had three medical schools and ten million non-whites had none, backed up by the size of King Edward VIII Hospital and the density of the African population in Natal, gave the Action Committee . . . and the University of Natal a strong case . . .'[21] After the war, this was reinforced by the NPA's declaration that it would also make available three acres of land adjacent to the province's largest 'non-European' hospital – the King Edward VIII Hospital – for the building of such a school, which could then be used as its teaching hospital.[22] Opened in 1936, this hospital's location on Umbilo Road provided easy access to black patients coming from central Durban, the industrial area around the Durban harbour, and to African and Indian residents coming from areas to the south, north and west of the city.

Representatives of the NUC, which was granted autonomous status and renamed the University of Natal in 1949, also strengthened Durban's case. E.G. Malherbe, the son of an Afrikaner *dominee* (a clergyman or minister) and one of South Africa's leading liberal educationalists, who had acquired postgraduate degrees from a number of leading American, British and European universities, and who had become the principal and vice-chancellor of the NUC in 1945 (a position he held for twenty years), did much to dispel one of the government's concerns.[23] During the mid-1940s, he produced statistical evidence to show that a sufficient number of qualified black matriculants existed and would be forthcoming to warrant the cost of establishing a separate school.[24] During this same period, the council of the NUC gave its public endorsement to the proposal to establish a black medical school under its control.[25] Finally, as a member of the Joint Action Committee, Malherbe also repeatedly highlighted the unique set-up of his university's separate-but-equal educational formula, which could easily accommodate a separate black medical faculty under its control.

Started in 1936, the NUC had established a separate 'Non-European Section' under the leadership of the indomitable Dr Mabel Palmer, a university-educated, English-born woman, whose feminist and leftist, Fabian, socialist political leanings made her a strong advocate for women's and workers' advancement through education.[26] In a context where many whites objected to having racially mixed classes, Palmer established and then acted as the organiser of the 'Non-European Section', providing, on a racially separate basis, a parallel but purportedly equal university education for black students. Often held at night, at first in Palmer's own home, and later, as the numbers grew, at the Sastri College buildings in the centre of Durban, classes were duplicated by lecturers for black students. As one newspaper article highlighted, 'Africans and Indians, many of them from remote country areas, came by trains and slept in doorways . . . to attend these classes, to train as teachers, lawyers, accountants, and other professionals'.[27]

The NUC's 'Non-European Section' segregation formula was a solid pull factor for Durban.[28] Malherbe made a convincing case that if the state enabled his university to provide black medical education, it would give this institution the chance to distinguish itself as 'a university centre for the general and medical training of non-Europeans in the Union and the whole of East Africa'.[29] A careful reading of various primary sources also suggests that the proposal to establish a black medical school in Durban was made more palatable to the Nationalists when they came into power in 1948 because a man from an Afrikaner family background was firmly seated at the helm of the NUC in a predominantly English-speaking province and university.[30] They would be disappointed in time as Malherbe, it turned out, would become a strong 'opponent of University apartheid, as well as of every form of interference with University autonomy', although some felt that, as a liberal, he did not go far enough in his policies whilst serving as principal.[31] Palmer and Malherbe's 'Natal Experiment' represented a compromised solution in a restrictive segregation and later apartheid context.[32]

Like McCord and Taylor, they aimed to provide equal education opportunities for black students, even if at first on segregated lines, which they regarded as one step forward until full integration was a feasible option.

Eventually, the breakthrough came in 1947, after considerable further pressure from a number of quarters. This included a strongly worded resolution supporting Durban that was passed by the Federal Council of MASA, the most powerful medical professional body in the country, and a promise by the Medical School Joint Action Committee to help raise £100 000 from the general public in Natal to assist with the building costs.[33] Moreover, it should be noted that in 1947, delegates from the Joint Action Committee made an appointment to see the prime minister to obtain his support. In a 1964 newspaper recognising the illustrious career and retirement of Taylor, it was reported that the endeavour to establish 'a medical school in Durban . . . [involved] a long fight, during which Dr Taylor, never one for half measures, went right to the top. He applied for and was granted an interview with General Smuts . . . The interview was a success. Smuts was impressed.'[34] In December 1947, the UP government agreed in principle to fund the building of a medical school in Durban under the auspices of the NUC.[35] It recognised that building this medical school would provide a national service and thus merited national support.

Unfortunately, implementation and government financing for the school's creation was delayed further the following year when the UP was defeated in the May elections, and power was transferred to the National Party (NP). Elected on the platform of 'apartheid' (meaning 'separateness'), successive NP governments, from 1948 until the party's election defeat in 1994, developed a political system that built on earlier racial segregation precedents. Many new legislative enactments tried to ensure the fuller segregation of African, Indian, coloured and white racial groups in South Africa in every facet of life.[36] In addition, the NP worked to reserve social, economic and political privileges for the country's white minority. This extended even to the educational opportunities and health-care services that different South Africans had access to.[37] The UP government's Gluckman Commission report was quashed and its far-sighted recommendations, recognised even by developed countries (such as Britain) as progressive for their time, were declared undoable by NP hardliners.[38] As a missed opportunity, this move would prove significant, and in time led to the worsening of provision of health-care services for black South Africans.

'Rising from the ground':[39] The opening of Durban's medical school

In a letter dated May 1954, Alan Taylor recorded how 'the matter rested' during 1948 and the first half of 1949 while the new government got settled.[40] After several months had passed and further delays, Dr A.J. Stals, the new minister of education and health in the NP government, reaffirmed the decision of its UP predecessors to subsidise the establishment of a medical school in Durban under the aegis of the newly inaugurated University of Natal. In August 1949 the government asked the University of Natal to appoint a subcommittee to draw up estimates of the cost of building, running and equipping such a medical school. Asked to head this committee, Taylor, who had just returned from furlough in the United States, was joined by a number of individuals representing members of the local medical profession and university including Professor E.G. Malherbe (principal); Dr Mabel Palmer and Professor S.F. Bush (faculty members); Professor Sidney L. Kark (head of the Institute of Family and Community Health); a number of doctors from the Durban branch of MASA, such as drs G.G. Campbell and J.A. Macfadyen; and Dr F. Cluver (deputy chief health officer of the Natal provincial health department).[41] Many of these individuals had liberal intentions, thus providing some continuity with previous-era UP ideologies and approaches.

While in the States, Taylor had used some of his time to collect expert advice from what he considered 'the best' black medical schools in the country, particularly Howard University College of Medicine in Washington, DC.[42] One of only two remaining black medical schools at the time – the other being Meharry Medical College in Nashville, Tennessee – which had survived the challenges of the reconstruction years after the Civil War, as well as stringent medical educational reforms and funding shortages through the early twentieth century, Howard Medical School provided a useful model for Taylor's Durban school. It had strong founder links to the Congregational Church of Washington, DC – the church Taylor was brought up in and whose approaches he continued to follow in South Africa – and it was in the vanguard for a number of reasons. By the 1940s, it had struggled and succeeded against the odds to provide thousands of the best and brightest African American students, including women, as well as those from poor socio-economic backgrounds, with high-quality biomedical undergraduate and postgraduate training opportunities in a wider US context marred by racial discrimination and inequalities.[43]

Following the insights gleaned from his stay in America, Taylor then purposively made trips to the universities of the Witwatersrand and Pretoria to better understand local medical school issues.[44] He also worked closely with a variety of architects to draw up the best possible plan for a 'very modern building'.[45] In March 1951, Taylor wrote to friends in Grand Rapids, Michigan:

> Fearing that future generations might cut me out as a lay man who rushed in where only Professors might tread without fear, in planning the buildings, we had three sets of plans drawn up and submitted to the Professors of the three Medical School faculties in the country for their consideration and criticism. In each case their criticisms were incorporated into the new design.[46]

This committee 'got [the] figures together', and submitted to the government the estimated cost of £207 000 for capital start-up, though it would be many more months before they were given the go-ahead. It was only in July 1950 that the NP government gave the university its first treasury approval to start building its new school.

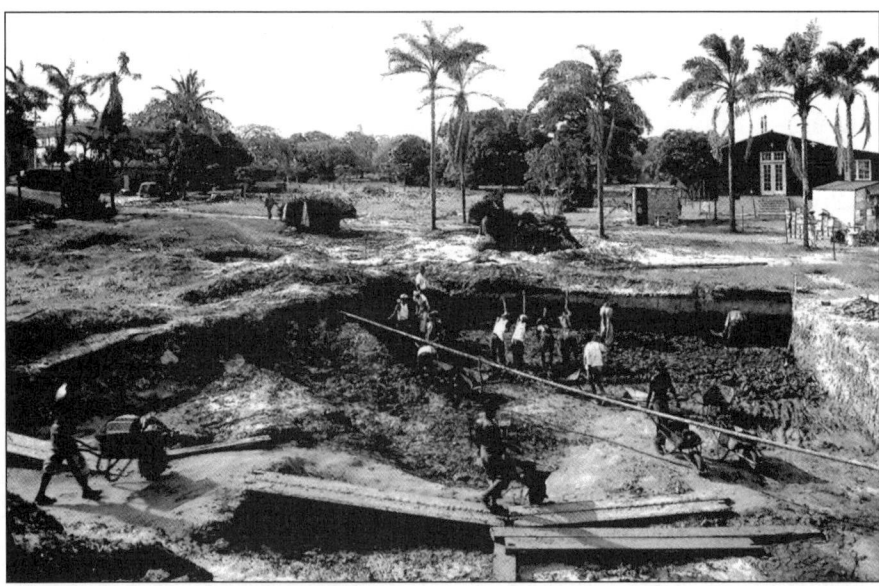

Photo 2.1 The medical school site, June 1952. (*UKZN Medical School Archives*)

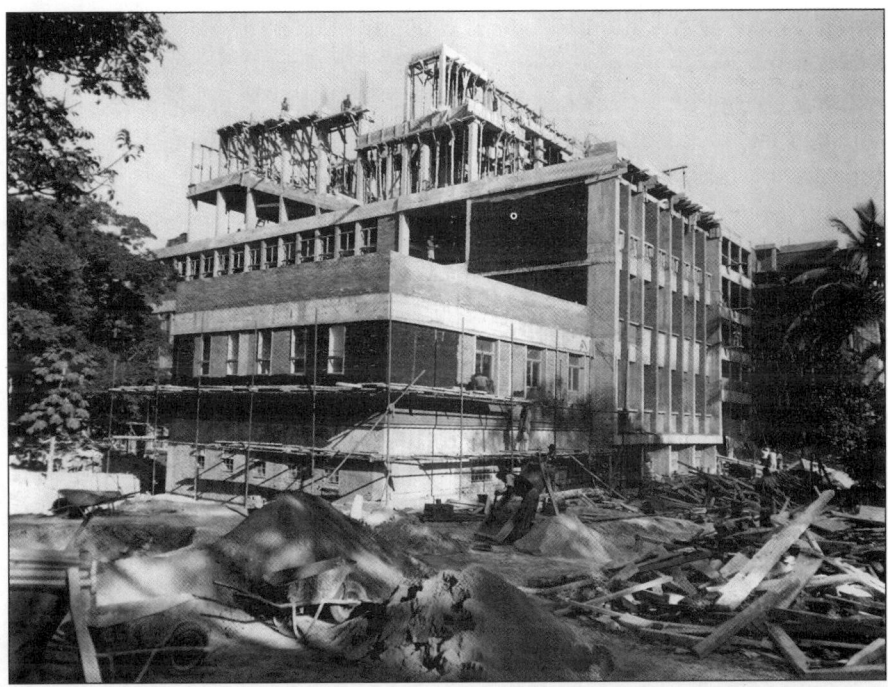

Photo 2.2 Durban Medical School building, *circa* 1950s. (*UKZN Medical School Archives*)

Following this, in August 1950, the university appointed Alan B. Taylor as the first acting dean and chairman of an acting board of the Faculty of Medicine, which was composed mostly of individuals who had been members of the subcommittee. Additional members were appointed as new staff joined the permanent staff from 1951, eventually resulting in the establishment of a permanent board in 1955.[47] Tasked with overseeing the building, equipment, early staff appointments, the syllabus and then the actual opening of the new school in 1951, Taylor was thrilled to accept the position as acting dean, despite his busy work schedule as medical superintendent at McCord Hospital.[48] In a 1958 letter to 'Friends in America', reflecting back on the developments in which he had played so central a part, he wrote with happiness, and using a Christian idiom, that he '. . . considered [his] cup full'.[49] This enabled him to see – finally – the successful implementation of the long-standing dream that had originally brought him to South Africa in 1921.

Thus, in 1951 – about 30 years after drs McCord and Taylor's failed attempt to establish a private school in Durban – the University of Natal's Medical School finally opened with its first cohort of 35 students, forming a 'multiracial' blend of African, Indian and coloured students, as well as a mixture of both men and women. Although the characteristics of the students who were admitted, as well as their training experiences, will be discussed in later chapters, it should be highlighted here that this school did prioritise from the very beginning the training of *African* students, whose communities were considered in greatest need of doctors. The school's admission committee attempted to accept proportionally, that is, in terms of places available, a majority of African students each year.[50] In addition, many African students who came from disadvantaged families in South Africa were not denied the opportunity to study at this school. The state supported such students with a specially set up bursary-loan scheme to finance their training on condition that they passed each year and agreed to either pay back their grants in full or work in government service for a stipulated number of years after graduating.[51] Money for this scheme was obtained by withdrawing bursaries that had previously been provided for African students at Wits Medical School.[52] It was hoped that this incentive would discourage African students from studying at this 'white' medical school and instead apply to study in Durban.

In recognition of Taylor's many efforts on the Joint Action Committee and then as the first acting dean, the university decided to name the medical school's first residence, located in the largely coloured suburb of Wentworth, about ten kilometres south of the Faculty of Medicine buildings, in his honour.[53] This was significant. Until the new Umbilo Road buildings adjoining the King Edward VIII Hospital were ready for occupancy in 1953 (at least the lower floors, for the teaching of anatomy and physiology, of what would become a multi-storey building), 'the Alan Taylor Residence *was* the Medical School in its early days', as one early graduate remembered, as students lived there and had most of their premedical (including preliminary and first-year) classes taught there.[54] Taylor's name was linked, therefore, to the medical school for many years, long after his retirement from McCord Hospital in 1964 and his death in 1969, and until after the residence closed in 1989 to make way for a new and improved building. Unfortunately, as time went on, his original humanitarian dreams of providing medical education for black students were forgotten or obscured

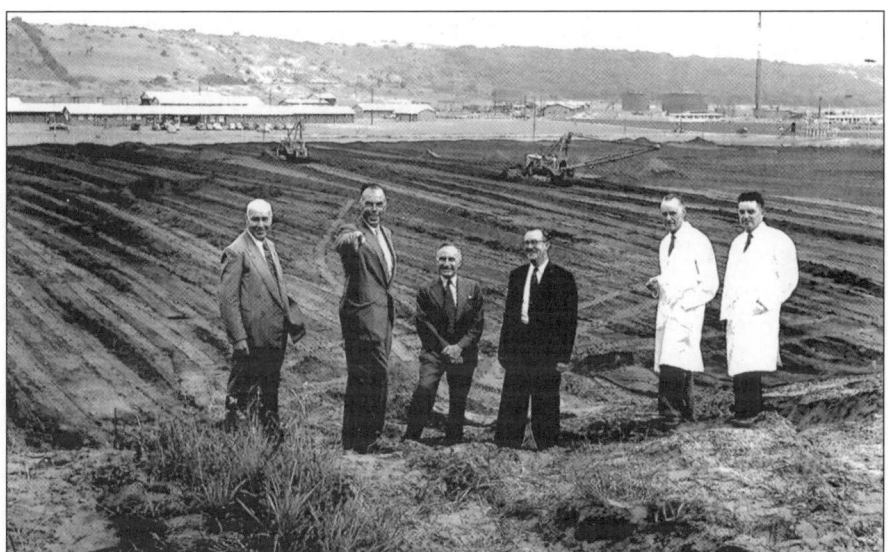

Photo 2.3   The students' sport field in construction in the foreground, the oil refinery in
the background, March 1953.
Left to right: Dr A.B. Taylor, Mr Kenney, Dr G.W. Gale, Mr Sedicum
(American Consul), Prof Keen, Mr Williams
(*UKZN Medical School Archives*)

by the inferior conditions that plagued this residence, which will form the
subject of chapters to come.

In March 1952, Taylor handed over the headship of the school to the
first full-time dean.[55] He was happy to step aside, having noted as early as
April 1950 the need for a full-time person who was committed to steering
the school through its difficult teething years:

> For a few years at least we need such a man to put his full time into getting
> things running smoothly. I will be pleased to be relieved of the responsibility
> because of the time it takes away from the hospital. This is my first love
> and I enjoy it most. It will give me more time with patients and the
> doctors.[56]

However, this was not the end of Taylor's association with the medical
school. He maintained 'a close connection' with the school by remaining an
active member of its faculty board and held an honorary teaching position
in obstetrics right through to his retirement in 1964.[57] Because McCord

Hospital was only a few kilometres away from the medical school, he also worked actively with other senior doctors on his staff to open his hospital to senior students for their clinical rotations. McCord Hospital became an important site for practical training in obstetrics and gynaecology, alleviating the congestion that beleaguered the overcrowded wards at the school's King Edward VIII teaching hospital.[58] And, when the first graduates completed their studies in 1957, it was one of the first hospitals to offer internship positions to black doctors graduating from the Durban Medical School. Furthermore, Taylor was awarded the highest award conferred by the University of Natal – an Honorary PhD – in March 1958 for his 'vision, struggle and foresight' which led to the provision of many years of medical services to 'non-European' peoples, and in particular for the leading part he played in the development of black medical education in South Africa.[59] It was a crowning achievement that saw him fittingly capped alongside the first twelve graduates of Durban's medical school.

Having had the pleasure of being – together with James McCord – the one to start things, Taylor considered George W. Gale an accomplished and worthy successor in whose capable hands he was leaving the medical school.[60] Born in Natal as the son of a missionary, Gale had qualified as a doctor at Edinburgh University in Scotland in 1927. He founded the Church of Scotland Hospital at Tugela Ferry in the northern Msinga district of Natal and served there as a missionary doctor from 1928 to 1936 until he entered the public health service, and worked his way up in Smuts's UP government to become secretary of the Department of Health in 1946.[61] By the late 1930s, he was one of the strongest opponents of the Medical Aid training scheme. As a person with liberal political leanings, he worked closely alongside Henry Gluckman for several years until Gluckman was replaced in 1948, and remained in this high-profile position until early 1952, when he finally resigned to escape the growing reactionary views and policies in a department, by then, firmly in the hands of NP officials. Thus Gale, like Taylor before him, came to the school in 1952 with a strong missionary, philanthropic background. Both had worked extensively with black patients, and both had considerable experience of conditions under which the majority of the medical school's black students would come to work once graduating. However, the founding years were not smooth ones, as many deep-seated contradictions and inequalities plagued the school's establishment and operation.

A showpiece of apartheid or an apartheid anomaly?: The difficult teething years

As founding deans, both Taylor and then Gale had to navigate a complicated working relationship with the apartheid state. As the state provided most of the finances to build, equip and run the medical school, it secured close ties to the institution's affairs right from the beginning.[62] A major effect of these 'financial strings' was the strict condition imposed on the university that it could admit only African, Indian and coloured students into its medical school.[63] Although this white-student exclusion clause was petitioned by the university, eventually leading to a proviso that white students could be admitted at the postgraduate level subject to ministerial approval, the university council was forced to accept 'the principles of apartheid' at the undergraduate level to continue receiving its annual subsidies.[64] The compromises these liberal stewards had to make to bring the dream of this medical school into reality are evident in a statement Taylor made in 1951:

> Out of evil sometimes comes good. While we don't accept the Government's policy of apartheid (compulsory separation of racial groups) we do appreciate the fact that having set its face against the admission of Non-European students to the European medical school in Johannesburg, the Government is heavily subsidizing Durban's Medical School for Non-Europeans.[65]

Accepting only 'non-European' students at the undergraduate level was a significant point of departure from the earlier recommendations made by the UP government and the Medical School Joint Action Committee to build a medical school 'primarily for non-Europeans', but also for those whites who intended to serve the needs of black patients. This admission restriction meant that white students who lived in Natal, or white students interested in studying medicine in Natal, could not be trained at what became officially classified as a 'non-European' medical school. The first white students were only admitted to the school in 1978 at postgraduate level and in 1995, in the post-apartheid period, at undergraduate level.

Still sensitive to international criticism during the early 1950s, which coincided with the early years of apartheid rule, officials in the Department of Health repeatedly stated on public occasions how the building and equipping of this school would be a positive 'showpiece of apartheid'.[66] While providing its students with the highest-quality MB ChB (Bachelor of Medicine and Surgery) degree, comparable to that of their white counterparts, this school would also fit well within the state's plans for creating separate education facilities for black and white students. Behind the scenes, however, the state's policy was one of financial stringency. Between 1952 and 1955, Gale and Malherbe struggled time and again to obtain sufficient capital outlay from the state for the school's building project.[67]

Both also fought hard to secure funding to construct competitive salary packages that would attract the highest-quality teaching staff, most of whom were white doctors in the early decades of the school's history.[68] Although more will be discussed in a later chapter about what motivated individuals to apply for teaching jobs in Durban, by 1956 the various disciplines in the Faculty of Medicine were headed by a number of esteemed scientists and medical professionals, many of whom had trained overseas or at UCT or Wits, such as Professor I. Gordon (pathology), Professor E.B. Adams (medicine), Professor S.F. Bush (zoology), Professor D. Crichton (gynaecology and obstetrics), Professor A.E. Kark (surgery), Professor S.L. Kark (social, preventive and family medicine), Professor J.A. Keen (anatomy), Professor T. Gillman (physiology) and Professor D.B. Hodges (physics).[69] Many of these professors had liberal political leanings and aimed to provide the highest standards of education, even if on a segregated basis, while some, like S.L. Kark, were even more progressive in their beliefs and actions and not always prepared to lie down quietly and accept the apartheid state's policy directives.

By early 1954, overspending on building and equipment costs brought Gale into direct conflict with state financiers.[70] By the end of 1957, total capital expenditure for the school in respect of buildings and equipment amounted to £503 600, way over the original sum budgeted in 1950/1, and producing a shortfall of £40 600 from the £463 000 the state had provided.[71] Thus, during the 1950s, the university was forced to go on a public fund-raising drive to meet the shortfall. As a result, state funding was supplemented by donations obtained from the Natal University Development Foundation (a non-profit organisation formed to collect money from the general public to advance the interests and development of the university), which, during the early 1950s, included wealthy members of the sugar and mining industries; the Transkei Bunga – or Governing Council – and professional and business people from a variety of racial groups. E.H. Brookes also discusses how a number of influential royal chiefs, including Paramount Chief Cyprian Bhekuzulu Nyangayezizwe ka Solomon (Zulu king from 1948 until his death in 1968), collected amongst themselves and their constituents nearly

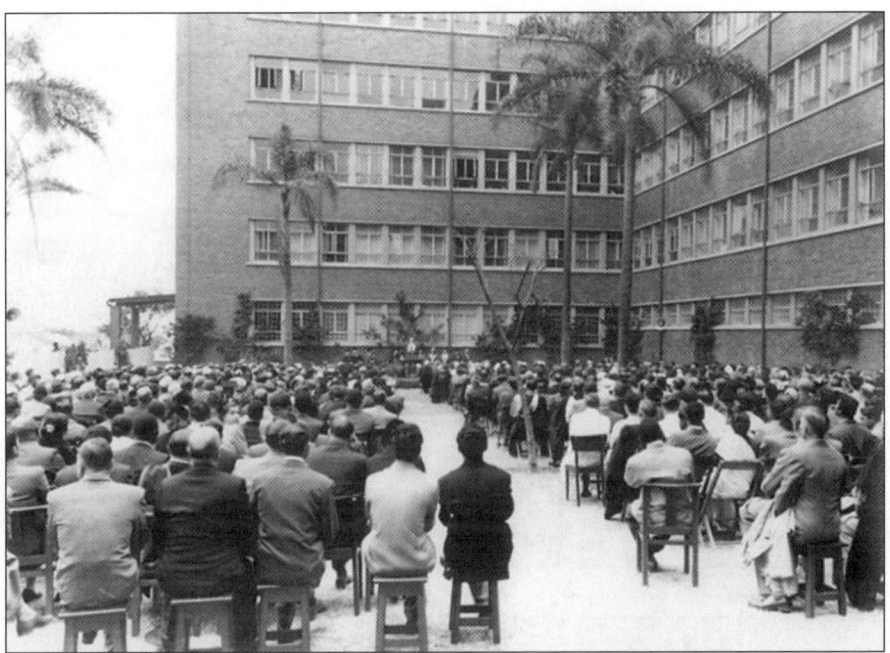

Photo 2.4 Opening of the medical school, Umbilo Road, 1955. (*UKZN Medical School Archives*)

£2 200, which they handed over to the university in a formal ceremony on 22 October 1954.[72]

Donations were not only received from wealthy or influential people, however. Many smaller donations were also obtained from working-class individuals scattered across the country. At the official opening of the new medical school buildings in 1955, the principal Malherbe, for example, acknowledged the 10/- note the university had received from an African women living in Alexandra Township, a not insignificant amount for a poor washerwoman who was prepared to make this financial sacrifice for something she believed in.[73] These donations imply that knowledge about the medical school's establishment was widespread during the 1950s. They also suggest that although the formation of the school was largely spearheaded by white liberals, there was keen interest shown by a variety of African and Indian South Africans in the medical school. It was a national institution that would produce doctors to care for the health needs of black communities, not only in Natal, but in the whole of South Africa, and was thus a worthy cause to support.

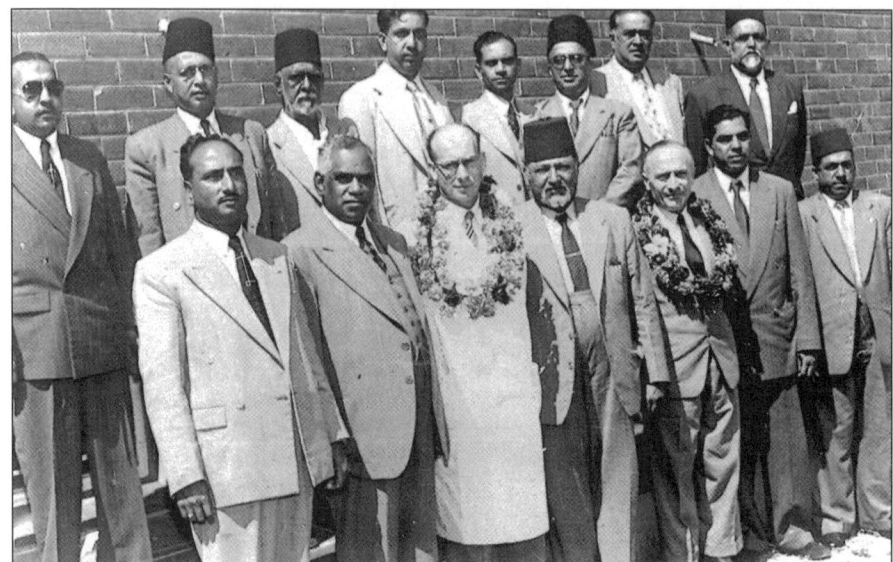

Photo 2.5   Farewell to Professor G.W. Gale (third from the right, front row) by leaders of the Indian community, 1955. (*UKZN Medical School Archives*)

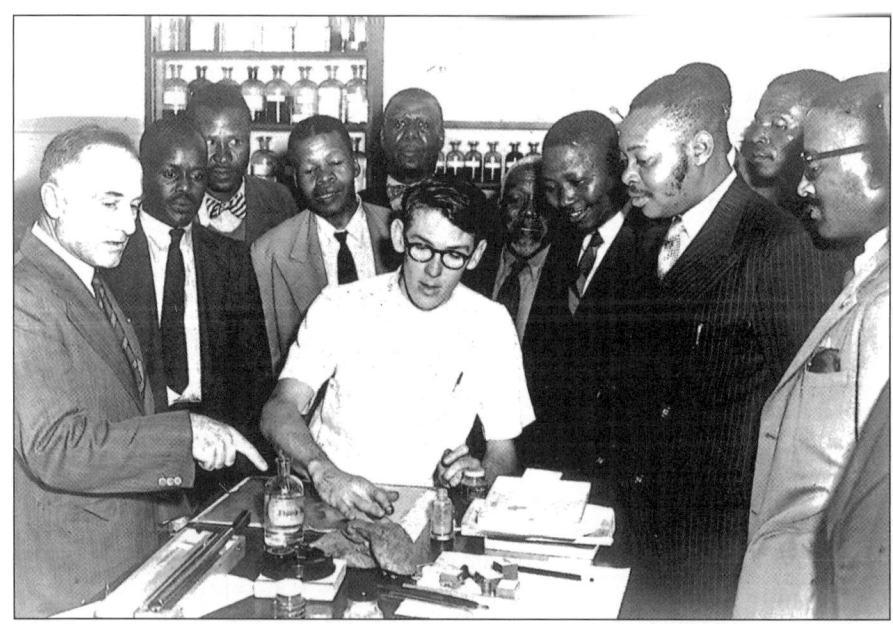

Photo 2.6   Visit of delegation of Paramount Chief Cyprian Bhekuzulu Nyangayezizwe ka Solomon, 1954. (*UKZN Medical School Archives*)

An extraordinary curriculum

The institution's new curriculum was another area to produce anomalies and to exacerbate relations between the school and the apartheid state. Unlike the professionally inferior Medical Aid training scheme provided for African students in earlier decades, Durban curriculum designers were determined that their school would produce doctors of the highest quality in line with international standards. Since the white academic staff's reputation would be made or broken by the quality of the doctors they produced, they aimed to train 'non-European' doctors comparable to those graduating from white medical schools. Thus, they had to balance carefully ideas for curriculum innovation with already long-established and well-accepted medical approaches. J.V.O. Reid, a South African-born, Oxford University-trained professor and for over twenty years head of physiology, and also dean of the Durban medical faculty in 1976 and 1977, said:

> [T]heir medical training was modelled closely on that of existing 'white' schools in the country if only because a departure from that practice would have carried too strong a connotation of something different, something inferior. It was a simple case of trying to put out doctors comparable to those produced from the other schools of the country, who [were] of high quality.[74]

All students considered for admission had to meet the minimum entrance requirement of matriculation, plus passes in mathematics and English as at other medical schools.[75] Since intake was limited due to space restrictions, only the best candidates stood a chance of being admitted. Originally built to accommodate about 40 students per year when it first opened, and increasing steadily to about 80 students per year by 1975 and 120 students by the early 1990s, there were always more applicants than places available, validating Malherbe's earlier arguments.[76] What made matters more difficult was that the selection committee also attempted – although this was not always possible – to maintain an admissions quota of 50 per cent African students per year.[77] In addition to being the country's most populous group, Africans had the lowest ratio of western-trained doctors to patients in the country, which the school hoped to address through its training programme. When places were available, a few students from neighbouring African countries, such as the Central African Federation (which includes today's regions of Malawi, Zambia and Zimbabwe), and from the British protectorates of Basutoland and Swaziland, which did not have medical schools in their own countries, were also accepted.[78] The remaining spaces available were occupied by Indian and coloured students, though Indian students always outnumbered coloured students, often because of their better class status and since Indians formed a more significant demographic grouping within the province of Natal.

In terms of maintaining high standards, the structure of the school's MB ChB degree had to meet the minimum requirements laid down by the South African Medical and Dental Council, the body responsible for registering all doctors to practise in the country.[79] As a result, the first to sixth years of the course followed a similar pattern to the six years of medical education offered at the white medical schools in the country. This required students to study the basic science subjects in the first three years, followed in the last three years with hands-on training in a number of clinical subjects, which required them to rotate through various departments at their teaching hospital.[80] After graduating and completing a further year's compulsory practical or internship experience in hospital ward work in a recognised teaching hospital, Durban medical graduates were then entitled to register to practise as doctors in South Africa in terms of the Medical, Dental and Pharmacy Act.

While being careful not to step too far beyond the established curriculum requirements of other medical schools, from the outset the medical school did, however, introduce two noteworthy curriculum innovations. The first involved an additional year of training – known as the 'preliminary year' or Year 0 – at the premedical level, extending the undergraduate medical degree programme from six to seven years.[81] Influenced by the problem of students applying for admission with inadequate primary and secondary school education, especially in key subjects like mathematics and science (which were taught, and often poorly so, at only a few of the state's segregated black schools), as well as English (which was stunted by the state's policy of teaching African students in their mother-tongue languages until high school), the addition of a preliminary year, or a 'bridging year' between high school and the first year, was considered essential from the outset.[82] Although the courses taught in this year were revised at various times to meet changing admission concerns, this additional year was a requirement for most black student applicants until its official abandonment in 1975, when higher costs and larger numbers of students making the entrance qualifications invalidated the need for it.[83] Sometimes, a few students who came from good private schools and had matriculation aggregates of 60 per cent and above, and at least 50 per cent in maths and English, were admitted directly into the first year. Occasionally, too, students who held approved degrees, such as BSc degrees, or had passed basic science courses at other recognised universities were permitted into second year.[84]

During the preliminary year, students were required to complete introductory basic science courses, which were to be studied more intensively in first year. It was hoped that this would make up for the shortcomings of many students' inadequate high school educations, and stimulate a higher pass rate overall. However, students were also required to complete courses in English (or Afrikaans), as well as history or sociology during this year, which flouted conventional medical curriculum norms at the time.[85] The 'language difficulty of many of the students and what could be done about it' was raised as a main issue for discussion at many board meetings. On 2 November 1962, Taylor wrote a letter to his adult children of these frustrations, having just attended a board meeting where these issues were hammered out again the day before.

> The lack of basic English has been thrown back into the laps of the University's English Dept. heads. Their solution seems to be to give them a course of reading including an anthology of poetry, two of Shakespeare's plays and some other good English books. We feel that more important is the giving to them of books to read that will inspire and interest them, books that are examples of good grammar and correct spelling of the terms they will use.[86]

During the 1950s, the introduction of social and human science subjects together with biological and physical sciences aimed to provide students with what Gale called 'a broader basis of general education before proceeding to more specialised professional training'. But more than this, and reflecting his Eurocentric perspectives which he shared with many of his white medical colleagues, he was very keen that his students gain a 'better mastery of western language . . . cultural values and . . . institutions' that influenced the development of the scientific medical paradigm and its code of ethics.[87] Furthermore, and controversially, as we shall see below, it aimed to encourage students to appreciate the wider societal, behavioural and cultural influences affecting human societies and their health, which was then built upon later in their clinical years in the Department of Social, Preventive and Family Medicine.

The second major curriculum innovation involved an in-depth and sustained training in social, preventive and community health medicine at the undergraduate level, which was not offered at other medical schools in the country at the time.[88] During the early 1950s, the fledgling medical school was formally affiliated to Durban's Institute of Family and Community Health (IFCH), which was established by Smuts's UP government as an outcome of the Gluckman Commission.[89] Under the leadership of a South African-born, progressive, Jewish, public health doctor, Sidney L. Kark, the work done at the IFCH was modelled on a successful, early-1940s, primary-level, community health centre experiment that married doctors Kark and his wife Emily had pioneered in Pholela, a poverty-stricken, rural, African 'reserve' area in the midlands of Natal.[90] Opened in 1945, this institute, situated in Clairwood (south of Durban) and affiliated with several health centres (including Pholela), aimed to provide both a theoretical and practical training, as well as research, in a variety of urban, peri-urban and rural socio-economic and cultural environments, for different categories of health workers who would staff the new nationwide network of primary-level health-care centres that were being established at the time. By the early 1950s, the IFCH and its health centres catered for a population of about 67 000 people, mostly Africans, both within and in surrounding areas of the city of Durban.[91]

Experts in the fields of family and community health, nutrition, environmental hygiene, health education, epidemiology, infectious disease control, psychology, dentistry and oral hygiene, laboratory work and health statistics were employed at the institute to provide postgraduate courses for doctors and nurses, and to train a new category of Community Health Worker (CHW).[92] These courses and the health services focused on providing a holistic 'social medicine' approach. Although social medicine was not an entirely new or an exclusively South African idea, as similar approaches had been and were being experimented on in the interwar and post-war years in other international locations, such as China and Britain particularly, the institute did press forward ideas and practices related to this approach.[93] Essentially, it highlighted the biological but also wider social and cultural aspects causing ill health, and actively promoted preventive and health educational approaches to improve the health of patients in communities outside the walls of expensive and overcrowded hospitals.

In the years leading up to the medical school's establishment, a handful of forward-thinking public health doctors, such as Henry Gluckman, George Gale and Sidney Kark, advocated something different. They felt that the provision of health-care services in South Africa required something more than simply training additional doctors to cure established diseases, as was the common pattern in the country and abroad at the time. As early as 1942, it was stated in a public health report that 'doctors should be trained as preserver[s] of health rather than as mender[s] of diseased bodies'.[94] In 1947, while still serving as secretary of health, Gale, reflecting on the training provided at the IFCH, argued that the IFCH's six-months' reorientation training for doctors provided at the postgraduate level came too late in a person's training when 'wrong emphases and outlooks inculcated over a period of six years' at medical schools were almost impossible to undo.[95] In addition, he asserted that the training offered at the IFCH needed to be an integral part of medical students' undergraduate curriculum to have the best effect. In 1951, just a few months before taking over as dean of the Medical School in Durban, Gale, having conferred with Kark (who was by this time a member of the initiating subcommittee of the medical school who had got involved through his relationship with Taylor),[96] wrote the following:

> We envisage that that majority of non-European doctors will go into general practice rather than hospital and we think it desirable that they should do so. For it is the general practitioner who first comes into contact with people in their homes, and it is in this sphere that the non-European doctor, with his more intimate knowledge of the outlook and language of his own people, will be able to make his most valuable contribution to their health needs . . . It is of particular importance that they receive adequate training in the practice of medicine outside as well as inside hospitals.[97]

During the early 1950s, as members of the acting board, Kark and Gale worked hard to convince other discipline heads, firstly, to support the design of a new curriculum that bucked the trend of increasing fragmentation and narrow specialisation in medical education at the time. Secondly, and more importantly, they encouraged training in curative, hospital-based medicine, *but also* in social and preventive aspects of medicine at the family and community levels.[98] Together, they also persuaded the faculty board to allow 'a fourth main clinical division, Family Practice and Community Medicine' to be included in the clinical years, alongside the usual divisions of medicine, surgery, and gynaecology and obstetrics.[99] By 1952, two years before clinical training was to commence, Gale and Malherbe together wrote to the Department of Health to determine the possibility of using the IFCH and its attached health-centre facilities as a practical teaching base for the school's medical students in a similar vein to that being negotiated with King Edward VIII teaching hospital.[100]

A key issue that concerned promoters of this approach was the apartheid state's increasing oppositional stance towards its predecessor's health policies. The UP government's nationwide, state-subsidised, health-centre-based approach made state officials nervous, as it did many in the white medical fraternity concerned about the loss of profits. Although a more conservative Afrikaner Nationalist political agenda was not entirely to blame for the eventual collapse by the early 1960s of Gluckman's approach, which was already hampered by staffing and financial cutbacks before 1948, the state's efforts to undermine what it considered leftist-leaning, 'socialist' health-care policies were essential after 1948. State budgetary cuts, which prevented the building of new health centres, reduced funding for existing centres, and open verbal attacks against the ideas and work of the social medicine practitioners at the roughly 40 health centres that were established by this point, but especially 'the nest of liberals' at the IFCH, were not idle threats.[101]

After 1948, finding himself at the centre of this storm in his position as secretary of health, the embattled Gale, who remained strongly supportive of Gluckman's social medicine, health-centres approach, worked determinedly to salvage what he could of this scheme. The Karks argue that it was Gale who played a pivotal role in convincing the Rockefeller Foundation to provide funding to support an affiliation of the IFCH with the Durban Medical School, to enable the teaching of its students in social medicine.[102] Renowned for its grants to universities and other research institutions to assist in the advancement of medical education, the foundation had shown an interest in supporting South Africa's experiment in social medicine since the Gluckman era. Anticipating a possible link between the IFCH and a medical-education institution, in 1947 and 1948 it had funded the advanced training of a number of IFCH staff members at leading social medicine institutions in the USA.[103]

Between 1952 and 1954, in his capacity as dean, Gale wrote many letters to the Rockefeller Foundation laying out his concerns and asking for financial assistance, as one letter highlights:

> [W]e are very anxious that the teaching of social medicine – or, to use terminology . . . which they [the apartheid state] favour, teaching in health centre practice as developed at the IFCH – should be incorporated in the medical curriculum from the very outset. Otherwise, so quickly do conservative influences become dominant in institutions, it is probable it will never be introduced at all.[104]

Convinced by Gale of the threat the growing conservative element in the Department of Health posed to the innovative work being done at the IFCH, in 1954 the Rockefeller Foundation agreed to work with the University of Natal to persuade officials in the department, with a substantial financial grant offer, to create an institutional collaboration between the IFCH and Durban's medical school to prevent its closure.[105] Although a complex series of negotiations between the various parties delayed the process further, between 1956 and 1960, a five-year arrangement was organised based on the Rockefeller Foundation's agreement to donate £42 400.[106]

This agreement facilitated the creation of a formal relationship between the institute and the Durban Medical School, and led to the formation of the new Department of Social, Preventive and Family Medicine (SPFM) headed by Sidney Kark, who had by this stage been invited to join the school as a permanent faculty member.[107] As part of this arrangement, the Department of Health and the Natal Provincial Administration (NPA), which by then had taken over administrative control of the IFCH, agreed not to close the institute or any of its health centres and to continue to meet the running costs of these facilities, as well as to pay the salaries of the non-academic staff.[108] A similar joint staffing agreement to that established between the university and the NPA, which allowed academic staff to have dual teaching and clinical care service responsibilities at the medical school and its King Edward VIII teaching hospital, was arranged.[109] The academic staff of the Department of SPFM, who also worked at the IFCH, was jointly appointed and paid by both the state and the university (subsidised by the Rockefeller grant). Their duties included teaching and research for the university, and health-care service responsibilities in the IFCH's health centres. This mutually beneficial arrangement aimed to provide the school with sufficient 'extra-hospital' teaching material for its students, who, in turn, would provide the state with doctors skilled in a more comprehensive curative and preventive form of medicine. Many would go on to work in the public health-care service.

Thus, during the 1950s, the newly established Durban Medical School committed itself to a different curriculum approach, which allowed it to develop along new lines.[110] Much thought was given to the design of the new curriculum to give more than merely lip service to the preventive and health educational aspects of medicine. Not only would it provide students with a sound curative, hospital-based training in the major subjects of medicine, surgery, and obstetrics and gynaecology, students would also gain special training in the family and community settings of patients served by the IFCH and its health centres.[111] In addition to providing a theoretical training via weekly lectures, seminars and demonstrations, the Department of SPFM enabled students, through their inclusion in health-centre teams that went out to the different health centres, to work one-on-one with patients under the close supervision of trained doctors and nurses.[112]

During 'family practice clerkships', students were each given carefully chosen, long-term, case studies. This was to provide them with a sense of continuity in dealing with the needs of a particular patient and his or her family in their community contexts.[113] A number of short-term clerking experiences were given to students too, to enable them to understand and treat many of the common health problems faced by their patients. Furthermore, students were taught to work closely with a variety of Community Health Workers (CHWs), who assisted the doctors and nurses and who were skilled in the promotion and preservation of health. Students would accompany CHWs into various home and community settings to survey and monitor factors influencing patients' health, spotting and encouraging early treatment for diseases, such as tuberculosis and sexually transmitted diseases, and preventing diseases by helping to devise and implement health education programmes to safeguard good health.[114] This training offered students a much more sophisticated and holistic understanding of the complex root causes of and treatments for diseases, as Kark argued in a 1980 interview:

We began a new approach in which we decided that we needed to know the people we were dealing with . . . This meant that we needed to meet them in various situations, not only in clinic, we had to visit homes, we had to meet them in the fields, we had to go to their schools . . . This gave us insight into their living . . . it also made the people realise that we were different kinds of creatures from the doctors they'd met before.[115]

While much has been written about the history of the community health experiment in South Africa during the 1940s and 1950s and its positive contributions to the country and even the world once these ideas expanded beyond South Africa's borders, much less has been focused on Kark and his team's controversial work at the medical school itself.[116] Here, the new department faced tough opposition from within the school from a number of academics who questioned the value of teaching SPFM subjects. Since these subjects were not offered at other medical schools at the time and, in addition, cut into the time available for training students in the other major clinical subjects, they were not regarded as a forward step at all by these individuals.[117]

Furthermore, careful analysis of interviews conducted with 1950s-era alumni also highlights students' resistance. During this period, strong concerns were voiced by many students about the extra work burden this subject would entail and whether it was a racially biased move exclusively associated with a black medical school. As Soromini Kallichurum remembered:

[Y]ou know, in the beginning, we as students were a bit worried about this because now instead of writing four major subjects [we] were going to write five . . . It was an orientation that wasn't present in other [schools] . . . and it was just an orientation that came from a . . . single medical school . . . We also wondered whether it was racially orientated to have this . . . being the only medical school with it.[118]

In a 1993 interview, Albertina Luthuli relayed how many students did not simply accept these curriculum changes. Instead, they gave Kark and his team a hard time and seriously questioned its value as individuals and as a group: 'We were up in arms as students. We thought this was not in our favour.'[119] Luthuli had also argued that many students felt it was yet another 'impediment they were putting there, because we were black, by the white lecturers and professors, [and] that they wanted to make it more difficult for us to become doctors'. She even remembered how students nicknamed the subject 'Spoof', as a play on the new SPFM department's acronym, but also because many did not take it seriously at first.

To alleviate these internal concerns, Kark had to work hard to explain and justify his social medicine approaches to his colleagues and students as cutting-edge innovations, based on the highest western-based, scientific medical-training standards. For example, while wanting his students to consider a variety of complex, biological, economic and sociocultural factors (including 'traditional' healing beliefs and practices) affecting health, in an apartheid socio-political context where indigenous beliefs and practices were considered inferior, and in a medical context where indigenous healing therapies were taboo, Kark and his team were careful to teach their students about these issues from a position that encouraged understanding of their patients' backgrounds, while promoting the superiority of biomedical perspectives and approaches.[120] Many of these Eurocentric perspectives, especially the sense of difference and opposition between indigenous and western forms of medicine encouraged by the lecturers, would trickle down and influence some of their students' views too.

In addition, Kark's 'genuine concern about the community and its problems', his passionate belief in the value of social medicine, the many dedicated hours he spent working with his students in various community settings, and the useful skills he and his team taught his students won many sceptical students over to this approach.[121] As Luthuli asserted, eventually, 'when we completed it, every one of us really, we all said, "you know, Spoof was a good thing". It equipped us with an attitude and something extra which we needed very much and we appreciated it in the end.'[122]

Although Kark was able to overcome most of the internal resistance, a damaging blow to his educational experiment was the loss of George Gale, who had been a promoter and protector of his vision and work. In April 1955, Gale, feeling under constant attack from the state over his supposed 'extravagance and irresponsibility' in overspending on behalf of the school, and concerned that his job was not secure, resigned as dean to take up a position elsewhere. In various letters written to defend his actions, Gale argued that he was not prepared to bow to the state's budgetary cuts on what he considered the minimum necessities to ensure good medical educational standards.[123]

While Gale (like Taylor before him) was certainly not a radical, and ultimately accepted that the medical education of black students would occur within the structural set-up of apartheid, he was determined to ensure that separate education for black students would be of equal quality to white students. However, his efforts were viewed as too progressive by the state and, as a result, he was ultimately pressured to resign. Although he gave up his fight as dean in Durban, Gale did not give up on his interest in social, preventive and family medicine.[124] Gale emigrated to Uganda, where he was actively encouraged to start a new Department of Preventive Medicine at Makerere Medical School. Later, he went on to Thailand and Malaysia to help develop departments of social and preventive medicine at various medical schools in these countries, before finally retiring in Britain in 1969.[125]

In a letter addressed to the new dean in May 1955, a disheartened Gale wrote how disappointed he was at being forced to resign from a position he had hoped to hold until retirement: 'I need not deny to you, that it is a very bitter thing to have to leave one's country and, at the same time, a lifetime's ambition unfulfilled.'[126] Some years later, in an autobiographical document penned during his retirement in 1976, reflecting on his many professional accomplishments but also his failures, Gale wrote about his great 'sorrow at having to leave my native land and School in the establishment of which I had so much to do over so many years'.[127] The only thing that assuaged his bitterness was the appointment of one of his colleagues, Isidor Gordon, as his successor. Gordon had sought employment at the school after achieving success as the senior government pathologist in the Department of Health and officer-in-charge of the state pathology labs in Durban.[128] Although he was an esteemed professor in his own right, and had assumed the position as head of the school's Department of Forensic Medicine and Pathology before becoming dean, he was also, more importantly, a man whom Gale felt 'shared my ideas and ideals for medical education'. Born into a Jewish family, he was sensitised to the many injustices in the world around him, including racism. Like Gale and Taylor before him, Gordon as dean would also find himself on many occasions in opposition with the state during the sixteen years he held this position, as he devoted himself to the advancement of black medical education.

However, it was not simply internal opposition or the loss of Gale's support that scuppered Kark's progressive teaching approach. What really damaged the work of the school's Department of SPFM was a more antagonistic apartheid government stance by the late 1950s.[129] Reflecting on why the state turned against this medical-education innovation, Kallichurum felt that her medical school's curriculum was becoming too 'radical' in their eyes:

[F]or one thing they were bringing to the surface the lot of black people . . . and I think they felt that they would have . . . an influence on students and maybe even the patients, the communities . . . You must remember also that no other medical school . . . had this subject and here [was] a black medical school that has [sic] this . . . special subject about social and community [health] and they could have seen it as a threat. You know, that they were training . . . activists and things like that.[130]

Increasingly, towards the end of the decade, Kark and his team were investigated for so-called communist activities in an era of heightened anti-communist rhetoric during the Cold War.[131] The state's association of 'social medicine' with 'socialised medicine' was based on Kark and his staff's free distribution of food and skimmed milk to poverty-stricken and malnourished patients who attended the IFCH's health centres. Although Kark and his team might not have regarded themselves as political activists at the time, their work had political undertones that advocated what medical historian Shula Marks has argued was 'a more liberal and liberating medical practice', which inspired many young medical students and the black communities they served.[132] The Department of SPFM's approach that emphasised bottom-up and holistic understandings of health care, focusing on the deeper socio-economic root causes of diseases as well as a philosophy of prevention and equal primary health-care services for all, represented a huge leap beyond the thinking of most government officials and many in the South African medical profession. What also worsened relations between those working at the Durban Medical School and the state and helped to undermine the school's social and community health curriculum experiment were the state's more conservative tertiary education policies.

'This is an institution worth fighting for': Defiance against the 1957 Separate University Education Bill

During the late 1950s, the state turned its gaze to universities to entrench complete racial segregation, seeking to augment what had already begun at primary and secondary schools with the Bantu Education Act in 1953. Apartheid hardliners in government wanted to halt racial fraternisation between students at the liberal universities and eliminate what they saw as potential political threats that could emerge from these institutions.[133] In 1957, the traditions of autonomy and academic freedom at South African universities were subjected to direct attack by the state's introduction to Parliament of the Separate University Education Bill. This bill proposed the closure of Wits, UCT and Natal universities to black students unless prior ministerial permission had been obtained, and outlined financial provision for the creation of a number of new separate, race- or ethnic-based and state-controlled university colleges for African, Indian and coloured students.[134] The aim of this bill was to provide training for 'non-European' students in their own separate, tertiary facilities, who would then graduate to provide skilled personnel to work in their own racial areas.

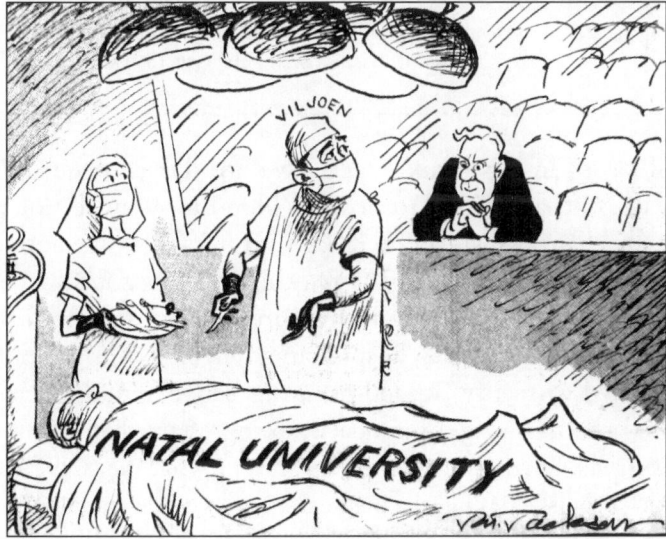

Figure 2.2 'Surgeon Viljoen: I know the patient shouldn't have this . . . but as Dr Verwoerd insists.' (*Cape Argus* March 12, 1957)

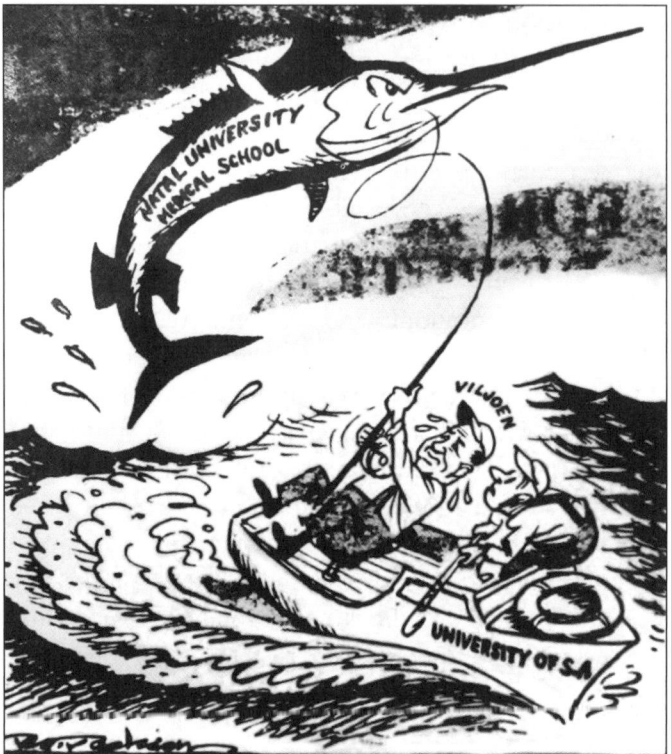

Figure 2.3 'In troubled waters . . . Do you want to put it in the party museum.' (*Cape Times* February 18, 1957)

This bill, if passed in this form, would have had dire consequences for the University of Natal as it aimed to close its 'Non-European Section', but also fundamentally change what had been achieved at its black medical school on Umbilo Road.[135] During the early 1950s, this area was zoned under Group Areas Act legislation as a white residential area, placing the medical school's buildings and adjacent teaching hospital in an incongruous position, which the state wanted to rectify. In addition, this school's multi-racial student body blurred the more rigid boundaries being established by the state at other institutions. Furthermore, the existence of what the state increasingly considered a 'socialist' trend in the medical school's undergraduate curriculum was a dangerous anomaly that had to be corrected. The bill stipulated that the University of Natal – like Wits and UCT – had to become a white university once again, and provided for the transfer of administrative control of its black medical school to the Department of Bantu Education, which aimed to make the long-distance, correspondence University of South Africa (UNISA) its examining body.

Much opposition emerged against the bill from those at and affiliated to the universities of the Witwatersrand, Cape Town and Natal, and other concerned individuals and organisations.[136] During 1957, strong public opposition was raised by outraged members of these universities' councils and senates, academic staff and students, the South African Medical and Dental Council, members of various branches of the Medical Association, various civic organisations such as the Black Sash and South African Institute of Race Relations, international medical schools and private individuals.[137] It was based largely on the grounds that the bill violated the long-standing sanctity of university autonomy that had successfully guided the operation of these universities for decades.

Unlike those objecting at Wits and UCT, however, the University of Natal's objections were carried out from a position of ambiguity, having for years before already bowed to the pressure of establishing racially separate facilities. This is evident in the public statements made by people like E.G. Malherbe. As principal, Malherbe was placed in a particularly difficult position. Despite objecting to what he considered the 'irrational' and 'unnecessary' drastic changes that the bill recommended, and the flagrant violation that state interference posed to his university's autonomy, he had to be diplomatic in what he said to prevent a loss of subsidies for his university.[138] Instead, he tried cleverly to use the state's own apartheid arguments against it. He also attempted to show that his university already carried out its academic functions on an apartheid basis, providing separate facilities for its black medical school, and ran separate but parallel classes for black and white students in other subjects. For example, in a February 1957 newspaper article, he asserted that the medical school had 'become the Government's best showpiece . . . built up with so much care, dedication and idealism by the University, and which gained the confidence and trust of the non-Europeans' and if the government went ahead with this bill, 'it will be a vital blow for the most successful experiment in University apartheid'.[139]

For many medical professionals, the attempt to remove the medical school from the aegis of the University of Natal was viewed as an attack on the country's medical standards.[140] In March 1957, Taylor wrote that when he heard about the bill, it was like 'a bombshell [had] burst . . . it [was] a shattering blow . . . for even with the best will in the world, such a department cannot run a medical school successfully', but will turn out graduates 'who will have a sense of inferiority because of the substandard training they will have received'.[141] What tipped the scales in favour of the medical school were the protest actions of its academic staff. On 18 March 1957, after a secret ballot, the school's academic staff adopted a resolution by 29 votes to two to resign en masse if the government refused to retract clauses related to the medical school from its bill.[142] In an exchange of correspondence with the secretary for education later that year, Malherbe wrote that his medical staff 'by refusing to cooperate . . . decline to be party to the carrying out of a death sentence on our Medical School, where they have so devotedly braved the difficulties and problems of the pioneering years'.[143]

In addition to threatening the university's autonomy and lowering the school's standards particularly, the staff also objected strongly to provisions in the bill that gave the state the power to control their appointments, conditions of service and dismissals for misconduct.[144] These conditions would have largely changed their status from university employees to government civil servants. Isidor Gordon, who played a central role as coordinator and leader of this protest action, captured the firm resolve of his staff, which was reported on in many local, national and international newspapers, to fight against this recommended change in policy:

> As resolved as the Government may be to convert our Medical School into a Government institution, so determined are we to remain in the University of Natal. In the space of a few years, the Durban Medical School has made great contributions in the field of medical education, medical research and medical services to non-white peoples . . . [This] is an institution worth fighting for and if the Government wishes to rob the University of Natal of its School, then it must carry out this assault without any assistance from us. We hope that the University of Natal's teachers, medical profession and general public in all parts of the country will continue to help us to resist the Government plan, and will support us in the bitter struggle, which must now inevitably ensue.[145]

The threat of mass staff resignations and the storm of public protests persuaded the government to back down, at least on its medical school plans. The state had sought to assume administrative control of the school, not close it down completely, which it feared would happen after doctors at the school and the medical profession more broadly had made it clear that they would refuse to cooperate to re-staff this institution. Nineteen fifty-eight was also an election year, and the National Party government could not afford to provoke too much opposition. Thus, the provisions relating to the medical school were withdrawn from revised versions of the bill in 1958.[146] In a letter to the minister of health in April 1958, Malherbe wrote triumphantly that 'the Dean and I repeatedly warned you and the late Minister that in this particular case you have to deal with a group of independent professional men who will not submit to threats of arbitrary governmental State institutions'.[147] When the final Extension of University Education Act No. 45 was passed through Parliament in 1959, the University of Natal maintained administrative control of its Faculty of Medicine.

The university, nonetheless, lost its right to admit 'non-European' students to its other disciplines as it had done in the past. In addition, both Wits and UCT, whose staff and students had also vehemently opposed the bill, were forced, owing to their reliance on state subsidies, to close their doors to black students unless prior ministerial permission was obtained. Although black students already registered at these universities were allowed to complete their degrees, and while a small number of Indian and coloured students did receive ministerial approval to study at Wits and UCT, especially if certain subjects were not offered at their 'own' campuses (African students did not receive ministerial permission until the late 1970s at Wits and the late 1980s at UCT), most new black student applicants were directed to apply to 'their own universities' that had been built and opened in the 1960s.[148] These included the University College of Zululand or Ngoye (for Zulu students), the University College of the North or Turfloop (for Tswana/Sotho students), the University College of Durban-Westville (for Indian students) and the University College of the Western Cape (for coloured students). After this law was passed, the University College of Fort Hare was reserved for Xhosa students.[149] In addition to establishing a more rigid apartheid order in higher education, these government restrictions contributed to a decline in the overall number of black medical graduates, but especially African graduates, until the late 1970s, when the Medical University of Southern Africa opened for African students, and when more reformist apartheid legislation allowed small numbers of African students to start registering at Wits and UCT once again.[150]

The demise of Durban's social medicine experiment

The early 1960s brought many changes for the Durban Medical School. While it is true that the state was not able to remove the black medical faculty from the white University of Natal, it was successful in undermining this school's innovative social and community health undergraduate teaching programme. When the Rockefeller Foundation's five-year funding scheme came to an end in 1960, the ministers in the state's Department of Health refused to provide the necessary funding to continue the joint teaching and service arrangement that had been set up between the medical school and the IFCH. Explaining some of the reasons why the Rockefeller Foundation refused to provide further funding for this educational experiment, Gale wrote:

> 1960 was the year of Sharpeville, and the Rockefeller Foundation, recalling with bitterness that the many millions of dollars it had contributed to development of the Union Medical College in Peking early in the century had not helped in any way to prevent the Communist take-over of China, and fearing that South Africa too was now set on a course towards totalitarianism, albeit of a right-wing variety, it was not prepared to risk a repetition of its experience with China.[151]

However, the writing was already on the wall by the late 1950s, as the state had steadily cut funding and slowly limited the supply of health personnel under state employment working at different health-centre locations across the country. In addition, a number of senior-level community health doctors, who experienced growing attacks on their social and community health-centre ideas and efforts during these years, were ultimately forced to resign to save their work, and emigrated overseas. Following Gale's lead, two other pivotal members of Durban's Department of SPFM emigrated from South Africa. Sidney and Emily Kark left for the United States in 1958, where Sidney had been invited to initiate a new Department of Epidemiology at the School of Public Health at the University of North Carolina at Chapel Hill. A year later, the Karks moved to Jerusalem, Israel, where they joined other doctors and nurses (some of whom had emigrated from South Africa) on the staff of the Hebrew University Hadassah Medical School.[152] Here they helped develop this medical school into an important international centre for social and community medicine training, research and service.

While the South African state and medical profession increasingly turned their backs on social and community medicine approaches from the 1960s, the Karks and many others who taught with them in the Department of SPFM and IFCH saw their work expand and their ideas achieve international recognition in a variety of countries more hospitable to their approaches. Their more open access to, and training of, students from around the world spawned many new social and community medicine projects similar to those the Karks and their team had started in Durban in the 1940s. This ultimately led to the development of what became popularly known from the 1970s onwards as the Community-Oriented Primary Health Care (or COPC) approach, which was officially endorsed by the World Health Organization in 1978 at the Alma Ata Conference as the most effective way forward to promote improved public health-care for people.

The demise of Durban's IFCH and health-centre approach was swift after the Rockefeller Foundation's funding dried up. In 1961 the IFCH was closed, and by the mid-1960s most of the remaining health centres in the country had either been forced to close or were handed over to provincial administrations for conversion to curative clinic services. Remaining doctors and nurses were transferred to curative facilities. Employees trained as Community Health Workers were either retrenched or used as hospital orderlies.[153] Moreover, while attempts were made to continue teaching aspects of COPC subjects from the Department of SPFM as a sub-speciality within the Department of Medicine in 1960 and 1961, by 1962 this sub-speciality was removed from the faculty's list of subjects taught to students.[154]

Thus, from the early 1960s, only a decade after its founding, Durban's innovative medical curriculum was brought into line with other white medical schools in South Africa. From the 1960s through to the 1980s, despite listing in 1976 a Community Health Department in the faculty handbook as a subject offering for its students, the Durban Medical School's focus remained overwhelmingly curative and hospital-based. The staffing of its Community Health Department remained 'vacant' until 1979, when Ian W.F. Spencer was employed as a professor to start building up a community focus and orientation once again at the Durban school.[155] Thus, until the mid- to late-1980s, when this department gained more staff and became more rooted at the school, the multiplicity of departments and specialities, which focused on curing established diseases (as was the case in other medical schools around the country), provided an undergraduate medical education little concerned with teaching students about prevention or health promotion. The state had been successful in purging the school of its anomalous and far-sighted social-medicine curriculum orientation. This move represented a great loss to South African public health-care services and medical education more generally, which, for decades to come, would remain vastly inadequate to address the majority of the country's health-care needs.

It took enormous courage and determination from its liberal pioneers over nearly half a century to bring the dream of a full medical education for black doctors to fruition. And it took even more effort and many struggles to keep it there. After 1948, the tertiary education sphere became a site of keen interest to, and constant intervention by, the apartheid state, as it worked to implement stricter racial segregation at the university level. On the other hand, while the state's policies strengthened and expanded from the 1950s onwards to incorporate and control many aspects of people's lives, the field of higher education came to provide a contentious minefield for government officials trying to entrench apartheid policies. During its fledgling years, the medical school's academic staff actively challenged the apartheid state, leading the way in many of these university educational struggles. Firstly, some of its staff developed an innovative social and community health teaching experiment not offered at any other medical school in the country. Secondly, its whole academic staff mounted a determined fight to oppose the state's efforts to take control of their medical school in 1957.

So contentious did these two sets of issues become that the state's praise of the medical school as a positive 'showpiece' of apartheid in the early 1950s was quickly muffled just a few years later. By the late 1950s, the school had become an anomaly whose staff and students did not simply fall into line with apartheid-state directives and policies. The difficulties of dealing with these issues would set a contradictory historical track record for Durban's medical school, as in the eyes of the state it became a highly contested educational space. Furthermore, these 1950s intrusions by the state would not be the end of its interference in the affairs of the school, and further attempts would be made to separate the medical school from the University of Natal.

However, from the late 1960s and through the 1970s and 1980s, it would be the school's students – not its academic staff – that would take up this oppositional role. Using a variety of sources, including interviews and autobiographical accounts of individuals who attended the medical school during the apartheid period, the chapters that follow continue to explore how the school came to exist as an ambiguous and contested space, but through the experiences of those who studied there.

Notes

1. *Report of the Committee on Medical Training in South Africa, UG 25 of 1939* (Pretoria: Government Printer, 1939); and Edgar H. Brookes, *A History of the University of Natal* (Pietermaritzburg: University of Natal Press, 1966), 80.
2. *The University of Natal Durban Medical School: A Response to the Challenge of Africa* (Durban: Hayne and Gibson, 1954), 7.
3. Henry Gluckman, *Abiding Values: Speeches and Addresses* (Johannesburg: Caxton, 1970), 435.
4. Gluckman, *Abiding Values*, 116. Also see Brookes, *A History of the University of Natal*, 81.
5. NAR UOD 1546, U3/40/4, Natal University College for Establishment of Medical Schools for Natives, 1945–48, 'Memo on the question of a fourth medical school' attached to letter from H. Gluckman (Minister of Health) to J.H. Hofmeyr (Minister of Finance), 1 October 1947.
6. Maurice G. Pearson, 'History of government hospitals in Durban, 1858–1945', *South African Medical Journal* (3 June 1961).
7. Gluckman, *Abiding Values*, 115–6; and NAR UOD 1546, U3/40/4, Natal University College for Establishment of Medical Schools for Natives, 1945–48, 'Summary of representations for the establishment of a fourth medical school (primarily for non-Europeans) at Durban', 1947.
8. Bruce K. Murray, *Wits the 'Open' Years: A History of the University of the Witwatersrand, Johannesburg, 1939–1959* (Johannesburg: Witwatersrand University Press, 1997), 28, 37–45.
9. George W. Gale, 'Medical schools in Africa: A short historical and contemporary survey', *Journal of Medical Education* 34, no. 8 (August 1959), 716.
10. NAR NTS 2862, 7/303 Part 5 Dr McCord's Mission Nursing Home 1944–49, 'Correspondence from McCord Zulu Hospital', 26 September 1948.
11. Interview with Soromini Kallichurum, Durban, 29 May 1999. For more on Kallichurum, see UKZNA MF3/1/1-8, 'Professor Kallichurum first female president of NIMDC', *MedNews: Faculty of Medicine Newsletter* (November–December 1995); and 'No stopping this doc of a "different" gender', *Mercury* (16 November 1995).
12. *Who's Who of Southern Africa, 1964* (Johannesburg: Wootton and Gibson, 1965).
13. Gail M. Gerhart, 'Edgar Brookes 1897 to 1979', in the *Dictionary of African Christian Biography*, http://www.dacb.org/stories/southafrica/brookes_edgar.html.
14. Brookes, *A History of the University of Natal*, 79.

15. UKZN MSA, 'Non-European medical school. Minutes of the meeting in the mayor's parlour, City Hall, Durban, on 13 November 1945'.

16. Brookes, *A History of the University of Natal*, 82; and Isidor Gordon, *Report on the Government's Intended Action to Remove the Faculty of Medicine from the University of Natal* (Durban: Hayne and Gibson, 4 March 1957), 6.

17. UKZN MSA, 'Non-European medical school. Minutes of the meeting in the mayor's parlour'.

18. UKZN MSA, 'Non-European medical school. Minutes of the meeting in the mayor's parlour'; and *The University of Natal Durban Medical School: A Response to the Challenge of Africa*, 9.

19. UKZN MSA, 'Biographies – Dr A.B. Taylor'; 'He founded a health corps', *Natal Mercury*, 22 June 1964; and Brookes, *A History of the University of Natal*, 80–2.

20. Gordon, *Report on the Government's Intended Action*, 6.

21. John V.O. Reid and Alexander J. Wilcot, eds, *Medical Education in South Africa: Proceedings of the Conference on Medical Education held at the University of Natal, Durban in July 1964* (Pietermaritzburg: University of Natal Press, 1965), 2.

22. *The University of Natal Durban Medical School: A Response to the Challenge of Africa*, 15 and 27.

23. For more on E.G. Malherbe, see Brookes, *A History of the University of Natal*, 58–62; and Ernst G. Malherbe, *Never a Dull Moment* (Southern and Eastern Africa and the UK: Timmins Publishers, 1981).

24. NAR UOD 1546, U3/40/4, Natal University College for Establishment of Medical Schools for Natives, 1945–48, Letter from E.G. Malherbe to H. Gluckman, 5 May 1947.

25. Gordon, *Report on the Government's Intended Action*, 5.

26. For more on this, see Sylvia Vietzen, 'Mabel Palmer and black higher education in Natal, 1936–42', *Journal of Natal and Zulu History* vi (1983); and Sylvia Vietzen, 'Beyond school: Some developments in higher education in Durban in the 1920s and the influence of Mabel Palmer', *Natalia* 14 (December 1984).

27. 'How non-European classes began at Natal University', *Natal Daily News* (15 March 1957).

28. 'New university applauded: Apartheid formula in Natal', *Cape Times* (21 February 1948).

29. 'Commission of natives: Medical school discussed', *Natal Mercury* (27 November 1947); and CC EGM File 463/4/1, KCM 56990 (17)c, 'Medical school history and establishment', *Natal Witness* (7 July 1955).

30. CC MPC File 35, KCM 18254, 'Minutes of fifth annual meeting of the Convocation of the University of Natal held at City Building Durban', 23 May 1953; and UKZNA BIO P 3/2/5, SP 6/12/5, Cuttings, E.G. Malherbe 3/10/76 – 13/5/81, 'Man behind the Broederbond file', *Daily News* (3 October 1976), and 'Malherbe's latest book exposes the great laager' (5 May 1977).

31. Brookes, *A History of the University of Natal*, 61.

32. CC EGM File 465/3, KCM 56990 (170), Letter from E.G. Malherbe to the editor entitled 'Commission of enquiry into separate university facilities for non-Europeans 1953-54', *The Times Educational Supplement* (12 May 1948); and CC EGM File 464/2, KCM 56990 (130), 'Higher education of non-Europeans in South Africa', *South African Outlook* 86, no. 1023 (2 July 1956).

33. 'Natal must contribute liberally: Government view on medical school', *Natal Mercury* (5 January 1948); and *The University of Natal Durban Medical School: A response to the Challenge of Africa*, 7.

34. UKZN MSA, Biographies – Dr A.B. Taylor, 'He founded a health corps', *Natal Mercury* (22 June 1964). Also see CC MH Mouldy Box Scans, Dr A.B. Taylor; From January 1946, 1947, pages 49–50, Letter from Dr Alan B. Taylor to Margaret and Duane Sprague, Vermont, USA, 26 July 1947 and Dr Taylor up to Dec 1958, page 158, Letter from W.B.D. Evans, Bridgman Memorial Hospital, Johannesburg to Dr A.B. Taylor, 8 May 1954.

35. NAR UOD 1546, U3/40/4, Natal University College for Establishment of Medical Schools for Natives, 1945–48, 'Government favours non-European medical school in Durban', *Natal Witness* (5 May 1948).

36. See, for example, William Beinart and Saul Dubow, eds, *Segregation and Apartheid in Twentieth-Century South Africa* (London and New York: Routledge, 1995) and Deborah Posel, *The Making of Apartheid 1948–61: Conflict and Compromise* (Oxford: Clarendon Press, 1991).

37. See, for example, Peter Kallaway, ed., *Apartheid and Education: The Education of Black South Africans* (Johannesburg: Ravan Press, 1984); Cedric de Beer, *The South African Disease: Apartheid Health and Health Services* (London: Catholic Institute for International Relations, 1986); and Anne Digby, *Diversity and Division in Medicine: Health Care in South Africa from the 1800s* (Oxford: Peter Lang, 2006).

38. Shula Marks has shown that for a variety of reasons these recommendations were already under threat before 1948, though the election of a new government sounded its final death toll. See Marks, 'South Africa's early experiment in social medicine: Its pioneers and politics', *American Journal of Public Health* 87, no. 3 (March 1997).

39. CC MH Mouldy Box Scans, Family Letters 50–55, page 205, Letter from Dr. A.B. Taylor 'To the kids', 5 August 1952.

40. Quoted in CC MH Mouldy Box Scans, Dr Taylor up to Dec 1958, page 158, Letter from W.B.D. Evans, Bridgman Memorial Hospital, Johannesburg to Dr A.B. Taylor, 8 May 1954.

41. UKZN EGML, 'Alan Boardman Taylor', *University of Natal Gazette* (June 1958), 4; CC MH McCord Hospital Board minutes, 8 September 1949, 27 July 1950 and 29 January 1951; and Sidney and Emily Kark, *Promoting Community Health: From Pholela to Jerusalem* (Johannesburg: Witwatersrand University Press, 1999), 177.

42. CC MH Mouldy Box Scans, Family Letters 40–50, page 145, Letter from Dr A.B. Taylor to 'Dear Family', written whilst on furlough in Auburndale, Massachusetts, 10 March 1949.

43. Earl H. Harley, 'The forgotten history of defunct black medical schools in the nineteenth and twentieth centuries and the impact of the Flexner Report', *Journal of the National Medical Association* 98, no. 9 (September 2006); Todd Savitt, 'Abraham Flexner and the black medical schools', *Journal of the National Medical Association* 98, no. 9 (September 2006); and 'A Short History', *Howard University College of Medicine*, http://medicine.howard.edu/about/history/default.htm. For more on the segregated nature of medical education in the USA, also see Wilbur H. Watson, *Against the Odds: Blacks in the Profession of Medicine in the United States* (New Brunswick, NJ, and London: Transaction Publishers, 1999).

44. CC MH Mouldy Box Scans, Family Letters 40–50, page 145, Letter from Dr A.B. Taylor to 'Dear Family', written whilst on furlough in Auburndale, Massachusetts, 10 March 1949; and page 109, Letter from Dr A.B. Taylor to Dr N.L. Mills, 1 September 1949.

45. CC MH Mouldy Box Scans, Dr Taylor up to Dec 1958, page 257, Letter from Dr A.B. Taylor to Dr E.M. Dodds, New Jersey, USA, 27 December 1957.

46. CC MH Mouldy Box Scans, Dr Taylor up to Dec 1958, page 70, Letter from Dr A.B. Taylor to Dr and Mrs E.A. Thompson, Congregational Church, Grand Rapids, Michigan, 27 March 1951.

47. Gordon, *Report on the Government's Intended Action*, 9.

48. CC MH Mouldy Box Scans, Tied Together, Dr Taylor Personal 1959–60, page 130, Letter from Dr A.B. Taylor to Professor Clifford Herman, University of Vermont College of Medicine, Burlington, Vermont, 5 April 1959.

49. CC MH Mouldy Box Scans, Dr Taylor up to Dec 1958, page 203, Letter to 'Our Friends in America', 1958.

50. B.T. Naidoo, 'A history of the Durban Medical School', *South African Medical Journal* 50, no. 41 (25 September 1976), 1627.

51. CC GP File 21, KCM 25878, 'Summary of conditions of the award of a bursary/ loan offered by the Government of the Union of South Africa at the University of Natal', n/d.

52. CC MH Mouldy Box Scans, Family Letters 40–50, page 109, Letter from Dr A.B. Taylor to Dr N.L. Mills, 1 September 1949.

53. See CC MH Aldyth Lasbery Papers, Box 8, Series II, 'Natal University Graduation Ceremony, Pietermaritzburg, 29 March 1958', *Isibuko* no. 23 (June 1958); and UKZN EGML, 'Alan Boardman Taylor', *University of Natal Gazette* (June 1958), 4.

54. Interviewee's emphasis. See Interview with Soromini Kallichurum in *Students in the Barracks: Memories of Alan Taylor Residence* (University of Natal, Durban: Audio-Visual Alternatives, 1989).

55. CC MH Mouldy Box Scans, Family Letters 50–55, page 227, Letter from Dr A.B. Taylor 'To the Kids', 4 March 1952.

56. CC MH Mouldy Box Scans, Family Letters 50–55, page 329, Letter from Dr A.B. Taylor 'To the Kids', 3 April 1950.

57. CC MH Mouldy Box Scans, Tied Together, Dr Taylor Personal 1959–60, page 130, Letter from Dr A.B. Taylor to Professor Clifford Herman, University of Vermont

College of Medicine, Burlington, Vermont, 5 April 1959. Also see CC MH Pretoria Disk 2 Doc 65 Annual Report of the Medical Superintendent of McCord Hospital, 1955 and CC MH Box 7 Series II Medical Superintendent Reports 1956 to 1962.

58. Gordon, *Report on the Government's Intended Action*, 16; and CC MH Mouldy Box Scans, Tied Together, Dr Taylor Personal 1959–60, page 137, Derk Crichton, 'The clinical work of the Department of Gynaecology and Obstetrics of the University of Natal during 1957: A brief review', reprinted from *Medical Proceedings* 4, no. 19 (20 September 1958).

59. 'Natal University Graduation Ceremony, Pietermaritzburg, 29 March 1958'. Also see CC MH Box 7 Loose Photocopies in Box, 'Citation as given by the Orator, Recommending an Award of PhD *Honoris Causa* to Dr Alan Boardman Taylor, 29 March 1958'.

60. CC MH Mouldy Box Scans, Family Letters 50–55, page 227, Letter from Dr A.B. Taylor 'To the Kids', 4 March 1952.

61. For more on Gale's background, see Michael Gelfand, *Christian Doctor and Nurse: The History of Medical Missions in South Africa* (Sandton: Mariannhill Mission Press, 1984), 135–8; and Shula Marks, 'Doctors and the state: George Gale and South Africa's experiment in social medicine', in *Science and Society in Southern Africa,* ed. Saul Dubow (Manchester and New York: Manchester University Press, 2000).

62. UKZNA H6/2/2 Medical School Advisory Committee, Estimates and Expenditure, 1955: 'University of Natal subsidy for a trifocal university', 2 April 1955; and Letter from E.G. Malherbe to the Secretary for Education, Arts and Science, re 'Non-European medical school', 7 January 1955.

63. See Gordon, *Report on the Government's Intended Action*, 31.

64. See above, 34; UKZN MSA, Prof. Isidor Gordon, 'The Durban Medical School 1951–197', 2; and Brookes, *A History of the University of Natal*, 83.

65. CC MH Mouldy Box Scans, Dr Taylor up to Dec 1958, page 15, Letter from Dr A.B. Taylor to 'Dear Friends', 3 February 1951.

66. See CC EGM File 465/6, KCM 56990 (215), E.G. Malherbe, 'The autonomy of our universities and apartheid', 1957; and File 463/4/1, KCM 56990 (15) b, Ernst G. Malherbe, 'Opening the non-European medical school', *The South African Outlook* 81, 966 (2 October 1951), 147; *University of Natal Durban Medical School: A Response to the Challenge of Africa*, 14; and Gordon, *Report on the Government's Intended Action*, 7.

67. NAR, UOD 56, U3/26/4/5, University of Natal Building Grants and Loans for Medical School Non-Europeans Durban 1949–53, Letter from E.G. Malherbe to the Sec. for Education, Arts and Science 'Re. Additional capital costs: Non-European medical school', 29 December 1953; CC GP File 13, KCM 25771, Letter from G.W. Gale to Dr E.G. Malherbe, 20 April 1954; and UKZNA H6/2/2, Medical School Advisory Committee Estimates and Expenditure, 1955, Letters from G.W. Gale to E.G. Malherbe, 1 March and 20 April 1955; UKZNA H6/1/1, Medical School – History, George W. Gale, 'The story of the Durban Medical School' (25 January 1976), 12.

68. CC GP File 13, KCM 25748, G.W. Gale, 'University of Natal memorandum on the financial needs of the medical school submitted to the UNDF', 15 April 1952.

69. To see a full list of the names of all the academic staff who were employed at the Durban Medical School during different years, see UKZNA *UN Calendars*, especially the Faculty of Medicine handbooks.

70. UKZNA H6/2/2, Medical School Advisory Committee Estimates and Expenditure, 'University of Natal subsidy for a trifocal university', 2 April 1955.

71. Gordon, Report of the Government's Intended Action, 9. *University of Natal Durban Medical School: A Response to the Challenge of Africa*, 27.

72. Brookes, *A History of the University of Natal*, 84; 'Zulu Chief Cyprian Bhekuzulu', *South African History Online*, http://www.sahistory.org.za/dated-event/zulu-chief-cyprian-bhekuzulu-born.

73. CC EGM File 463/4/1, KCM 56990 (13), E.G. Malherbe Medical School History and Establishment, 'Address at Medical School Opening July 1955', 3.

74. UKZN EGML, John V.O. Reid, 'The concept of the medical school', *Concept: Convocation of the University of Natal* 7 (June 1976), 3–4. For more on Reid's background, see 'Honoris Causa II: Laudations spoken in presenting honorary graduands in the University of Natal, 1968–80 by the university orator, J.V.O. Reid (Durban: University of Natal, 1984). Similar arguments were also made in Interviews with Y.K. Seedat, Durban, 7 July 2003, J.V.O. Reid, Plettenberg Bay, 16 June 2002; and Sam Fehrsen, Pretoria, 22 August 2003.

75. UKZN MSA, 'Information for students seeking admission to the Faculty of Medicine of the University of Natal', n/d, 4; and CC GP File 21, KCM 25878, 'Report of screening committee appointed to consider application for admission in 1956'.

76. See graphs in appendices of student registrations between 1951 and 1994.

77. W.R.G. Branford, 'Examination systems and selection: The experiences of the admissions committee of the Board of the Faculty of Medicine, University of Natal', in *Medical Education in South Africa: Proceedings of the Conference on Medical Education held at the University of Natal, Durban in July 1964*, eds John V.O. Reid and Alexander J. Wilcot (Pietermaritzburg: University of Natal Press, 1965), 191.

78. CC GP File 18, KCM 25863, Letter from H.S. van der Walt, Secretary for Education, Arts and Science to the High Commissioner of Southern Rhodesia, 5 November 1953; and CC MH Mouldy Box Scans, Tied Together, Dr Taylor Personal 1959–60, page 120, Letter from I. Gordon to Dr Paul Dudley White, Boston, Mass, USA, 22 May 1959.

79. *University of Natal Durban Medical School: A Response to the Challenge of Africa*, 14.

80. Isidor Gordon, 'Experience in the establishment of a medical school for non-white undergraduate students in South Africa', and S.F. Oosthuizen, 'The intern year', both in *Medical Education in South Africa: Proceedings of the Conference on Medical Education held at the University of Natal, Durban in July 1964*, eds John V.O. Reid and Alexander J. Wilcot (Pietermaritzburg: University of Natal Press, 1965), 301, 377–80.

81. CC GP File 17, KCM 25841, 'Minutes of the meeting of the curriculum sub-committee, 20 June 1952'; and CC GP File 17, KCM 25826, 'Notes on proposed curriculum for subcommittee meeting, 13 September 1954', 1–2.
82. Branford, 'Examination systems and selection', in *Medical Education in South Africa*, 195–6.
83. Gordon, 'Experience in the establishment of a medical school for non-white undergraduate students in South Africa', 302; and 'End to course causes anger', *Natal Mercury* (27 June 1973).
84. UKZN MSA, 'Information for students seeking admission to the Faculty of Medicine of the University of Natal', 4; and Gordon, 'Experience in the establishment of a medical school for non-white undergraduate students in South Africa', 302.
85. Branford, 'Examination systems and selection', 191.
86. CC MH Mouldy Box Scans, 56–63, Folder 1 [S], page 90, Letter from Dr A.B. Taylor 'To the Kids', 2 November 1962.
87. See Gale, 'Medical schools in Africa', 717; and George W. Gale, 'The Durban Medical School: A progress report', *South African Medical Journal* (7 May 1955), 437. Also see Alan B. Taylor, 'Presidential address' in *Medical Education in South Africa: Proceedings of the Conference on Medical Education held at the University of Natal, Durban in July 1964*, eds John V.O. Reid and Alexander J. Wilcot (Pietermaritzburg: University of Natal Press, 1965), 3.
88. Sidney L. Kark, 'Family and community practice in the medical curriculum: A clinical teaching program in social medicine', *Journal of Medical Education* 34, no. 9 (September 1959).
89. For more on the history of the IFCH, see Kark and Kark, *Promoting Community Health*, chapter 7; and Alan Jeeves, 'Delivering primary care in impoverished urban and rural communities – South Africa's Institute of Family and Community Health in the 1940s', in *South Africa's 1940s: Worlds of Possibilities*, eds Saul Dubow and Alan Jeeves (Cape Town: Double Storey Books, 2005).
90. For more on the Karks and Pholela, see Maya Scholtz, 'Mervyn Susser and Zena Stein: Pioneers in community health and their Jewish identity as an orienting factor in their contribution' (Honours thesis, University of Natal, 1999); and Sidney L. Kark, 'Health centre service: A South African experiment in family health and medical care', in *Social Medicine*, ed. Eustace H. Cluver (Johannesburg: Central News Agency, 1951).
91. 'The Institute of Family and Community Health (Union Health Department): Summary of the report of the Medical Officer-in-Charge, for the year ending 30 June 1950', *South African Medical Journal* (24 November 1951), 870. Also see Eva J. Salber, *The Mind is Not the Heart: Recollections of a Woman Physician* (Durham and London: Duke University Press, 1989).
92. For more on CHWs, see Louise Vis, 'We Sow the Seed: Perspectives of Health Educators at the Institute of Family and Community Health in Durban in the 1940s and 1950s' (Master's diss., University of KwaZulu-Natal, 2004).

93. For more on this international context, see Marks, 'South Africa's early experiment in social medicine'; and Shula Marks, 'Social medicine in South Africa in the mid-twentieth century: The international context' (Seminar Paper, WISER, Johannesburg, 17 July 2006).

94. NAR GES 2957, PN 5, Native Medical Aids, 'Report of the committee of enquiry on the medical training of natives to the Minister of Public Health', 15 June 1942, 8.

95. Letter from G.W. Gale to J.B. Grant, 27 September 1947, quoted in Marks, 'Social medicine in South Africa in the mid-twentieth century', 15.

96. Kark and Kark, *Promoting Community Health*, 177.

97. NAR GES 1831, 68/30, Medical and Dental Training for Natives, 1948–1958, George W. Gale, 'The functions of the Institute of Family and Community Health (Clairwood) with particular reference to the Durban Medical School', 7 November 1951, 1.

98. CC GP File 1, KCM 25662, 'University of Natal Report of the sub-committee appointed by the Acting Board of the Faculty of Medicine to draft a proposed curriculum for the training of African medical students', 1 September 1950; and CC GP File 17, KCM 25841, 'Minutes of the meeting of the curriculum sub-committee', 20 June 1952.

99. Kark and Kark, *Promoting Community Health*, 178.

100. UKZNA H6/2/3 Correspondence concerning Establishment of the Department of Family Practice, 1953–55, 'Letter from E.G. Malherbe and G.W. Gale to Dr Bremer, Minister of Health', 14 August 1952.

101. See Derek Yach and Steve M. Tollman, 'Public health initiatives in South Africa in the 1940s and 1950s: Lessons for a post-apartheid era', *American Journal of Public Health* 83, no. 7 (July 1993); and Marks, 'Doctors and the state', 189.

102. Kark and Kark, *Promoting Community Health*, 178.

103. James Trostle, 'Anthropology and epidemiology in the twentieth century: A selective history of collaborative projects and theoretical affinities, 1920–70', in *Anthropology and Epidemiology*, eds Craig R. Janes et al. (Dordrecht: Reidel Publishing, 1986), 64; and Marks, 'Social medicine in South Africa in the twentieth century', 2–3, 7–14.

104. UKZNA H6/2/3 Correspondence concerning Establishment of the Department of Family Practice, 1953–55, 'Durban Medical School project for a department of family medicine', 6. Also see 'Arguments against closure of the Institute of Family and Community Health', in the same file.

105. UKZNA H6/1/1 Medical School – History, Letter from Flora M. Rhind (Secretary, Rockefeller Foundation) to Dr E.G. Malherbe, 24 September 1954.

106. UKZNA H6/2/3 Correspondence concerning Establishment of the Department of Family Practice, 1953–55, 'Letter from G.W. Gale to Dr Le Roux, Secretary for Health', 8 November 1954; G.W. Gale, 'University of Natal Faculty of Medicine Department of Family Practice', 16 November 1954; and 'Letter from Prof. I. Gordon to W.A McIntosh', 2 June 1955; and Gordon, *Report on the Government's Intended Action*, 17.

107. 'Department of Social, Preventive and Family Medicine, University of Natal: Appointment of Professor Sidney L. Kark', *South African Medical Journal* 10 (March 1956), 250.

108. UKZNA H6/2/3, Correspondence concerning Establishment of the Department of Family Practice, 1953–55, 'Memorandum by the principal of the university to the Minister of Health the Hon. Dr T. Naude re. Negotiations with the Department of Health regarding the establishment of a department of family practice at the Clairwood Institute of Family and Community Health', 13 April 1955.

109. CC GP File 23, KCM 25927 UN Medical School Miscellaneous, G.W. Gale, 'Recognition of hospitals by the SAMDC', 5 January 1955; and Gordon, *Report on the Government's Intended Action*, 8–9 and 35–37.

110. Vanessa Noble, 'A medical education with a difference: A history of the training of black student doctors in social, preventive and community-oriented primary health care at the University of Natal Medical School, 1940s–1960', *South African Historical Journal* 61, no. 3 (September 2009).

111. UKZNA H6/2/3, Correspondence concerning Establishment of the Department of Family Practice, 1953–55, Letter from G.W. Gale to E.G. Malherbe re 'Establishment of a department of general or family practice: Durban Medical School', 12 July 1954; and Kark, 'Family and community practice in the medical curriculum', 905–6.

112. For more on specific subjects taught by the Department of SPFM, see UKZNA *UN Calendar 1957*, Faculty of Medicine: Information for Students, 418; and Kark and Kark, *Promoting Community Health*, 181–6.

113. UKZNA H6/2/3, Correspondence concerning Establishment of the Department of Family Practice, 1953–55, Sidney L. Kark, 'Family health and medical care: The need for training a family doctor', 26 May 1954; and UKZN EGML, Sidney L. Kark, 'A university department of social, preventive, and family medicine', *University of Natal Gazette*, iii, no. 1 (June 1956).

114. Sidney L. Kark and Emily Kark, 'A practice of social medicine', in *A Practice of Social Medicine: A South African Team's Experiences in Different African Communities*, eds *Sidney L. Kark and Guy Steuart* (Edinburgh and London: E. and S. Livingstone, 1962), 38–9; and Kark, 'Family and community practice in the medical curriculum', 909.

115. Interview with S. Kark and I. Gordon on the 'Facts and Aspects of our Medical School which are not Recorded', by S. Cameron-Dow, December 1980, 11. This interview was conducted by a University of Natal public relations officer who was collecting oral memories about this school leading up to its 30th anniversary.

116. See, for example, Jack H. Geiger, 'Community-oriented primary care: The legacy of Sidney Kark', and Mervyn Susser, 'A South African odyssey in community health: A memoir of the impact of the teachings of Sidney Kark', both in *American Journal of Public Health* 83, no. 7 (July 1993); Yach and Tollman, 'Public health initiatives in South Africa in the 1940s and 1950s'; and Steve M. Tollman, 'The

Pholela Health Centre – the origins of community-oriented primary health care: An appreciation of the work of Sidney and Emily Kark', *South African Medical Journal* 84, no. 10 (October 1994).

117. UKZNA H6/1/1, Medical School – History, Interview with Kark and Gordon, 20–2.

118. Interview with Soromini Kallichurum, Durban, 29 May 1999. For similar views, see Interviews with Fatima Mayet, Durban, 4 June 1999, and S.B. Pitsoe, Durban, 17 July 2003. Also see J.H Abramson, 'Natal medical students' attitudes to the social and preventive aspects of medicine', *South African Medical Journal* (25 March 1961).

119. Padraig O'Malley Interview with Albertina Luthuli, 10 January 1993, http://www.nelsonmandela.org/omalley/index.php/site/q/03lv00017.htm.

120. John Cassel, 'Cultural factors in the interpretation of illness: A case study', in *A Practice of Social Medicine: A South African Team's Experiences in Different African Communities*, eds Sidney L. Kark and Guy Steuart (Edinburgh and London: E. and S. Livingstone, 1962); Trostle, 'Anthropology and epidemiology in the twentieth century', 63–4; and Kark and Kark, *Promoting Community Health*, 61–5.

121. Interviews with Fatima Mayet, Durban, 4 June 1999, Soromini Kallichurum, Durban, 29 May 1999, and S.B. Pitsoe, Durban, 17 July 2003; and Abramson, 'Natal medical students' attitudes'.

122. Padraig O'Malley Interview with Albertina Luthuli, 10 January 1993, http://www.nelsonmandela.org/omalley/index.php/site/q/03lv00017.htm.

123. CC GP File 13, KCM 25771, Letter from G.W. Gale to E.G. Malherbe, 20 April 1954. Also see UKZNA H6/2/2, Medical School Advisory Committee Estimates and Expenditure, 1955, Letters from G.W. Gale to E.G. Malherbe, 1 March 1955 and 20 April 1955.

124. CC MH Mouldy Box Scans, page 56, Family Letters 50–5, Letter from Dr A.B. Taylor 'To the Kids', 8 February 1955.

125. UKZNA H6/1/1, Medical School – History, Gale, 'The story of the Durban Medical School', 15.

126. UKZNA H6/2/1, Medical School, Letter from G.W. Gale to I. Gordon, 2 May 1955.

127. UKZNA H6/1/1, Medical School – History, Gale, 'The story of the Durban Medical School', 15.

128. UKZNA BIO-S-506/1/1 Gordon, Isidor Prof., 'Admission of Emeritus Professor I. Gordon as an Honorary Fellow of Forensic Pathology in the Faculty of Forensic Medicine of The College of Medicine of South Africa at a Special Admission Ceremony in Durban on 4 July 1984', *Transactions of The College of South Africa* 28, no. 2 (July–December 1984), 60.

129. Marks, 'South Africa's early experiment in social medicine', 455.

130. Interview with Soromini Kallichurum, Durban, 29 May 1999.

131. Yach and Tollman, 'Public health initiatives in South Africa in the 1940s and 1950s', 1047–8.

132. Marks, 'Doctors and the state', 198–9; Interview with Mervyn Susser and Zena Stein, Durban, 4 June 1999.

133. Wits SAHA South African Political Materials 1964–1990s, The Karis-Gerhart Collection, Part III: Political Documents, NUSAS, Folder 575, Graeme C. Moodie, 'The state and the liberal universities in South Africa: 1948–90', *Higher Education* 27 (1994), 7; and CC EGM File 465/5/1 KCM 56990 (194), 'University apartheid in South Africa', reprinted from *Nature*, 180 (30 November 1957).

134. UKZN EGML, J.D. Krige, 'Nature and significance of the attack on university autonomy', *University of Natal Gazette* 4, no. 1 (June 1957); and Murray, *Wits the 'Open' Years*, 115 and 291–3.

135. For more on this issue, see I. Gordon's three reports: *Report on the Government's Intended Action* (4 March 1957); *Further Report on the Government's Intention to Remove the Faculty of Medicine from the University of Natal* (Durban: Hayne and Gibson, 4 May 1957); and *Third Report on the Government's Intention to Remove the Faculty of Medicine from the University of Natal* (Durban: Process Printers, 25 February 1958).

136. For more on the arguments and protest activities that took place at Wits and UCT against this bill, see Murray, *Wits the 'Open' Years,* especially chapters 9 and 10.

137. 'The proposed transfer of the Durban Medical School', *South African Medical Journal* (23 March 1957), 289; Gordon, *Further Report on the Government's Intention,* 6, 11, 23, 33; Gordon, *Report on the Government's Intended Action,* 22–3, 41; 'University in the bundu', *Natal Daily News* (11 February 1957); CC EGM File 465/5/1, KCM 56990 (202), 'University apartheid', *The Lancet* (30 March 1957); and 'Editorial: The Non-European Medical School', *South African Medical Journal* (27 April 1957), 400.

138. 'Malherbe says age-old rights are taken away', *Natal Mercury* (5 March 1957); CC EGM File 465/5/1, KCM 56990 (206), 'Malherbe attacks state's use of "power of the purse"', *Natal Daily News* (3 October 1957).

139. 'Drop medical school plan: Request made to minister', *Natal Daily News* (20 February 1957). Also see CC EGM File 463/7/2, KCM 57009 (12), Letter from E.G. Malherbe to Mr Op't Hof, Secretary for Education, Arts and Science re 'Transfer of medical school' (8 April 1958).

140. 'Medical school move: Fears of fall in standards', *Cape Argus* (11 March 1957); 'Medical school issue put to medical council', *Natal Daily News* (11 March 1957).

141. CC MH Mouldy Box Scans, 56–63, Folder 1 [S], page 18, Letter from Dr A.B. Taylor 'To the Kids', 5 March 1957.

142. 'Threat of medical staff boycott', *Natal Mercury* (15 March 1957); and UKZN Board of the Faculty of Medicine minutes, 'Resolutions taken at special meeting of the full-time members of the academic staff of the Faculty of Medicine', 18 March 1957.

143. Gordon, *Third Report on the Government's Intention*, p. 10.

144. CC EGM File 465/5/1, KCM 56990 (202), 'University apartheid', *The Lancet* (30 March 1957), 676; and Gordon, *Report on the Government's Intended Action*, 42–3.

145. Gordon, *Third Report on the Government's Intention*, 12. Also see 'Natal Medical School issue: Professor attacks government move', *Natal Mercury* (12 March 1957); 'Natal Medical School head warns on state control', *Cape Argus* (14 March 1957); CC EGM File 465/5/1, KCM 56990 (202) 'University apartheid', *The Lancet* (30 March 1957).

146. Brookes, *A History of the University of Natal*, 91.

147. CC EGM File 463/7/2, KCM 57009 (12), Letter from E.G. Malherbe to Mr Op't Hof, Secretary for Education, Arts and Science re 'Transfer of medical school', (8 April 1958), 3.

148. See Saleem Badat, *Black Student Politics: Higher Education and Apartheid, from SASO to SANSCO, 1968–90* (New York and London: Routledge, 1999), especially chapter 2.

149. Badat, *Black Student Politics*, chapter 2; and Murray, *Wits the 'Open' Years*, chapters 9 and 10.

150. P.V. Tobias, 'Apartheid and medical education: The training of black doctors in South Africa', *The Leech* 60, no. 1 (March 1991).

151. Gale, 'The story of the Durban Medical School', 16–7.

152. UKZN MSA, 'Israeli social health project run by Natal doctors', *Natal Mercury* (November 1959). For more on this subject and on those working with the Karks who also emigrated, spreading South Africa's social medicine ideas internationally, see Kark and Kark, *Promoting Community Health*, especially chapters 13 and 14.

153. D. Harrison, 'The National Health Services Commission, 1942–4: Its origins and outcome', *South African Medical Journal* (September 1993), 682. For more on the effects on CHWs, see Vis, 'We sow the seed'.

154. See UKZNA *UN Calendar*, Faculty of Medicine handbook sections, 1960–2.

155. For more on the hardships encountered during the start-up phase of this Department of Community Health, see Ian Spencer, *Hope Beyond the Shadows* (Kloof: Forest Publishers, 1992).

CHAPTER 3

The difficult journey to medical school

'My life and education have been a struggle.'
— Mamphela Ramphele

Veronica Wilson was an early 1970s graduate of the Durban Medical School and one of only a handful of women trauma surgeons working at the medical school's King Edward VIII teaching hospital. She recalled the great anguish she experienced during her final high school year as she contemplated her uncertain future. Having done well academically at school, she hoped to become a doctor, but financial difficulties were a serious obstacle to her aspirations:

> As a young girl it was actually very difficult because my mum was a domestic [worker] and, you know, I actually came from a very poor background . . . So it was actually very difficult for my mum to make ends meet . . . And then I actually finished matric and . . . I got, you know, good results . . . But then my mum had said to me . . . 'You're crying for the moon!' when I said I wanted to become a doctor.[1]

During the apartheid era, medicine was viewed as a prestigious and highly paid profession that offered students and their families the possibility of a more secure financial future and the ability to help their communities. For many students, however, the journey was not an easy one. Racial inequalities, financial obstacles and gender discrimination made advancement through high school an extremely difficult and unlikely possibility for most black students. Only a tiny and determined few successfully struggled to reach tertiary level with high enough matriculation passes to gain admission into the University of Natal Medical School.

Students applying for admission to the Faculty of Medicine came from a variety of family backgrounds. The majority who gained admission came from African and Indian families.[2] African applicants came from across the whole of South Africa, while Indian applicants were mainly from Natal, where the majority of Indian South Africans lived.[3] The numbers of students coming from racially mixed, coloured families always remained low, rarely exceeding five or six per year. Until more restrictive apartheid university legislation was imposed by the state in 1959, a handful of African students also applied and were accepted from a few neighbouring countries, such as Zimbabwe, Lesotho, Zambia, Malawi and Swaziland. However, these students were accepted only when there were insufficient numbers of qualified local African applicants available to make up the selection committee's admissions quota of 50 per cent African students per year.[4] This skewed admissions quota system, as the next chapter will show, produced much contention amongst the school's students over the years.

Certain socio-economic and family background characteristics were shared amongst students. Two sociological studies of medical students studying in Durban during the 1950s through to the early 1970s found that the majority surveyed came from urban home backgrounds, and that there was a greater urban bias in trends as the years continued.[5] Moreover, they revealed that most students had parents, usually fathers, with an above-average education (at least a Grade 8 or Standard 6 high school education), thus showing a pattern of selective recruitment from amongst higher-educated families.[6] Some students' parents had studied further, obtaining tertiary-level qualifications. In another study, University of Natal researcher J.W. Macquarrie found that educated occupations such as lawyers, teachers, nurses, clerks, ministers and businessmen were well represented among the parents of African university students in the 1950s and 1960s.[7] Some even had doctors as parents.[8]

Obtaining a high school education was a significant achievement in a racially oppressive context where most black South Africans attending school only completed primary level. Many who were able to continue their education had parents with higher-paying and skilled jobs,[9] with a few Indian applicants even 'coming from homes where the father is well-to-do', as Alan B. Taylor noted after a selection committee meeting in 1959.[10] It was even found in these studies that many siblings of medical students had matriculated too, and were white-collar workers, further highlighting how families of these students were 'not drawn from a complete cross-section of the African or Indian population'.

Being born to educated parents in South Africa was a key factor, as sociologist Leo Kuper has argued. It could enhance people's life chances, 'raising them above the general level of the . . . communities' and permitting 'qualitative differences in their style of life', including improved educational opportunities.[11] Reflecting on her life growing up in a small village in the northern Transvaal in the 1950s and 1960s, Mamphela Ramphele noted that her parents were both primary schoolteachers – 'a position of relative privilege in their social environment at the time, which placed me in a better position to survive and thrive than most of my contemporaries'.[12] Thus, certainly in the earlier generations of Durban Medical School graduates, coming from a higher socio-economic class background would have assisted a number of students in a variety of ways – particularly in facilitating opportunities for better primary and secondary education, which gave these students a greater chance of gaining admission to tertiary institutions.

What's more, many early generations of African and coloured students who came to study medicine in Durban had parents who belonged to recognised Christian denominations,[13] and many of these graduates came from missionary-administered high schools. For example, S.B. Pitsoe, an early 1960s graduate of the school and an obstetrics and gynaecology specialist, came to Durban from St Peter's Anglican High School in Rosettenville in Johannesburg, while Veronica Wilson came from Little Flowers, a Catholic boarding school for coloured girls in Ixopo, Natal.[14] Even black consciousness leader Steve Biko, who started his medical studies in 1966, came from completing his matriculation year at St Francis College in Mariannhill, Natal.[15] Other common missionary high schools that Durban Medical School graduates attended during the 1950s and 1960s included the Inanda Seminary, Adams College, Lovedale and Healdtown, to name but a few. These mission schools generally provided a better quality of academic education and thus the opportunity for young people to aspire towards a higher-earning professional career. They also instilled in many students 'western' Christian religious principles and cultural values, which their parents espoused too as a way to improve their families' lives in South Africa's discriminatory socio-economic context. This provided an important basis for further class differentiation amongst different black families.[16] In his 1969 study, Watts found that although the majority of Indian students had parents who were not Christians, professing instead to be practising Hindus or Muslims, a selective socio-economic basis affected Indian students too. Most were found to have come from English- or Gujerati-speaking families. He noted:

> [B]earing in mind the language distribution of Indians in South Africa, this quite clearly shows a definite economic selection from the wealthier Indians. Working-class Indians such as Tamil, Telegu and Urdu-speaking, are notably absent from the ranks of the Indian medical students, despite the fact that they form a large proportion of the Indian population of the country.[17]

'The path to a medical career had a number of major hurdles.'
— Mamphela Ramphele

While a large number of medical students' parents might have been better educated or in higher-paying skilled jobs, as black South Africans, most would have been racially discriminated against under apartheid conditions. They would have been paid salaries lower than those of their white contemporaries with the same education levels or for doing the same jobs, and it would still have been difficult for them to afford to send their children to university.

The woes of getting a student to the medical school would have been exacerbated for those who lived in another province, or for those who had only one parent to support them. B.T. Naidoo, one of the first graduates of the school, who later became a specialist paediatrician, remembered the 'uphill task' his family suffered 'to get me through' when he lost his father, the primary breadwinner, in his second year of study.[18] Many African families could not even afford the cost of a train ticket to send their children to medical school, not to mention covering the University of Natal's tuition and accommodation fees for a seven-year training programme. In her autobiography, *Across Boundaries*, Mamphela Ramphele recorded how the death of her father in May 1967 was a devastating blow emotionally and also financially for her family, making her journey to the medical school at the start of 1968 a very difficult one:

The level of material deprivation which I had to endure in the late 1960s and 1970s seems unbelievable even to me looking back. Train fare for a second-class return ticket was simply beyond the means of my family income at the time. My mother, the only breadwinner, was earning R86 per month as a teacher. I had to appeal to [my aunt] to lend me R55, which enabled me to buy a ticket from Johannesburg to Durban, shop for some provisions, and gave a bit of pocket money over to see me to the medical school doors.[19]

The situation would have been worse for those students whose parents were uneducated or employed in the lowest-paying, unskilled forms of work, such as domestic workers, manual labourers, drivers and night watchmen. Maila J. Matjila, who graduated in 1976 and specialised in community health, reflected that '[t]he pressures . . . come [sic] from . . . financial concerns . . . And where do you get the resources? . . . You depend on a parent who's a domestic worker or a poorly paid [labourer] . . . supporting a family . . . [and] you have to buy books [and pay your tuition] and all these other things.'[20]

Most of the students who applied for admission to the school from 1950 onwards were also products of the townships or rural 'reserves'. Although many came from families with higher-education achievements and some with a parent or parents in better-paying jobs, this would not have protected them from the harsh, discriminatory laws implemented by the apartheid state.[21] They would have been forced to live side by side with their poorer and less-educated or uneducated neighbours in state-approved 'non-European' areas, which were often located at a distance from 'white' urban areas, and were overcrowded and poorly serviced.[22] Their racial classification, not their class status, determined their subordinate positions in South African society. The negative effects of grand and petty apartheid laws that were introduced systematically from 1948 onwards affected all black South Africans, but were particularly severe on poor African families. Jerry Coovadia, who completed his postgraduate training in paediatrics at the medical school in the late 1960s and lectured at the school during the 1970s, eventually becoming head of the Department of Paediatrics from 1990 to 2000, remembered with exasperation the degree of hardships some of his African students experienced: '. . . you take a black [African] kid who grows up in the township, who doesn't have lights, doesn't have enough food.

There can't be equity, you know. How can he expect to perform when he goes to school?'[23]

As the apartheid years continued, particularly from the late 1960s onwards, greater numbers of students who applied to the University of Natal's medical school did not apply from high-quality missionary high schools, but from inferior, segregated and government-funded 'Bantu Education' schools. The apartheid state's system of Bantu Education came into operation in African schools in 1955, and in coloured and Indian schools in 1964 and 1965 respectively, having a profoundly negative effect on the educational advancement of black children.[24] On the one hand, it aimed to bolster job-reservation legislation to protect the skilled occupations of whites; on the other, it provided education and training for black populations to ensure their subordinate status as manual and semi-skilled workers. The state built new public schools in black areas for this purpose and targeted missionary schools for takeover or closure to undermine what it viewed as too liberal and 'bookish' an education taught at these institutions, which was not considered appropriate for the subservient roles black South Africans were destined to occupy under apartheid.

Discriminatory conditions made it difficult for most black pupils to succeed at school. From the mid-1950s onwards the state's provision of racially separate and unequal education affected black children the most. African schools received the lowest amount of state financial support for their running costs,[25] were notorious for being poorly constructed and overcrowded, and were run by too few, often poorly qualified and inadequately paid teachers.[26] They also lacked essential supplies, such as furniture, books and laboratory equipment. In addition, only a small number of black secondary schools in the whole of South Africa included the teaching of mathematics and science subjects as part of their syllabi: essential requirements for admission to medical school.[27] May Mashego, who attended the medical school between 1976 and 1982, becoming a general practitioner after qualifying, described with frustration how she had to move schools during her high school years in the early 1970s, which meant leaving her friends and her family and studying in another province, just so that she could study mathematics to gain entry into medical school:

> [F]or you to be able to . . . go into these careers like medicine or engineering, you had to do maths, but there was no maths in Mpumalanga at that time.

So I had to come to . . . Natal to do a bridging class called Pre-Form 4 so
that I could do maths . . . [in] Form 4 and Form 5 [which were the Grade
11 and] . . . matric classes . . . [Once] I got my skills backed up, only then I
could choose to do medicine.[28]

Some even recall being sent by their parents to do part or all of their
secondary schooling in missionary high schools in neighbouring British
protectorate countries, such as Swaziland, where they hoped they would
receive a better education.[29]

Under the apartheid education system, African schools were also
organised as far as possible 'on a fragmented . . . "tribal" basis . . . [and] were
"Bantu-ised" in personnel' to fit into the separate-development or Bantustan
homeland policies being pursued by the state.[30] At least until Grade 8, the
vernacular languages were promoted as the medium of instruction. Switching
to English (the language of university instruction) at secondary level meant
that pupils were expected to continue their education in a second or even
third language, stepping up the level of difficulty in satisfying the pass mark
requirements.[31]

While the government claimed that its Bantu Education system was a
positive step that increased the number of subsidised educational facilities
available for black children, thus increasing the overall number of black
students being educated in South Africa, the expansion of public schooling
was concentrated on the lower primary school level and produced a high
drop-out rate between primary and secondary school.[32] Very few pupils
reached Grade 12, the matriculation level. The statistics speak for themselves.
By 1969–70, whereas most white children would complete primary school
and about a quarter would go on to complete secondary school, about
70 per cent of African children would leave after four or less years of
schooling. Only about 4 per cent of African children reached secondary
school, and only 0.1 per cent completed the five years to successfully
matriculate.[33] Indian and coloured student figures lie in between these
extremes. During these years, it was found that 24.3 per cent of Indian
children were in high school and only 1.6 per cent in Grade 12. Around
11 per cent of coloured children were in high school and only 0.4 per cent in
Grade 12. Even fewer black school-leavers passed with high enough marks
for a Matriculation Exemption Certificate to enable them to apply to

universities, while even less achieved passes in the mandatory mathematics and science subjects to enter medical school.

In February 1959, Alan B. Taylor, who was a member of the medical school's selection committee, captured in a letter the story of one of the African applicants he interviewed. His life story touched Taylor deeply. It is quoted at length here to draw attention to the ordeal some students had to undergo to enable them to apply to study medicine in Durban:

> One feels very humble and ashamed after such interviews. Humble because one has accomplished so little with all of the advantages that one has had and ashamed that others have to struggle so hard for what should be every man's opportunity . . . [One] stor[y] stand[s] out. Mrs X had eight children. About the time the last was born her husband became an invalid from rheumatism. She carried on with her washing, supported her invalid and the children, inspired for at least some to go on to become teachers, a nurse and a prospective doctor. She must have given the latter real inspiration for he has really struggled to get thus far. For his junior high work he travelled twenty miles night and morning by bus to his high school from Alexandra Township. In the township he lived with an uncle under conditions not conductive to study, six families about a single small courtyard, noisy, crowded, unhygienic, lawless. His last two years were spent in a boarding school as a boarder, yet here when a teacher resigned and couldn't be replaced he was compelled to study by himself for his Matric exams. Yet he came through with a good second class pass and should get into medicine . . . A second class pass under the conditions which many have studied means a first class mind.[34]

Between 1960 and 1990, even after the expansion in the provision of ethnic or racial university facilities for black students, the number of students per 1 000 of the population who attended university was still fewer than three for Africans compared to over 30 for whites, although Africans constituted over 70 per cent of the total South African population.[35] These educational discriminations made advancement for most black students to the tertiary level an extremely difficult and unlikely possibility, and a great accomplishment achieved by only a tiny and determined few.

Although the negative effects of apartheid, and particularly the Bantu Education system, would have been felt by the 1960s by the admissions officers tasked with sorting through and granting admission to students at the Durban Medical School, the effects on later-created institutions were to be severe from the start. The Medical University of Southern Africa (MEDUNSA) was created as a segregated apartheid university in Ga-Rankuwa in the homeland territory of Bophuthatswana, some 35 kilometres north of Pretoria.[36] When it opened for classes in 1978, it offered courses that led to a variety of qualifications, such as doctors, dentists, veterinarians and nurses, as well as allied and paramedical workers. It was prepared, and indeed required, to lower its entrance qualifications to meet its mandate to train more African doctors to meet the growing shortage in the country.[37] This institution, which received much criticism in the media for promoting lower entrance requirements, did so to give opportunities to promising African students whose disadvantaged educational backgrounds would have disqualified them from admittance to other medical schools.[38] By providing many mentoring and remedial academic programmes, including extra training in maths and science subjects, and extending, where necessary, the time allotted to students to complete their degrees, many African medical students successfully graduated from 1982 onwards, with degrees fully recognised by the South African Medical and Dental Council.[39]

Furthermore, in addition to being subordinated in the racial and class hierarchy of apartheid South Africa, black students could also find themselves locked in the gender trap on the journey to medical school. Gender stereotyping remained 'deeply entrenched' during the apartheid years. Many girl children were expected to grow up to become homemakers, with their primary goals to become wives and mothers.[40] Girls could often encounter disapproval from family, neighbours or members of their communities if they tried to buck established societal norms. Fatima Mayet was one of the first women to attend and graduate from the Durban Medical School in the 1950s. She went on to specialise in internal medicine and became head of the Department of Medicine at R.K. Khan Hospital in the early 1970s. In 1999 she recollected how

> my family was ostracised because I was attending high school [and later when I applied to medical school] because girls, and particularly Muslim girls, didn't go to high school. They stopped after Standard 4 or 5 [Grade 6 or 7]. This is why my [older] sister was stopped from going to school and became a homemaker.[41]

111

This was the attitude shared by many Muslim and Hindu families, especially in the 1950s and 1960s. Another Indian doctor who trained in the 1960s and who wished to remain anonymous, said that members of her family expressed their disapproval by saying that 'medicine wasn't a good profession for a woman to go into'; that women should 'just stay at home' and not waste their time pursuing medicine as a career 'because it was very difficult for a woman to do'.[42]

Sociologist Cherryl Walker argues that during the apartheid period, many Indian South African women faced a great deal of subjugation. Generally, she said, 'both Hindu and Moslem religions sanctioned an extreme form of submission and passivity among women. Prejudice from within the Indian community against women participating in any form of activity outside the home was deeply rooted.'[43] Although attitudes to the education of young Indian girls would slowly change over time as industrialisation and urbanisation processes helped to loosen educational and work constraints on women, during the earlier apartheid years young Indian girls were not expected to remain at school beyond primary level. With the onset of puberty, it was felt that they should be cloistered in their family homes until marriage. Marriage and motherhood were viewed as their primary duties in life.[44]

Many of these patriarchal ideas were shared within African communities too. Nkosazana Dlamini Zuma, who studied in Durban in the early 1970s, but was forced to complete her degree in exile in Britain in the late 1970s, recalled with clarity her days of growing up in rural Zululand when a male community member actively tried to dissuade her father from allowing her to attend medical school in Durban. He argued that she would 'get married sooner [rather] than later' and then leave the medical profession, wasting what skills she had acquired.[45] However, it was not only African men who were discouraging of women's educational progress. Women also tried to dampen the educational and professional aspirations of other women. Mamphela Ramphele reminisced with frustration and some disbelief about a Mrs Jwili, the mother of a fellow student whom she met whilst waiting to catch a train to Durban to start medical school in January 1968:

> Mrs Jwili was clearly very proud of her son, who had earned a Masters degree from an American university after having completed his BSc at Fort Hare University in the Cape. She had misgivings about my intention of

being in the same class as her son and Khoadi Molaba, who also had a Fort Hare BSc. She mercilessly set out to whittle away any remnant of self-confidence I had. How could I, a female and lacking as well the head start of a degree which the other two possessed, hope to make my way at Medical School? Another vote of no confidence.[46]

As it turned out, her son did not make a success of his medical studies and was excluded in his third year.

Reinforcing these negative societal perspectives, educational disadvantages worked to restrict the number of girls who advanced to and then through secondary school. Black families were more likely to devote limited financial resources to educate their sons, as their sons, not their daughters, were viewed as the future breadwinners of families. Support for their careers was regarded as paramount.[47] Girl children were thus given greater domestic responsibilities in the home that distracted them from their studies. Moreover, for the tiny number of girls who actually reached secondary school, and in the few Bantu Education schools where maths and science subjects were even offered, teachers also worked to channel girls into what were considered more suitable 'feminine' subjects to prepare them for lives as housewives, or for less ambitious careers such as teaching, or more caring professions like nursing, which also provided students with a small income whilst they were training.[48] Recalling his matriculation class of 1968, Maila J. Matjila emphasised this point:

> T]here were few girls who . . . did science subjects. They were encouraged to do other subjects . . . [like] domestic science . . . In my . . . matric class, there were only two girls out of a class of 48, only two girls who did maths . . . In African communities . . . higher education for girls was not encouraged. Very few of them went [far and those who did] . . . went more into the nursing area . . . [or] into teaching; 'soft' jobs like those and not into the hard sciences.[49]

Gender discrimination worked as a real obstacle to black women's entry into the medical field. Career guidance was 'non-existent during our school days', according to Ramphele, and 'one's horizons were not widened beyond the known'.[50] There were also few positive role models for high school girls beyond the professions of teaching and nursing. Although women were not prevented from applying to South African medical schools on the basis of their gender, as their international counterparts had been – in fact, it can be argued that they benefited from the many earlier battles that women had fought to gain entry into overseas medical schools – cumulative racial, social and educational disadvantages worked to restrict the number of women who were sufficiently qualified to apply.[51] For those black men and women who were able to push their way through inequalities and discrimination to reach medical school, however, most came from families that would not have been able to afford the costs the long training would have entailed.

Financial obstacles

A large number of African students born in South Africa could not have realised their dreams of becoming doctors without the assistance of the government's bursary-loan scheme. Recognising that most applicants came from families who could not afford to pay the fees, as well as the need to train more African doctors to address the desperate shortage in the country, when the medical school opened in 1951, the state made available fifteen bursary-loans every year for selected candidates in each of the seven years of study to cover their academic and residence fees. These funding packages were awarded primarily to African students (usually those who had obtained the highest matriculation marks), and only occasionally were they awarded to needy Indian or coloured students when suitable African candidates were not available.[52]

During the 1950s, the bursary-loans given to students amounted to £150 per annum for the first two years and £200 per annum for each of the subsequent five years, resulting in the large total of £1 300 at the end of seven years for the average student.[53] However, while these grants – half of which was an outright bursary and half of which was a loan – assisted students to pay for their medical studies, they indebted them to the government. Students granted these bursary-loans had to agree to confine their work after graduating to 'non-European' patients exclusively, and to practise only in areas approved by the state where they would be 'in the service of the Government for a period . . . of at least one year for every 200 pounds allocated to the candidate'. Graduates who refused to enter government service were required to repay the entire amount once they completed their internship year, and with an additional 4 per cent interest.

The conditions attached to these bursary-loans formed an integral part of the apartheid state's separate-development plans. They worked to channel the economic advancement and social mobility aspirations of African professionals into state-sanctioned 'non-European' Group Areas and the Bantustans.[54] One African graduate aptly summarised the contentious political strings attached to accepting a state bursary-loan:

> [W]e were given bursaries that were government-sponsored, but they were government-sponsored in the sense that they served the policies of apartheid. So basically, when you finished, the government should decide where you must go and practise and they normally decided to send you where they thought you belonged ethnically. So as much as it helped you as a student, it helped you with a purpose that was directed towards the policy of the government.[55]

Comparatively, many MEDUNSA students who grew up in the latter years of apartheid would have faced similar financial hardships and would have relied on state bursary-loans that were made available to them as well. In 1982 F.P. Retief noted that 66 per cent of MEDUNSA's undergraduates received bursaries, with approximately 48.7 per cent sponsored by the state and 51.3 per cent by other funding raised by MEDUNSA and also through private individuals and institutions. Those students sponsored by state bursaries were also obligated to repay them by working for a fixed period in rural homeland areas where doctors were desperately needed.[56] Despite being aware of these conditions, however, many African students in Durban and Ga-Rankuwa did not have another choice if they wanted to advance their careers and were forced to accept the state's bursary-loan stipulations. In his 1969 Natal study, H.L. Watts found that '95% of our sample of Africans received this State Loan Bursary, while two-fifths of them relied on it entirely'.[57]

For students who did not qualify or who were not eligible for state bursary-loans (that is, most Indian and coloured students, but also some African students), the financial path was even less secure. Some students managed to obtain private scholarships which assisted them to pay for their studies.[58] For instance, Veronica Wilson's financial worries were alleviated by an unexpected benefactor who fortuitously came her way towards the end of her matriculation year:

> [W]e were in OK Bazaars [a supermarket] in Vereeniging . . . and one of the ladies that I met was a nurse and she told me about this Muslim man . . . [who] sponsored needy students. So my mother and I . . . [found him in] a very dark little shop . . . And then he asked me for my symbols and I gave him my symbols. And, you know, it was amazing. He said, 'The first thing that we need to do is to send the university a telegram and tell them you're coming.' So we got into his rickety van and we went to town, sent a telegram . . . And that's how I actually ended up [at medical school] . . . [T]his gentleman helped me first year and then second year, then occasionally [thereafter].[59]

Others sought the help of their families. While a few Indian students over the years could rely on money from their well-to-do families to pay for their studies, as observed earlier, many students who were not granted a state bursary-loan were burdened with 'serious financial worries'.[60] They often did not know where the money would come from to cover their annual expenses. As mentioned earlier, B.T. Naidoo, who lost his father during his second year at the medical school, put enormous financial strain on his mother and his older working siblings who were then required to 'pitch in' to get him through until he was later awarded a couple of small private scholarships.[61] Over the years, parents sacrificed much to give at least one of their children the chance to become professionals. Bank loans that had to be repaid were sometimes taken out by family members to help students meet their costs.[62] Some parents worked longer hours or extra jobs to help pay for their children's studies, hoping that their children would do better career-wise than they had themselves and that their efforts would help secure a higher standard of living for their children and their families. Watts found in his 1969 study that employed older siblings often helped subsidise the costs of their younger siblings.[63] One graduate remembered relying on regular 'pocket money' that was given to him from his older brothers who helped pay for his many sundry costs, such as transport, clothes, toiletries and stationery, which his state bursary-loan did not cover.[64]

Some students also worked over weekends and during holiday periods to help pay for their studies, as one highlighted in an interview in 2003: 'I always actually worked during the holidays, summer holidays, to actually supplement, in terms of buying clothes for myself and whatever small things I needed.'[65] Fatima Mayet, who trained in Durban during the 1950s, worked as an assistant in her father's general-dealer shop during weekends and holidays too.[66] Some students even worked for months, if not years, in either white-collar or manual-labour jobs to earn sufficient money to pay for their studies, before applying to study medicine. Medical historian Anne Digby highlights how one of UCT's early coloured medical graduates – Ralph Hendrickse – worked as a labourer on the docks in Simonstown before starting his medical courses in 1943.[67] A Durban graduate had a similar experience: 'I worked . . . in the Rosslyn industrial area next to Pretoria where I was doing menial [factory] jobs. But I was prepared to do that because I was determined that I wanted to come here [to Durban] . . . I had spent a year outside [working] after Matric.'[68]

Tellingly, Watts found that only two-thirds of the Africans surveyed, in contrast to four-fifths of Indians, went from high school straight to medical school. The average age of entering the medical school amongst the 1957-to-1970 black graduates surveyed was 23 years for Africans and 20 years for Indians. Watts argued that his African respondents' older age 'partly reflects some who worked before entering the medical school, but also reflects the older age of African matriculants, at least in part due to their culturally deprived home environments'.[69] Similarly, many of MEDUNSA's early students were 'very mature', as one professor remembered, with 'an average age of 28 years'.[70]

These figures also reflect students who had attended other universities, where they had taken courses or completed whole degrees prior to being accepted in Durban or Ga-Rankuwa, because they could not gain entrance to medical school on their first attempt.[71] A number of graduates over the years, including illustrious alumni, entered the Durban Medical School in this way. For example, Frank T. Mdlalose graduated from the Native College of Fort Hare with a BSc degree in 1952 before studying medicine at the University of Natal, while Mamphela Ramphele completed her pre-medical chemistry, physics, botany and zoology subjects at the University of the North in 1967 before proceeding the following year to Natal.[72] While for some, studying elsewhere before coming to Durban reflected a change in career choice, initial tertiary studies in these subjects enabled them to improve their chances of admission to medical school.

'Literally the brightest children did medicine': Student motivations

Despite the many difficulties that black students endured to reach the tertiary level, for the small number who did, there were a number of factors that motivated them to study medicine as a career. Many students who applied to Durban's Faculty of Medicine had been academic achievers at their local high schools. Malegapuru Makgoba, who trained in Durban between 1970 and 1976, later going on to specialise as a molecular immunologist at the University of Oxford, asserted this point strongly in his autobiography. Referring specifically to the excellent grades one of his colleagues at the medical school was renowned for, he wrote the following about his rural northern Transvaal high school experience:

> ... [T]he teachers were inspired and determined to make an African success out of the students [at his Hwiti High School] ... [They] were desperate to obtain first class passes that could compare Hwiti with Setotolwane (Dr Ramphele's school), Pax and Motse Maria. In fact Mamphela had set such high standards in the district [of Pietersburg], that she was the reference point for all aspiring bright students.[73]

Jerry Coovadia felt that often it was 'literally the brightest children [who] did medicine', while Maila J. Matjila said that his matriculation 'results were among the top . . . in the country in both maths and science', which inspired him to study medicine.[74] Some high performers also remembered that specific teachers were among those who encouraged them to opt for medicine as a career. Since there were far fewer professional career choices open to 'non-European' students in the apartheid era than there are today – with courses in architecture, dentistry, engineering and accountancy, for example, not even available for study in the 1950s and 1960s – medicine was one of the limited professional choices on offer.[75] Another African graduate said: 'Basically, it sort of felt like a given thing in that if one did well at school . . . you had A-grades in maths and [science], then everyone would say you must go to Wentworth [Durban] . . . because it was either become a doctor or a lawyer or a teacher or a nurse . . .'[76]

Studying medicine had significant social status implications. Medicine was one of the most difficult professions to gain entry into and was regarded within black communities as prestigious. The few black medical practitioners who actually succeeded were highly respected. The idea that doctors became powerful individuals with the training and intellect to make life-and-death decisions for their patients was essential, and even moved them to the peak of their communities' social hierarchies.[77] For example, doctors were accorded preferential treatment and even given places at the most important tables at community functions, such as weddings or meetings, with other highly respected community leaders. Bongiwe Bolani, a nurse who trained at King Edward VIII Hospital during the 1950s and became matron of McCord Hospital in the 1980s, recollected with clarity how African communities were proud of their African medical students and doctors. She also noted how 'they were watched very keenly by the communities'. People generally took a keen interest in their personal lives, often treating them like celebrities. 'I believe young people who saw them wanted to be like them,' Bolani remarked.[78]

A medical education also fostered the opportunity to escape the common fate of impoverishment facing most black South Africans. Although salaries paid to black doctors in public service were lower than those paid to whites, they were comparatively higher than the salaries earned by most black workers at the time.[79] Those choosing to enter private practice after graduating could earn a good living through patient fees, depending, of course, on the area in which they chose to start their businesses. This could provide greater financial security. This higher earning potential was attractive in a discriminatory context where the few class and social privileges that accompanied this rare professional achievement helped soften the harsh consequences of racial inequalities under apartheid. Max Price, a community health-trained doctor who studied with a handful of black students at Wits Medical School during the late 1970s, felt that many black students went into medicine

> to escape poverty or because they saw it as an opportunity to escape maybe their living environment . . . And for most students growing up in townships, the only big houses they would ever have seen in the townships were the ones belonging to doctors. So they would have identified that as a way out . . . And part of the evidence for that is that most of them went straight into private practice after qualifying.[80]

Bloke Modisane, an African journalist and writer who grew up in Sophiatown,[81] remembered how the 'bold and majestic' house of A.B.

119

Xuma, one of the first black doctors to practise in this area from the late 1920s,[82] had been a role model for him. Although Modisane did not become a doctor himself, as a child growing up he had aspired to become a doctor, which he described in his autobiography:

> Dr William Modisane, I love the sound of the title, the respectability and security it would have given our family and eased the handicap of being black in South Africa. Money and social position would have compensated for this, maybe even bought us acceptance; I was not particularly concerned with the groans of suffering humanity, was not dedicated to wiping out malnutrition, malaria, or dysentery, I had no pretensions to such a morality, I wanted solely, desperately . . . only to pull my family up from the mud level of black poverty.[83]

For many graduates, improving their social positions and enhancing the financial security of their families were essential motivators. K.P. Naidoo, a student at the time, who had returned to complete his studies after he had dropped out of the Durban Medical School in the 1980s, said that many of his fellow students gave everything they had to come to the medical school. They were driven by the desire to help their families once they graduated, but also wanted to gain more respect as professionals within apartheid South Africa:

> In your family, in your village, wherever you come from, everybody is so poor, you are now one of the masses, thousands, and there's nothing for you. There's only some hope in UNB [University of Natal Black Section] and there's [limited] . . . seats there. You must all try and get in . . . [as] you always have some better life as a professional. So all these people were clamouring for these pos[itions] to come in here. [And] they know they can go back and . . . share their wealth with their families, make it a better life for them.[84]

Although financial rewards and prestige certainly influenced some students' decisions to enter medicine as a career, others were inspired by altruistic motives. For many black South Africans born and brought up in the harsh apartheid conditions of the townships or rural reserves, the desire to serve their communities and help alleviate the suffering of those around them was strong.[85] Some were inspired by the specific and deep sadness caused by the loss of loved ones who had died prematurely from various illnesses. For instance, Maila J. Matjila's father died from pneumonia when he was ten years old and his mother died when he was seventeen from cardiac failure. Matjila said he felt 'cheated and robbed for losing my parents at a very early age and in fact there is something that hopefully I could do in response to help those who . . . needed me'.[86] Others were motivated by their broader concern with the lack of adequate health-care services in their own communities. For Breminand Maharaj, who completed his undergraduate degree in Durban in 1977, then worked his way up to become a professor and principal specialist in the Department of Clinical and Experimental Pharmacology, studying and then practising medicine gave him 'the greatest opportunities to influence people's lives . . . [and] to look after people. I've always wanted to look after people and I don't think you can get closer to a human being than as a doctor.'[87]

Having supportive family members was certainly an essential motivating factor too. Some students had family members, including parents or siblings who had trained and worked as doctors, who inspired them to study medicine. This was the case with Y.K. Seedat, who came from a family of doctors and himself went on to become a professor and head of medicine at the University of Natal from 1978 to 1994.[88] Soweto-born Diliza Mji had parents who were both trained as medical doctors and who encouraged him. He studied in Durban in the 1970s, becoming the SASO president from 1975 to 1976 and, more recently, ANC treasurer in KwaZulu-Natal.[89] Others had parents who were not doctors, but wanted the best for their children and supported their choices. Malegapuru Makgoba has also written extensively about being born into a family with educated parents who promoted professional ambitions in their children. In his autobiography he discusses at length the influential role played by his father, a schoolteacher and headmaster, as well as his mother, who was 'revered for her intelligence' but was forced to give up her studies after Standard 6 because of family responsibilities. For Makgoba, inspiration to become a doctor came from a unique blend of his parents' 'love of knowledge' and his experiences as a young shepherd tending goats and sheep whilst growing up on a rural farm:

> My father had a mini-zoo of birds and animals . . . [Observing] these provided the first lessons in science . . . Therefore, my foundation and orientation towards the sciences were well established in the village and

countryside where nature in its totality was a big laboratory . . . As a shepherd and through my father's influence, I fell in love with animals and the natural environment . . .[90]

Having a parent with unconventional views was essential as well. For example, in her autobiography Ramphele describes how both her maternal and paternal grandparents took enormous risks by parting with their 'traditional' lifestyles to become Christian evangelists within the Dutch Reformed Church. Her parents had also deviated from their generational counterparts by studying in mission schools to become primary school-teachers, which provided them with more open opinions about what their children could achieve.[91] Ramphele learnt much from her mother, whom she described as a woman who lived her life 'through a combination of creativity, hard work and courage in standing up for her rights'. Nkosazana Dlamini Zuma reiterated a similar point, highlighting the open-mindedness and courage of her father, qualities which enabled her to enter a career not usually considered appropriate for women:

> I was fortunate because my father had a very different view. He just said, 'All children are equal' and if there was anything to be discussed in the house we all took part . . . He got trained as a teacher . . . He wasn't very traditional though we lived in a rural area . . . My father's attitude was that he doesn't want to choose who he educates, but if he had to choose it would be the girls because in his experience the girls tend to be the ones who suffer most because they tend to remain in marriages because of financial dependence.[92]

Finally, possessing determination and a firm conviction in their individual abilities could do much to persuade hesitant parents to support their children's unusual career choices. This point was highlighted by Fatima Mayet. Speaking of her own experiences, she said:

> . . . we were four sisters and a brother . . . My brother was a teacher, the oldest was a sister, she had to go into the house, and do house duties. My parents realised that I was determined to go on, so I was allowed to matriculate and go ahead.[93]

Having a strong, independent and even defiant personality in a male-dominated society and profession was helpful too, as May Mashego remembered of Nkosazana Dlamini Zuma, one of her female role models:

> [She was] a person who had already proven herself . . . For you as a woman to ultimately get into medicine, you've done so well that you've left the fold of women . . . [S]o you're regarded as quite an exceptional woman . . . [They] would be so outspoken . . . were strong women . . . [and were] much more vociferous . . . [T]hey were the type of women who were not easily intimidated.[94]

Being your own boss in private practice brought greater freedom for black South Africans in apartheid South Africa, and the challenging and stimulating nature of medical work did much to encourage some students to study medicine as a career.[95] As Mamphela Ramphele argued strongly in her autobiography:

> The little I had heard about doctors suggested that medicine could offer me the greatest professional freedom and satisfaction. It was not the desire to serve which influenced my career choice, but the passion for freedom to be my own mistress in a society in which being black and a woman defined the boundaries within which one could legitimately operate.[96]

While not wanting to undermine the earnestness of graduates' altruistic explanations for entering medicine, one should consider other complexities surrounding the issue of motivations. Anne Digby paints a more complicated picture, and highlights two deep tensions in the motives driving these early physicians.[97] The first entailed the inherent tension these professionals faced between selflessly serving the health needs of 'their own people' versus pursuing profitable, private-practice careers. Digby found that given the financial hardships experienced by these individuals and their families to get them to and then through medical school, 'it was predictable to find that [both] profit as well as service figured largely in . . . [their] careers'. Secondly, she argued, we need to appreciate the 'multiple ambiguities involved in African professionalism', including the 'regulatory constraints' that the state placed upon black medical careers. Although many black doctors might have argued or implied that they had entered medicine to help serve the health needs of 'their own communities', this should be considered in the light of strong apartheid structural constraints that limited their choices, particularly where they could practise, which ultimately restricted their autonomy. For Digby, it is important to understand how working in impoverished black rural and urban communities was usually more a career necessity – regulated by a racially segregated and unequal health-care system in South Africa – than a strictly individual choice.

Most who applied to study medicine in Durban during the apartheid era really had no other choice. It was increasingly difficult to gain admission to the UCT and Wits medical schools during the 1950s, but especially after 1959, when the government passed the Extension of University Education Act, making it mandatory for black doctors to apply for ministerial permission. A good example of this is Fatima Mayet, who was born in Natal. Despite receiving a six-monthly, renewable permit to complete a Bachelor of Arts degree at Wits in Johannesburg in the late 1940s, her inter-provincial government permit was revoked in 1951 when she wanted to start studying for a medical degree. Like many other black students, she was forced to apply to the University of Natal in 1951:

> I was told by the government that there is a . . . medical school in my own province, and they refused to give me a permit . . . [O]nce the [Durban] Medical School opened I had no choice but to come here . . . I got exempted from the preliminary year . . . So I went into first-year medicine . . . in '52 . . . [But] I was very reluctant to come to this medical school because the perception was that it's going to be a 'tribal' medical school and we would be sort of second grade, with our qualifications not gaining any recognition.[98]

Although anxieties about the school's academic standards would decrease as the years went on and the school proved itself academically, for early generations the issue of education quality provided in this apartheid-created institution was a major concern. Consequently, while application in Durban was not a first choice for some students, it did provide an opportunity for many students who originated from Natal and who might not have been able to afford to travel elsewhere to study medicine.[99]

However, while a tiny numbers of Indian and coloured students did manage to obtain ministerial permission to study at Wits and UCT after 1959, for African students the situation was worse. The Extension of University Education Act eliminated the possibility of studying at Wits, which in the 1950s had been the only alternative to the University of Natal. As a result, apartheid laws determined where African students were allowed to study, and after 1959 until the late 1970s, when MEDUNSA was opened and Wits once again accepted token numbers of African students, the Durban Medical School was the only one that was available for Africans. As one graduate emphasised: '... it was not a matter of choice ... I mean, it was *the only* medical school that was open where blacks [Africans] could be admitted.'[100] May Mashego emphasised this point too:

> If you chose to do medicine, at that time the only medical school was in ... Natal ... And everybody knew that. So if you go and do medicine, your teachers would give you, 'This is the address'. So you write and apply. That was the only medical school for blacks ... so there was nothing like you had to go and think. There was no thinking. If you're going to do medicine, *this is the address.*[101]

The Natal Medical School was, however, not the most accessible geographically for many students, nor was it financially viable for others. The great geographical distances that potential students had to travel from their home province to Natal was a serious deterrent for many cash-strapped families.[102] One African graduate found himself in just such a situation, but managed to overcome his difficulties by receiving bursaries to cover his expenses. He summarised this problematic situation for many potential medical students: 'So medicine ... you could only do it at the medical school in Natal. I couldn't go to Wits although it was nearer my home, only about 200 kilometres, and I had to come 850 kilometres as an eighteen-year-old to come and study medicine.'[103] The only alternative was to make the ultra-long journey overseas to study medicine in the USA, the UK or India, for example, where the high costs and long-distance separation from their families were serious deterrents for most.

Of course, the initial motivations that drove individual students to enter medical school could also be re-prioritised, compromised or changed once he or she had reached medical school, based on interactions with different people and experiences they had there. They could also be altered at a later stage, after students had graduated and found themselves out working in black hospitals doing their internship training, or once they were out working in the public or private sector.

The personal stories captured in this chapter seem to paint a romanticised narrative of heroic struggle of young individuals and their families to overcome many obstacles thrown their way. While the quotations cited seem genuine and the historical circumstances suggest that the obstacles black students faced under apartheid were certainly significant, the fact that these narratives are structured in similar ways of triumph against adversity also shows how they have been crafted to fit within the broader struggle-against-apartheid narratives that have been keenly promoted by the ANC government in the post-apartheid period. Whether these constructions were done consciously or not, they do highlight the importance of the socio-historical rootedness of memories. They also speak to the importance of producing memories that are part of something bigger than an individual, which in turn gives deeper meaning and relevance to individual lives. Thus, settling on what probably amounted to a multifaceted amalgam of private and structural motivations is perhaps the safest bet when considering what inspired different black students to become doctors at Durban's Medical School during the apartheid years.

Furthermore, we should not forget that the passage of time could also have played havoc with individuals' memories, especially of those who had studied medicine over 40 or 50 years ago. Certainly, this does not in any way undermine the level of hardships some students experienced in getting to the medical school. However, we need to consider the ways in which nostalgia and distorted and selective memories can influence an individual's memorialisation of the past. Shifting priorities in the tellers' present, as well as the desire to tell audiences things they believe they want to hear, are imperative to understanding the narratives told about the experience of the past.

A careful analysis of different types of sources highlights the varied nature of students' experiences leading up to acceptance at the Durban Medical School. Many racial, financial and gendered difficulties influenced the journeys of different black students through primary and secondary school. The ability to reach the tertiary level was a rare accomplishment few achieved, while from this group only a tiny and determined minority made it into medical school. Numerous factors motivated different students to study medicine, which was considered an esteemed profession offering them social status and financial hope in a discriminatory apartheid context. While some of the students who arrived in Durban to study medicine were reluctant to be there, as the apartheid state removed their choice of institutions, others were delighted with the opportunity the medical school afforded them. For this latter group of students, it was better to have a segregated and geographically distanced training facility within which they could work to achieve their medical goals, than to have no institution available at all.

Having persevered and struggled for years to overcome the obstacles to reach medical school, however, the hardships in their quest to pursue their medical studies were only just beginning. A whole host of unequal and discriminatory experiences awaited them once they had reached the medical school in Durban. Furthermore, securing one of the limited places available at the school did not simply cause students' differences to vanish. It is to the complex positive and negative social and educational experiences of black students who successfully gained admission to this complex institution that the next chapters turn.

Notes

1. Interview with Veronica Wilson, Durban, 6 November 2003.
2. See graph in appendix showing Faculty of Medicine first-year registrations broken down by race.
3. In a study conducted of a random sample of 101 students (from a total of 413 students) registered in Durban in 1969, sociologist H.L. Watts found that one-third of the African students spoke Zulu as their mother tongue, and another third spoke Tswana, Tonga or Pedi. The rest spoke a mixture of other languages. He also found that 51 per cent of Indian students spoke English as their home language, followed by Gujerati (27 per cent). See H.L. Watts, 'Black doctors: An investigation into aspects of the training and career of students and graduates from the medical school of the University of Natal. Part I: The students' (Durban: University of Natal, Institute for Social Research, 1975), 5.
4. CC GP File 18, KCM 25863, Letter from H.S. van der Walt, Secretary for Education, Arts and Science to the High Commissioner of Southern Rhodesia, 5 November 1953; and John V.O. Reid, 'A study of second-year examinations', in *Medical Education in South Africa: Proceedings of the Conference on Medical Education held at the University of Natal, Durban in July 1964*, eds John V.O. Reid and Alexander J. Wilcot (Pietermaritzburg: University of Natal Press, 1965), 184.
5. These two sociological studies, which were led by H.L. Watts, were conducted by researchers at the University of Natal's Institute for Social Research. See note 3 above for more on the first study. Watts, 'Black doctors. Part I: The students', 4–5,

44. In 1970, the views of 80 African, Indian and coloured doctors who had graduated between 1957 and 1970 were surveyed. Africans made up 46 per cent of respondents. See H.L. Watts, 'Black doctors: An investigation into aspects of the training and career of students and graduates of the medical school of the University of Natal. Part II: The graduates' (Durban: University of Natal, Institute for Social Research, 1976), 4–5. The first study found that only one-fifth of Africans surveyed came from rural home backgrounds, while only one-tenth of Indians and coloureds came from rural homes.

6. See Watts, 'Black doctors. Part I: The students', 6, and Watts, 'Black doctors. Part II: The graduates', 5.

7. J.W. Macquarrie, 'The sociological background of the African university student', in *Medical Education in South Africa: Proceedings of the Conference on Medical Education held at the University of Natal, Durban in July 1964*, eds John V.O. Reid and Alexander J. Wilcot (Pietermaritzburg: Natal University Press, 1965), 226.

8. Wits SAHA South African Political Materials 1964–1990s, The Karis-Gerhart Collection, Part I: Interviews, Folder 23, Mji, Sikose (conducted by Victoria Butler, Lusaka, February 1988).

9. In his study of graduates, Watts found that two-thirds of respondents 'had a father who was a white-collar worker' and, in nearly all the cases, the mothers were either 'a housewife or a white-collar worker (usually a teacher or a nurse)'. Watts, 'Black doctors. Part II: The graduates', 5. Also see Watts, 'Black doctors. Part I: The students', 6–7.

10. CC MH Mouldy Box Scans, 56–63 Folder 2 Loose Papers[S], page 148, Letter from Dr A.B. Taylor 'To the Kids', 6 February 1959.

11. Leo Kuper, *An African Bourgeoisie: Race, Class, and Politics in South Africa* (New Haven, CT, and London: Yale University Press, 1965), 7.

12. Mamphela Ramphele, *Across Boundaries: The Journey of a South African Woman Leader* (New York: Feminist Press, 1995), 1.

13. In his studies, Watts found that two-thirds of Africans surveyed were from major Protestant denominations, one-eighth from the Roman Catholic Church, and one-tenth from other minor western religious sects. Only 8 per cent of the students had parents belonging to 'Bantu separatist churches'; 3 per cent stated that they had parents whose religion was 'traditional ancestor worship', and 2 per cent had parents who were said to be agnostic or atheistic. See Watts, 'Black doctors. Part I: The students', 5–6; and Watts, 'Black doctors. Part II: The graduates', 4.

14. Interviews with S.B. Pitsoe, Durban, 17 July 2003, and Veronica Wilson, Durban, 6 November 2003. Macquarrie, 'The sociological background of the African university student', 226.

15. Lindy Wilson, 'Bantu Stephen Biko: A Life', in *Bounds of Possibility: The Legacy of Steve Biko and Black Consciousness*, eds Barney Pityana, Mamphela Ramphele, Malusi Mpumlwana and Lindy Wilson (Cape Town, London and Atlantic Highlands, NJ: David Philip and Zed Books, 1991), 19.

16. Kuper, *An African Bourgeoisie*, 73–4.

17. Watts, 'Black doctors. Part I: The students', 5. For similar statistics amongst medical graduates studied in 1970, see Watts, 'Black doctors. Part II: The graduates', 4. Hindus (72 per cent), Muslims (19 per cent).

18. Interview with B.T. Naidoo, Durban, 15 September 2003.

19. Ramphele, *Across Boundaries*, 51. For more on her achievements, see http://www. whoswhosa.co.za/mamphela-ramphele-4739.

20. Interview with Maila J. Matjila, Durban, 11 July 2003. Also see Macquarrie, 'The sociological background of the African university student', 226.

21. J.H. Abramson, 'Natal medical students' attitudes to the social and preventive aspects of medicine', *South African Medical Journal* 35 (25 March 1961).

22. Steven D. Gish, *Alfred B. Xuma: African, American, South African* (London: Macmillan Press, 2000), 58–9.

23. Interview with Jerry Coovadia, Durban, 24 June 2003. For more on his achievements, see http://www.whoswhosa.co.za/jerry-coovadia-2890.

24. Frank Molteno, 'The historical foundations of the schooling of black South Africans', and Pam Christie and Colin Collins, 'Bantu education: Apartheid ideology and labour reproduction', both in *Apartheid and Education: The Education of Black South Africans*, ed. Peter Kallaway (Johannesburg: Ravan Press, 1984), 88, 94, 161–2, 171–3, 182; A.L. Behr, *New Perspectives in South African Education* (Durban: Butterworths, 1978), 205–39; and Muriel Horrell, *Bantu Education to 1968* (Johannesburg: South African Institute of Race Relations, 1968), 151.

25. See Phillip Tobias, 'Apartheid and medical education: The training of black doctors in South Africa', *The Leech* 60, no. 1 (March 1991), 97.

26. Macquarrie, 'The sociological background of the African university student', 226; Molteno, 'The historical foundations of the schooling of black South Africans'; and Christie and Collins, 'Bantu education: Apartheid ideology and labour reproduction', 89, 165, 178–9.

27. Tobias, 'Apartheid and medical education', 97; and I. Gordon, 'Experience in the establishment of a medical school for non-white undergraduate students in South Africa' in *Medical Education in South Africa: Proceedings of the Conference on Medical Education held at the University of Natal, Durban in July 1964*, eds J.V.O. Reid and A.J. Wilcot (Pietermaritzburg: University of Natal Press, 1965).

28. Interview with May Mashego, Durban, 7 October 2003.

29. Wits SAHA South African Political Materials 1964–1990s, The Karis-Gerhart Collection, Part I: Interviews, Folder 23, Mji, Diliza (conducted by Gail Gerhart, New York, 2 June 1987).

30. Molteno, 'The historical foundations of the schooling of black South Africans', 86; and Christie and Collins, 'Bantu education: Apartheid ideology and labour reproduction', 160.

31. W.R.G. Branford, 'Examination systems and selection: The experiences of the admissions committee of the Board of the Faculty of Medicine, University of Natal', and Macquarrie, 'The sociological background of the African university student', both in *Medical Education in South Africa*, 195–6 and 227.

32. Christie and Collins, 'Bantu education: Apartheid ideology and labour reproduction', 176–7.

33. Baruch Hirson, *Year of Fire, Year of Ash: The Soweto Revolt: Roots of a Revolution?* (London: Zed Press, 1979), 13, 60; and *South African Statistics*, 1972 (Pretoria: Department of Statistics, 1972), quoted in Peter Cooper, *The Need for Doctors in South Africa* (Cape Town: South African Medical Scholarships Trust, 1974), 3.

34. CC MH Mouldy Box Scans, 56–63 Folder 2 Loose Papers[S], page 150, Letter from Dr A.B. Taylor 'To the Kids', 13 February 1959.

35. John Dreijmanis, *The Role of the South African Government in Tertiary Education* (Johannesburg: South African Institute of Race Relations, 1988), 120–2; Cooper, *The Need for Doctors in South Africa*, 3; and Branford, 'Examination systems and selections', 195–6.

36. For more on MEDUNSA's history, see UWC MAC MEDUNSA, 1984, 'MEDUNSA – Where medical history is in the making', *Citizen*, 1 February 1978; F.P. Retief, 'The Medical University of Southern Africa after five years', *South African Medical Journal* (27 November 1982); and 'Medical varsity to train 200 black doctors', *Natal Witness* (17 October 1983).

37. During the 1980s onwards, a few white students were also accepted into various postgraduate programmes at MEDUNSA. See, for example, MA, MEDUNSA Annual Report, 1980, 11.

38. See, for example, UWC MAC MEDUNSA, 1984, 'Motlana hits at "bush medical school"', *Star* (8 October 1980) and Victor Mallet, 'Black medical school wins over skeptics', *Los Angeles Times* (25 November 1983).

39. MA *MEDUNSA Brief* (April/May 1984), 13, and Yearbook, 1994/95, 'MEDUNSA – the background', 11; UWC MAC MEDUNSA, 1989; 'Prof. rides the "white elephant" to glory', *Pace* (April 1988); and 'MEDUNSA has vital role in producing black doctors: Critics praise college "founded on apartheid"', *Star* (6 September 1988).

40. Ramphele, *Across Boundaries*, 43. Also see Belinda Bozzoli, 'Marxism, feminism and South African studies', *Journal of Southern African Studies* 9, no. 2 (April 1983); Cherryl Walker, ed., *Women and Gender in Southern Africa to 1945* (Cape Town: David Philip, 1990).

41. Interview with Fatima Mayet, Durban, 4 June 1999.

42. Interview with MA, Durban, 23 September 2003. For similar views, also see K. Goonam, *Coolie Doctor: An Autobiography* (Durban: Madiba Publications, 1991), 25. Some interviewees preferred not to have their names used.

43. Cherryl Walker, *Women and Resistance in South Africa* (London: Onyx Press, 1982), 106.

44. For more on the subject of Indian women and gender, also see, for example, Belinda Bozzoli, 'Marxism, feminism and South African studies'; Goonam, *Coolie Doctor*; and Thembisa Waetjen, 'Kitchen publics: *Indian Delights*, gender and culinary diaspora', *South African Historical Journal* 61, no. 3 (2009).

45. Wits SAHA, South African Political Materials 1964–1990s, The Karis-Gerhart Collection, Part I: Interviews, Folder 41, Zuma, Nkosazana Dlamini (conducted by Gail Gerhart in London, 3 July 1988), 16.
46. Ramphele, *Across Boundaries*, 51.
47. Rowena Martineau, 'Women and education in South Africa: Factors influencing women's educational progress and their entry into traditionally male-dominated fields', *The Journal of Negro Education* 66, no. 4 (Autumn, 1997).
48. For more on feminine career channelling for girls, see Shula Marks, *Divided Sisterhood: Race, Class and Gender in the South African Nursing Profession* (London: Macmillan Press and New York: St. Martin's Press, 1994); Ramphele, *Across Boundaries*, 43–4; and Catherine Burns, 'A man is a clumsy thing who does not know how to handle a sick person: Aspects of the history of masculinity and race in the shaping of male nursing in South Africa, 1900–50', *Journal of Southern African Studies* 24, no. 4 (December 1998).
49. Interview with Maila J. Matjila, Durban, 22 September 2003. He is currently a professor and head of the University of Pretoria Medical School.
50. Ramphele, *Across Boundaries*, 44.
51. Beryl Unterhalter, 'Discrimination against women in the South African medical profession', *Social Science and Medicine* 20 (1985); 'Shattering the male monopoly: The history and struggle of female doctors', *The Leech* 62, no. 3 (November 1993); Liz Walker, ' "Conservative pioneers": The formation of the South African Society of Medical Women', in *Social History of Medicine* 14, no. 3 (2001); and Liz Walker, 'The colour white: Racial and gendered closure in the South African medical profession', in *Ethnic and Racial Studies* 28, no. 2 (March 2005).
52. CC GP File 8 KCM 22571, 'Minutes of meeting of Acting Board of Faculty of Medicine held on 1 September, 1954'; CC MH Mouldy Box Scans, Family Letters 50–5, pages 56 and 288, Letters from Dr A.B. Taylor 'To the Kids', 30 January 1950 and 8 February 1955; and Edgar H. Brookes, *A History of the University of Natal* (Pietermaritzburg: University of Natal Press, 1966), 86.
53. CC GP File 21, KCM 25878, 'Summary of the conditions of the award of a bursary-loan offered by the Government of the Union of South Africa at the University of Natal'.
54. Saleem Badat, *Black Student Politics: Higher Education and Apartheid, from SASO to SANSCO, 1968–90* (New York and London: Routledge, 1999), 50–5, 63.
55. Interview with MM, Durban, 28 July 2003.
56. Retief, 'The Medical University of Southern Africa after five years', 844; UWC MAC MEDUNSA, 1984; Victor Mallet, 'Black medical school wins over skeptics', *Los Angeles Times* (25 November 1983); and 'MEDUNSA – former Verwoerdian project turned into a success', *Star* (26 April 1988).
57. Watts, 'Black doctors. Part I: The students', 11.
58. For example, May Mashego received an Anglo American scholarship. See Interview with May Mashego, Durban, 14 October 2003. Also see Ramphele, *Across Boundaries*, 52; and Interviews with M.B. Kistnasamy, Durban, 26 August 2003, and Breminand Maharaj, Durban, 10 June 2003.

59. Dr Wilson also managed to secure a Natal Provincial Administration (NPA) loan in her later years which she had to pay back. Interview with Veronica Wilson, Durban, 6 November 2003.

60. Watts, 'Black doctors. Part I: The students', 12; and Watts, 'Black doctors. Part II: The graduates', 18.

61. Interview with B.T. Naidoo, Durban, 15 September 2003.

62. Watts, 'Black doctors. Part I: The students', 40; B.T. Naidoo, 'The first twenty-five years', *Natal University News*, no. 2 (Autumn 1976), 9; and Interview with K.P. Naidoo, Durban, 4 June 2004.

63. Watts, 'Black doctors, Part I: The students', 6.

64. Interview with TM, Pretoria, 21 August 2003. Similar points were raised in Interviews with Maila J. Matjila, Durban, 11 July 2003, and B.T. Naidoo, Durban, 15 September 2003.

65. Interview with TM, Pretoria, 21 August 2003. Also see Watts, 'Black doctors. Part I: The students', 11.

66. Interview with Fatima Mayet, Durban, 4 June 1999.

67. Anne Digby, 'Early black doctors in South Africa', *Journal of African History*, 46, no. 3 (November 2005), 436.

68. Interview with Maila J. Matjila, Durban, 11 July 2003.

69. Watts, 'Black doctors. Part II: The graduates', 4.

70. Ina van der Linde, 'MEDUNSA at twenty', *South African Medical Journal*, December 1996, 1508. In MEDUNSA's annual report of 1984, it was reported that 51 per cent of its students were 25 years and older. See MA MEDUNSA Annual Report, 1984, 5.

71. Watts, 'Black doctors. Part I: The students', 38.

72. Wits SAHA South African Political Materials, 1964–1990s, The Karis-Gerhart Collection, Part I: Interviews, Folder 22, Mdlalose, Frank (conducted by TK, 24 May 1977); Frank T. Mdlalose, *My Life: The Autobiography of Dr Frank T. Mdlalose* (Wierda Park: Action Publishers, 2006), 33–42; and Ramphele, *Across Boundaries*, 46–8.

73. Malegapuru W. Makgoba, *Mokoko: The Makgoba Affair: A Reflection on Trans-formation* (Florida Hills, RSA: Vivlia Publishers, 1997), 29–31.

74. Interviews with Jerry Coovadia, Durban, 24 June 2003, and Maila J. Matjila, Durban, 11 July 2003.

75. Kuper, *An African Bourgeoisie*, 234. Also see CC MH Mouldy Box Scans, 56–63 Folder 2 Loose Papers[S], page 152, Letter from Dr A.B. Taylor 'To the Kids', 20 February 1959.

76. Interview with KM, Durban, 14 November 2003.

77. Kuper, *An African Bourgeoisie*, 122–5, 154, 244; Digby, 'Early black doctors', 436; Interviews with B.T. Naidoo, Durban, 15 September 2003, and May Mashego, Ashburton, 18 October 2003.

78. Interview with Bongiwe Bolani, Durban, 1 May 1999.

79. Kuper, *An African Bourgeoisie*, 7, 96, 239; and Watts, 'Black doctors. Part II: The graduates', 5.

80. Interview with Max Price, Johannesburg, 19 August 2003. Max Price is the current vice-chancellor and principal at UCT. Also see Interview with May Mashego, Durban, 7 October 2003 and Watts, 'Black doctors. Part I: The students', 9.

81. Then an African township just outside the city of Johannesburg.

82. In the 1940s, Xuma became president of the African National Congress (ANC).

83. Bloke Modisane, *Blame Me on History* (New York and London: Simon & Schuster, 1986), 33–4.

84. Interview with K.P. Naidoo, Durban, 4 June 2004.

85. Watts found that 22 per cent of Africans, 32 per cent of Indians and 40 per cent of coloureds surveyed mentioned the opportunity to serve others as a primary reason for studying medicine. Watts, 'Black doctors. Part I: The students', 9. Also see Raymond Tunmer, 'Vocational aspirations of African high-school pupils', in *Student Perspectives on South Africa*, eds Hendrik W. van der Merwe and David Welsh (Cape Town: David Philip, 1972), 146–9.

86. Interview with Maila J. Matjila, Durban, 11 July 2003.

87. Interview with Breminand Maharaj, Durban, 10 June 2003.

88. Interview with Y.K. Seedat, Durban, 7 July 2003; Y.K. Seedat Curriculum Vita, http://www.hospice.co.za/site/files/5600/CURRICULUM%20VITAE%201%20 pageProf%20Seedat.doc and Watts, 'Black doctors. Part II: The graduates', 9.

89. Wits SAHA South African Political Materials 1964–1990s, The Karis-Gerhart Collection, Part I: Interviews, Folder 23, Mji, Diliza (conducted by Gail Gerhart, New York, 2 June 1987) and Mji, Sikose (conducted by Victoria Butler, Lusaka, February 1988).

90. Makgoba, *Mokoko*, 14–5.

91. Ramphele, *Across Boundaries*, 12–4.

92. Wits SAHA South African Political Materials 1964–1990s, The Karis-Gerhart Collection, Part I: Interviews, Folder 41, Zuma, Nkosazana Dlamini (conducted by Gail Gerhart in London, 3 July 1988), 16.

93. Interview with Fatima Mayet, Durban, 4 June 1999.

94. Interview with May Mashego, Durban, 7 October 2003.

95. Watts, 'Black doctors. Part I: The students', 9–10.

96. Ramphele, *Across Boundaries*, 44. Also see pages 72–3, 181.

97. Digby, 'Early black doctors in South Africa', 446–7.

98. Interview with Fatima Mayet, Durban, 4 June 1999. Jerry Coovadia was also denied a study permit to go to UCT Medical School where he had been accepted during the 1950s. Interview with Jerry Coovadia, Durban, 24 June 2003.

99. Interviews with Soromini Kallichurum, Durban, 29 May 1999; M.B. Kistnasamy, Durban, 26 August 2003; and B.T. Naidoo, Durban, 15 September 2003.

100. Interview with Maila J. Matjila, Durban, 11 July 2003. Interviewee's emphasis.

101. Interview with May Mashego, Durban, 7 October 2003. Interviewee's emphasis.

102. Tobias, 'Apartheid and medical education', 96.

103. Interview with MM, Durban, 28 July 2003.

CHAPTER 4

Alan Taylor Residence and the challenges of studying medicine in Durban

'Medical school was a culture shock.'

— B.T. Naidoo

From 1951 onwards, some of the brightest African, Indian and coloured students travelled from across the country to study in Durban for their medical degrees. However, the institution at which they were enrolled, for which they and their families had sacrificed so much, would prove to be a setting full of contradiction and ambiguities. While the Durban Medical School offered its students the rare chance to enter one of the most sought-after, prestigious and highly paid professions in apartheid South Africa, its anomalous set-up as a black faculty within the white University of Natal forced its students to suffer many racial discriminations and inequalities. Coming from diverse family backgrounds had a significant influence on different students' experiences and helps to explain some of the tensions that arose in the student body. While some experiences on the medical school campus were positive and reaffirming, others were deeply hurtful as a result of racial oppression and humiliations that students were forced to endure on a daily basis. And, by the late 1960s, these difficulties would lead to the political radicalisation and mobilisation of many students in their attempt to improve the situation.

From its inception, and owing to the Natal medical faculty's close working relationship with the state, the medical school was caught up in and perpetuated many racially discriminatory and segregationist ideologies and practices. The campus was created a couple of kilometres distant from the university's main Howard College campus, out of sight and out of mind of white students registered at the University of Natal.[1] In a 50th anniversary celebration speech given in 2000, Soromini Kallichurum, who was part of the first graduating cohort of students in 1957 and at the end of 1983 became the first black dean of the medical school, recalled her experiences of studying on a segregated campus: 'We were told as soon as we began our academic studies that Howard College campus, with all its faculties, academic and sporting, was out of bounds for us. It is understandable therefore that we did not identify with the university with whom we were registered.'[2] Black medical students were even forbidden from wearing the university's colours and blazers, to prevent easy identification with their white counterparts.[3] Most medical graduates had never set foot upon the main campus and had no contact with their white contemporaries, despite spending many years studying at the same institution.

Another doctor, who was a lecturer and later a professor and head of the Department of Medicine in the late 1970s through to 1994, argued that 'many whites in Durban didn't even know of the existence of the medical school . . . [although] it was very well known in the black community . . . So we were living in different worlds.'[4] Zweli Mkhize, who completed his medical studies in Durban in 1982, also remembered the deep sense of separation students felt by the segregated and inferior residential arrangements they were forced to endure at their black residence. For him, the medical school was 'a school within a school'.[5] Although as registered students they were officially part of the University of Natal, they never felt they belonged at this institution. Instead, he argued, they felt 'separated, isolated, hidden away in the black students' residence, a third-world ghetto, which is part of the first world, [the] main white campus, miles away, with different staff, different students, [and] a different culture'. In addition to feeling almost like pariahs within the University of Natal, many other hardships came to define medical students' experiences in Durban.

'This could not be my "dream Wentworth"!': The Alan Taylor Residence

The creation of the university's 'non-European' residence proved controversial from the start. Although the University of Natal received permission to build its medical school on Umbilo Road – an area that had been zoned a white residential area in the early 1950s – so that it could stand adjacent to its King Edward VIII teaching hospital, this was achieved only after heated opposition was raised by many 'race conscious' members of the Durban City Council.[6] During one of the debates, E.G. Malherbe, the principal of the University of Natal at the time, remembered how a council member had stood up and called on him to 'promise to build a 10 ft wall on the pavement of Umbilo Road to shut off the medical school should it be built there'.[7] Eventually, persistent lobbying secured approval for this site, but the university was prevented from building its students' residence on land in the same area.[8] This was forbidden by the Durban City Council, acting in accordance with apartheid Group Areas Act residential zoning laws. While it was prepared to let black students study in a white area, it was not prepared to allow them to live there.

Instead, and after much negotiation, the state made available to the university on long-term lease a Second World War-era military barracks in the suburb of Wentworth, about ten kilometres away from the Umbilo Road school buildings and about fifteen kilometres from central Durban.[9] It cost the university R46 000 to adapt the buildings for its residential and academic purposes. In addition to providing accommodation for its black students, sections of the complex were also used for many years as classroom facilities to provide space for the school's premedical (preliminary and also first-year) training.[10] Situated in a location many kilometres south of Durban, the residence represented an ambiguous space, as one African doctor recalled: '[The] residence was a special zone . . . it was in an odd area too. It was in an industrial area [near to a] coloured residen[tial area], and as Africans we should not have been there according to apartheid laws. Even Indians shouldn't have been there. So I'm saying it was a special zone in that sense.'[11]

The residence was named after Alan B. Taylor – McCord Hospital's medical superintendent who had lobbied so hard during the 1940s to open a medical school in Durban, and the school's first acting dean. The Alan Taylor Residence (ATR), however, did not live up to the high ideals of its namesake. Instead, it proved inferior and inadequate from the start. And, problems extended well beyond the complaints about poor food quality in university residences.[12] Koleka Mlisana, a specialist microbiologist by training, who came to study in Durban from her hometown in the Transkei in the early 1980s, remembered how the high expectations she had of her new residence in Wentworth were dashed when she first set eyes on its buildings:

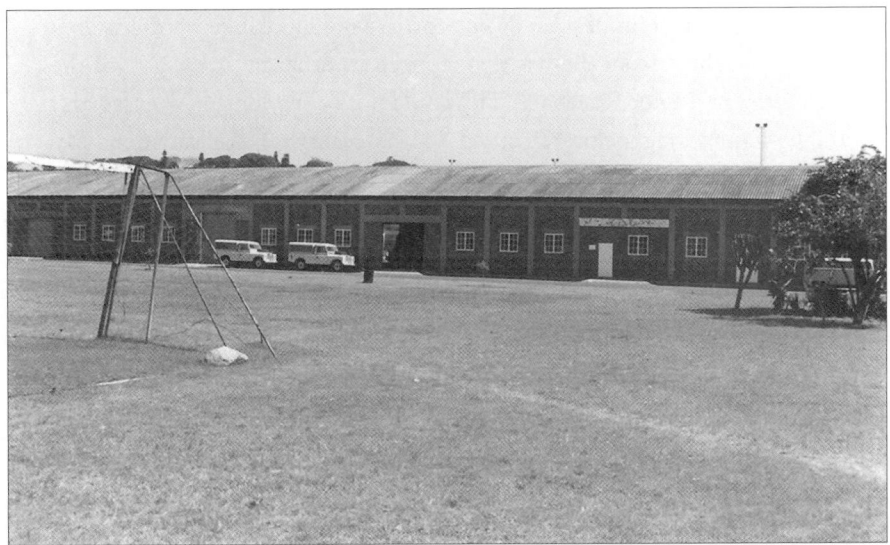

Photo 4.1 Wentworth Medical School, April 1978. (*UKZN Archives*)

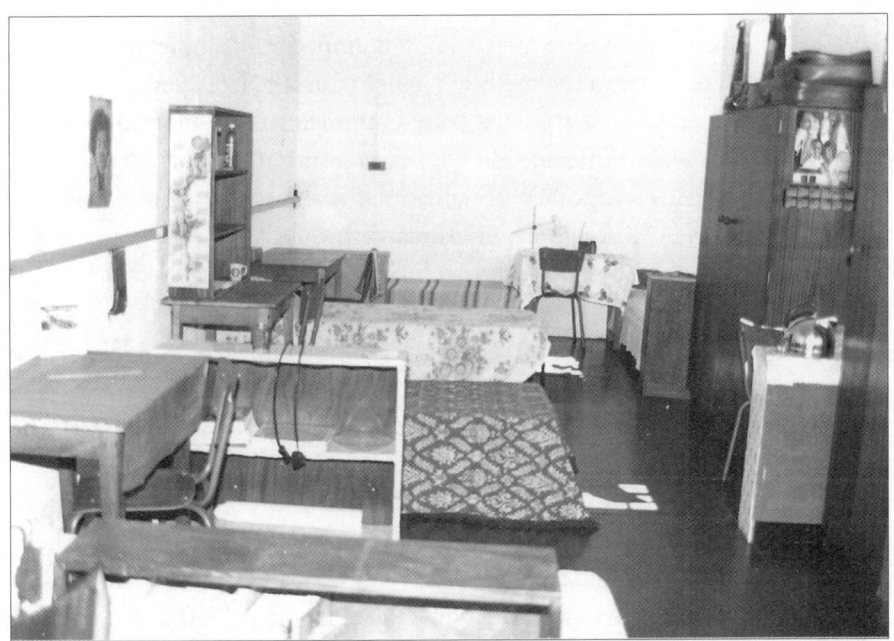

Photo 4.2 A cramped dormitory room at ATR. (*UKZN Archives*)

> My rich imaginations of what 'Wentworth' would look like were shattered before I alighted from the bus that stopped to drop me at the gate of the shabby Alan Taylor Residence. This could not be my 'dream Wentworth'! . . . It wasn't long before I settled to the reality of the situation. My country town high school dormitory was not too bad compared with [this place].[13]

The barracks-like, simple, brick, dormitory structures had asbestos roofs and cement floors, making them hot in summer and cold in winter, and communal bathrooms which lacked privacy.[14] B.T. Naidoo also described in detail the inadequate conditions at the residence, including the small size of the rooms:

> Our accommodation consisted of three blocks with dormitories housing three to seven students in each . . . Each of the rooms had . . . beds with an equivalent number of tables and chairs and single-door cupboards which housed all our possessions, including our books. It was difficult for more than one person to dress at a time.[15]

This accommodation became increasingly cramped and subdivided as more students were admitted to the medical faculty from the late 1960s onwards.[16] For example, in 1969 four students were crammed into double rooms, and bunk beds were placed in common rooms to house more students. During the 1970s and 1980s temporary prefabricated structures were also built on the ATR premises. Although negotiations with the state were started in the early 1980s to enable the university to build a new and larger residence for its medical students, the new residence (named the Albert Luthuli Hall), which eventually did come to fruition, was only opened in 1990 in the transition period leading up to the democratic elections.

What made matters more uncomfortable for the students was the pollution they experienced at this site. This was caused by ATR's nearest neighbours, the Standard Vacuum (later known as Mobil and then Engen) Oil Refinery, and later the Durban airport. A lecturer remembered how 'planes came over the huts to land on the runway and the oil refinery was belching out fumes all day and night'.[17] During the 1950s, the medical school's newsletter, *The Amoeba*, published a series of complaints by students

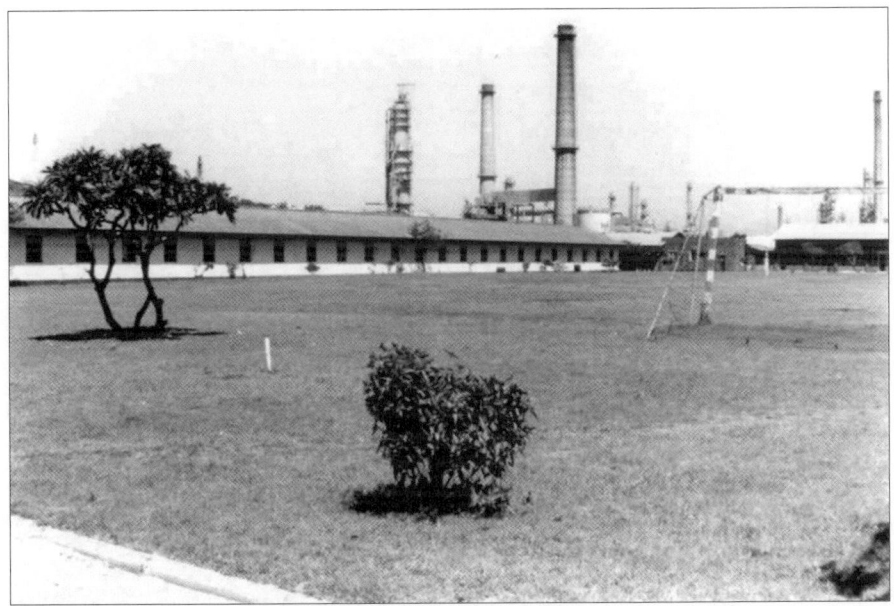

Photo 4.3   Soccer field at ATR, with oil refinery smoke stacks nearby. (*UKZN Archives*)

about the refinery, dealing particularly with the issue of noise pollution. One student wrote with frustration about the great mental strain residence students had to endure as they were required to put up with the constant and monotonous 'hum drum' from the oil refinery.[18]

Two doctors, thinking back on their experiences at ATR, also highlighted the polluted conditions students had to tolerate during the 1960s through the 1980s: 'The conditions were actually horrible . . . There was a huge, stinky oil refinery next door and the fumes were always suffocating us, especially in the afternoon.' 'The level of pollution from the oil refinery was such that one could see traces of soot when one blew one's nose, and the bed-linen would be covered with a black layer of dust if one left a window open on a windy day.'[19] It was even argued that the location of ATR was so bad that not only did it compromise students' health, causing headaches, asthma and nausea, but emissions from the refinery also interfered with the laboratory apparatus housed there for teaching purposes, causing rubber and fabrics to perish through prolonged exposure.[20]

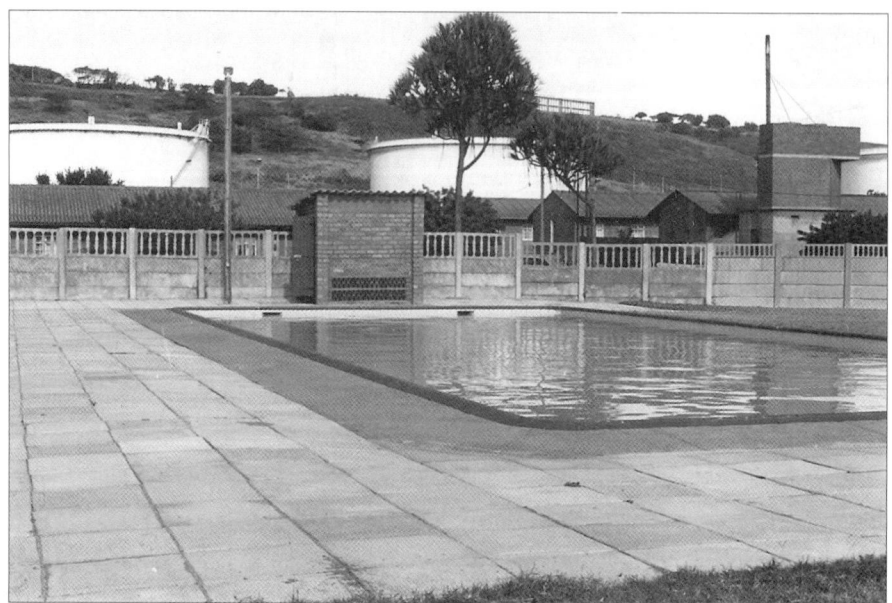

Photo 4.4   ATR swimming pool with oil refinery tanks in the background. (*UKZN Archives*)

Transport proved a major problem too for students living at ATR. Until the 1980s, when the University of Natal arranged free bus transportation for medical students between the residence and Umbilo Road, those staying at ATR had to find their own way to cover the approximately ten kilometres to and from the medical school. For most students, this was 'a daily affair at our own cost'.[21] Although municipal and private bus company services – which transported black residents living in the Durban south area to and from the CBD for work purposes – were available for use by students, many could not afford the additional transport costs. Limited financial resources were a serious problem for some students, as Hugh Philpott, who became the head of the Department of Obstetrics and Gynaecology in the 1970s, and later dean of the medical school in the early 1980s, recalled:

> We used to get students who had been doing well and then suddenly the marks came down. And then we tried to find out what's going wrong here. And we found out the student eats once every three days, saved their

money to pay for the bus from Alan Taylor Residence up to the medical school, things like that.[22]

Poorly maintained municipal and private bus services also meant passengers had to contend with regular breakdowns. Competition with neighbouring black residents for limited seats on segregated buses was another problem, while students often watched in frustration as empty buses reserved for whites passed them by:

> [S]ometimes what used to be very, very frustrating is that in the mornings, you're rushing to come to . . . medical school . . . and the non-white buses would be full with all the people from Wentworth going to work and you'll find . . . this [white] bus going past with maybe one white passenger, or sometimes it would be absolutely empty.[23]

A lucky few had bicycles or motorbikes to ride to and from the medical school, but over the years many were forced to walk the distance to get to their classes.[24]

For students who set out on foot in the early mornings and after finishing classes in the evenings, safety proved a great concern as well. Students waiting on the side of the road for buses were at greater risk for attacks. The Austerville area in Wentworth was notorious for being a 'rough' and violent place with high levels of crime. In this environment, 'gangsters' and 'thugs' used to patrol the streets to harass and steal from easy targets, including students.[25] In addition, over the years, many ATR students felt cut off from friends and family living in township areas around Durban because of the remote location of their residence. Travel for entertainment or recreational purposes, including watching movies in town, going to the beach or visiting friends and relatives, was an expensive and difficult endeavour.[26] African students also had the extra burden of worrying about the consequences of violating apartheid curfew laws, which restricted the movement of Africans on Durban streets after 9:00pm at night.[27] Furthermore, African students had to carry passes to explain their presence in the Durban area if stopped by the police. Police harassment and arrest was a constant threat for these students. In an interview in September 2003, B.T. Naidoo told me about the stressful and embarrassing experiences that some of his African friends had to endure on a regular basis:

You know, we used to go to the . . . movies with our black [African] friends [in Durban], and we used to take the bus to [get back to] Jacobs [an area near Wentworth] and walk up the hill, and if it was past 9 o'clock, these guys would hide behind the trees when they saw a car coming and you wondered why it was . . . And they'd say, 'This is . . . curfew.' And the guys would be picked up . . . if they caught them . . . and spend the night in jail.[28]

Another concern stemmed from the many wasted hours spent commuting. While this was raised as an issue by students staying at ATR,[29] the situation was even worse for those students who lived off-campus in distant townships. According to H.L. Watts's 1969 study of registered medical students studying in Durban, about two-fifths lived off-campus.[30] Of this figure, about two-thirds were Indian students, as many either came from or stayed with family members who lived in the Durban area. Fatima Mayet provides a good example of this. Whilst studying at the school during the 1950s, she lived off-campus and commuted long distances daily to and from the medical school and her family's home in an Indian-zoned residential area:

[We] had to catch a bus all the way in . . . it was restrictive because by the time we got home, and the time at which you had to leave [in the morning] to go . . . wasn't easy. And if you finished work . . . [and left the school] late, the buses were full already when we had to go home . . . so we had to stand in queues in order to catch your buses and by the time we got home it was dark.[31]

In addition to wasted time that could have been used for study, many students living off-campus in family homes also endured the hardships of township life. For some, this included cramped and noisy living situations, and inadequate study conditions created by poor lighting. Many students were required to help out with domestic responsibilities, which reduced their study time.[32]

These conditions were similar to those experienced by the small numbers of black students who studied at Wits and UCT. These students were forced to make their own arrangements as accommodation and transport were not provided for them in what were classified as white residential areas.[33] Conditions of hardship emerged in submissions made by black doctors to the hearings of the Wits Health Sciences' Internal Reconciliation Commission in 1998. Many submissions recounted the racially discriminatory experiences the students had had at Wits. Some discussed the cramped, noisy and poorly serviced housing conditions they had to live with in the townships, as well as the enormous expense and wasted time they were forced to endure in travelling between the university and their township homes.[34]

When considering what life would have been like for black students living at ATR and in family homes in Durban and elsewhere, it is also vital to highlight one further issue. These students were not protected from the daily experience of petty racial discrimination experienced by all black South Africans.[35] For example, they experienced many restrictions on what municipal amenities they could use, such as public toilets, as well as what facilities they could dine in or socialise in, not to mention where they could shop.[36] The frustration of living as a second-class citizen was still clearly remembered by an African graduate who studied in Durban during the early 1980s. She recalled the embarrassment she and her partner experienced when he tried to take her out on a date for a meal at a restaurant:

I remember one time, you know, when [I was] going out with my husband we went to this . . . restaurant over there at the beachfront and, shame, he was taking me out and he wanted to buy me [something] . . . and this one day that we came there they told us, 'No, [you] can't sit down. If you want to buy anything then you must order takeaway' . . . So we left.[37]

Hardships were not limited to Africans. B.T. Naidoo poignantly summed up his difficulties as an Indian student and later doctor in apartheid South Africa, and the restrictions he endured:

[W]hen you take your child into town and she wants to sit on . . . a park bench, and you say, 'No, you can't' . . . [i]t hits you hard, it hurts you. It cost you no money to sit on a bench but you were not allowed to. Or if you had to use the toilet urgently, you had to walk . . . yards to find it, you know, whilst there are toilets right there saying 'Whites Only'. Or . . . if you go to a post office . . . [the] white side of the counter used to be empty, and here you stood in queues that went into the road and the guy who was serving at that [white] counter wouldn't [serve you] . . . [T]hose were the sort of things that really hurt you . . . being a professional.[38]

Being a designated 'non-white' person in apartheid South Africa was often a humiliating and degrading experience. As students, these graduates recall not being spared, despite studying medicine at university and aiming to enter one of the most prestigious professions. May Mashego, whose testimony was touched on in chapter 3, captured this situation powerfully:

> [I]n the black community to be a doctor [resulted in] . . . a high status . . . But within the white communities, I think for a white person black was black, okay. It didn't matter . . . I mean, it didn't matter that you [were] a black doctor. It didn't mean that your doors will be open[ed] . . . Where it [was] written 'non-white', it was 'non-white' . . . [T]he laws affect[ed] you like they affect[ed] everybody else, which is why I think the more you are educated, the more you feel the pinch . . . [Y]ou remained a black person . . . [and] you still got the hit of the fact that you were black.[39]

These memories of studying and living at ATR provide valuable information on the challenges students faced whilst training in Durban. However, as highlighted in chapter 3, these memories also point to the common narratives constructed by alumni to make sense of their lives. They serve as a way to assign meaning to hardships experienced both in the past and today. They help validate difficult, apartheid-era experiences that are often brushed aside by the powers that be. Moreover, the construction of individual memories in line with common 'triumph-in-adversity' narratives in the post-apartheid period serve to alert audiences to black doctors' hardships and successes within the larger and triumphant struggle of black South Africans against their apartheid oppressors.

Nevertheless, while they may be insightful, common triumphalist memory narratives also hide a great deal. During the apartheid era, students' experiences were not easily generalisable. They were complicated by diverse race, ethnic, class and gender differences. Simply focusing on the heroic and celebratory narratives, which dovetail so well with the grand narratives of struggle prevalent in post-apartheid South Africa, hides the enormous complexity of the medical school's history. It also clouds an understanding of the rich diversity of experiences and interactions that occurred amongst its students who lived through this very difficult historical period.

Students' interactions

Despite offering its students inferior and geographically distant facilities, ATR was a unique space for black students living in apartheid South Africa. Unlike racial zoning laws that worked to separate different race groups from living and studying together in other parts of the country, the University of Natal's ATR anomalously brought together African, Indian and coloured students, as well as men and women, in the same residence. For many students, their acceptance into Durban's medical faculty was their first opportunity to study with students from different social, cultural and educational backgrounds. This situation allowed some students to bond across state-designated racial groupings, as well as class and gender lines, and laid the foundations for some genuine and enduring friendships.[40] This had significant implications for student anti-apartheid political mobilisations, as we shall see in later chapters.

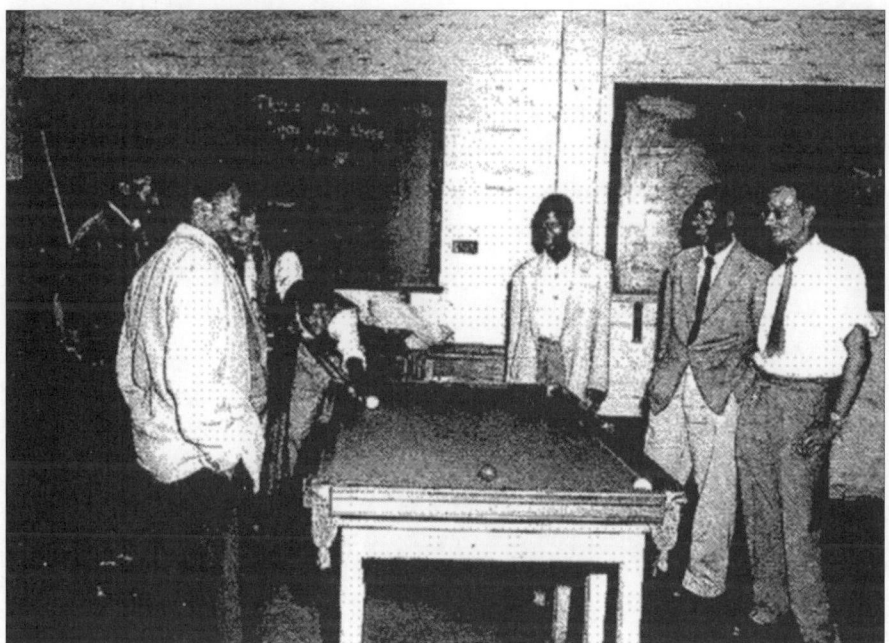

Photo 4.5 Medical students playing pool at ATR. (*UKZN Archives*)

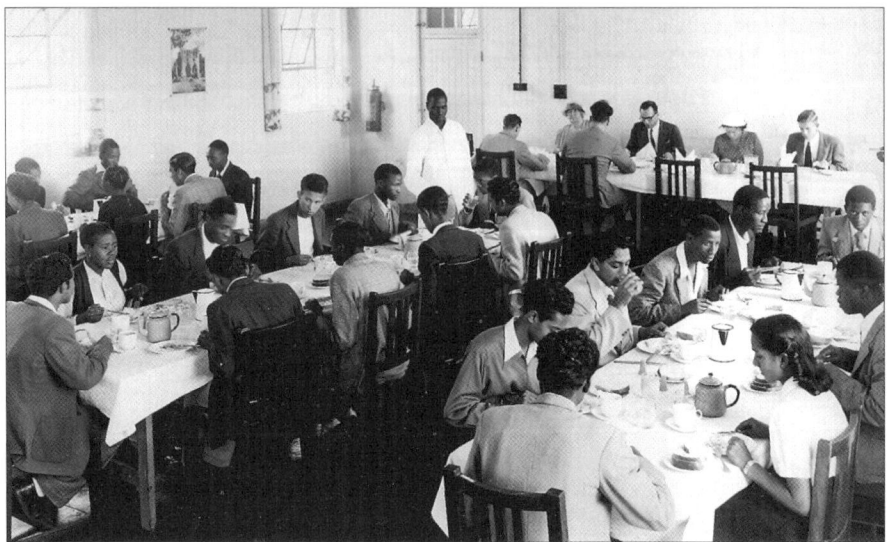

Photo 4.6   Non-European dining hall in the 1950s. (*UKZN Archives*)

This was not the only outcome of these interactions, however. Being at ATR was a situation that caused stress for many students, especially those who came from other provinces, and for those whose lives had not brought them into much contact or meaningful interaction with people of other racial or ethnic groups. Two graduates, one African and the other of Indian descent, summed up the difficulties some students experienced when they came to study in Durban:

> As a first-year student from the rural Transkei . . . it's your first time in the university, in a big city, and you go to your first class . . . [and] it's this huge class, with Indians. You've never had, you know, Indians and coloureds [in your classes before]. You've never associated with them.

> [W]hen you came into the university medical school it was a culture shock really . . . because you never mixed with . . . [Africans] or coloureds . . . And when you came together, you know, you suddenly realised there was this . . . big group of black people, you know . . . I mean, until then I was

leading a fairly sheltered life . . . you went to your own schools, we took our own buses and we lived in our [own] areas.[41]

Bringing students of different backgrounds to live and study together produced difficulties and also tensions within the student body, sometimes flaring up around issues as diverse as food preferences, different religious backgrounds, cultural practices and languages. A number of graduates, when reflecting on their student days, maintained:

> [T]here was very little social contact between Indian and African students
> . . . As a group, I think we sort of fairly kept to each other, you know, kept
> apart. I don't think there were many Africans that had close Indian . . . or
> coloured friends . . . I think it was institutionalised in terms of our upbringing
> . . . [S]o, you know, everybody sort of tended to keep to themselves.[42]

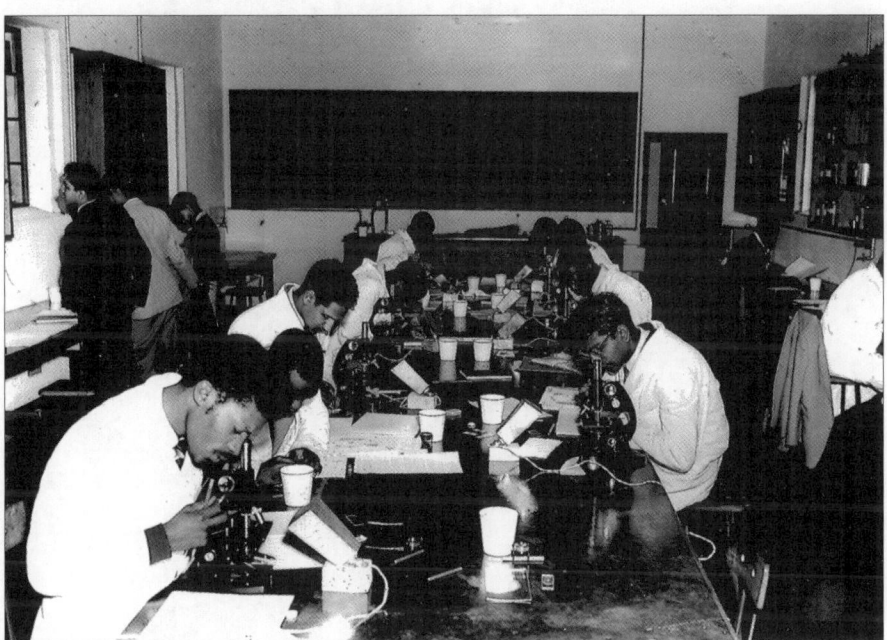

Photo 4.7 Students at work in the physics laboratory during their pre-medical training at Wentworth, 1952. (*UKZN Medical School Archives*)

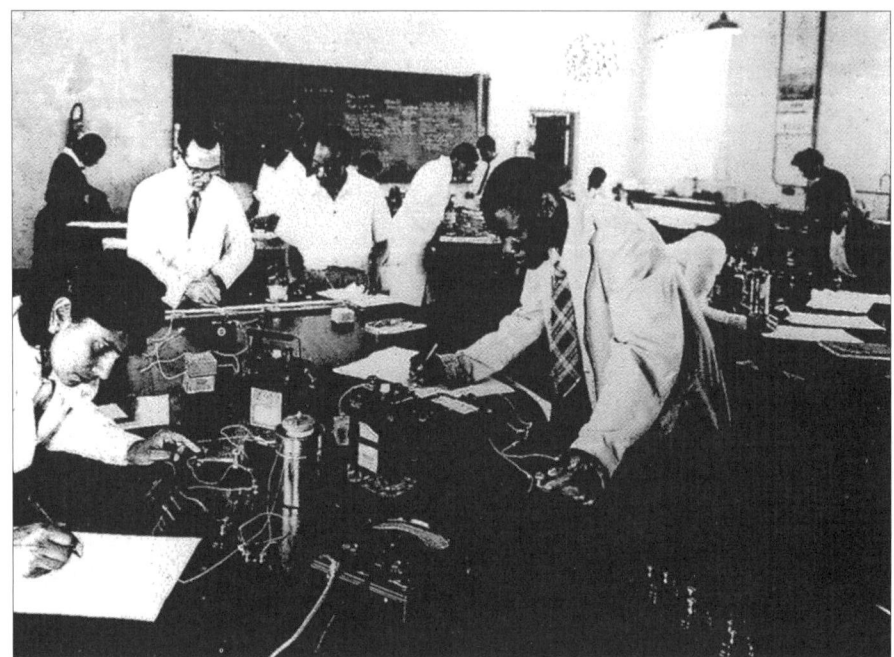

Photo 4.8   Physics lecture, first-year students, 1951. (*UKZN Medical School Archives*)

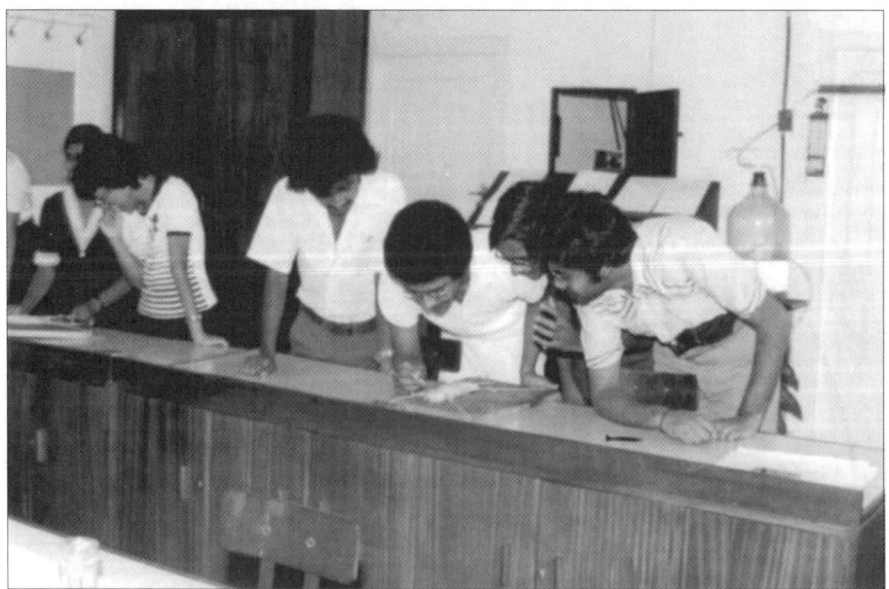

Photo 4.9   Dissecting mice, Wentworth Medical School, April 1978. (*UKZN Archives*)

Watts's two sociological studies of students in the 1950s and 1960s found that many students from different racial backgrounds did not mix easily, that friendships often occurred along 'group lines', and that friction or apathy between students from these different groups was common.[43] Although this was not necessarily the 'truth' or everyone's experience, many students could not forget where they had originally come from, or the difficulties they had encountered getting to the medical school. Unequal racial privileges, an outcome of the apartheid state's 'divide-and-rule' political strategies, were crucial here. If, for example, some socio-economic privileges – such as slight educational advantages – were given to Indian and coloured minority groups with the aim of dividing them from the African majority, this led to the production of tensions amongst students.[44]

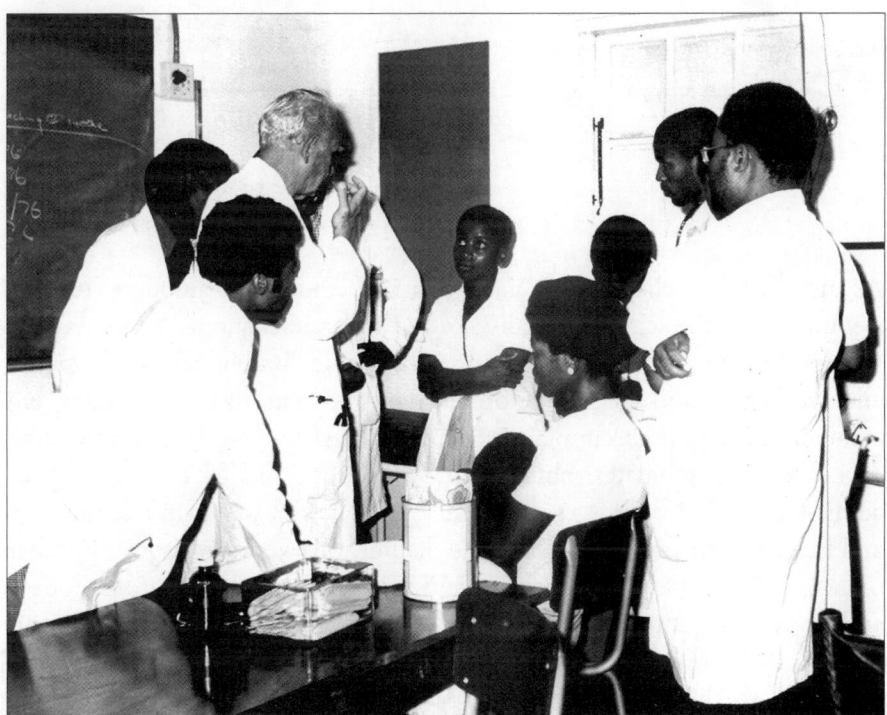

Photo 4.10   Students in a tutorial. (*UKZN Archives*)

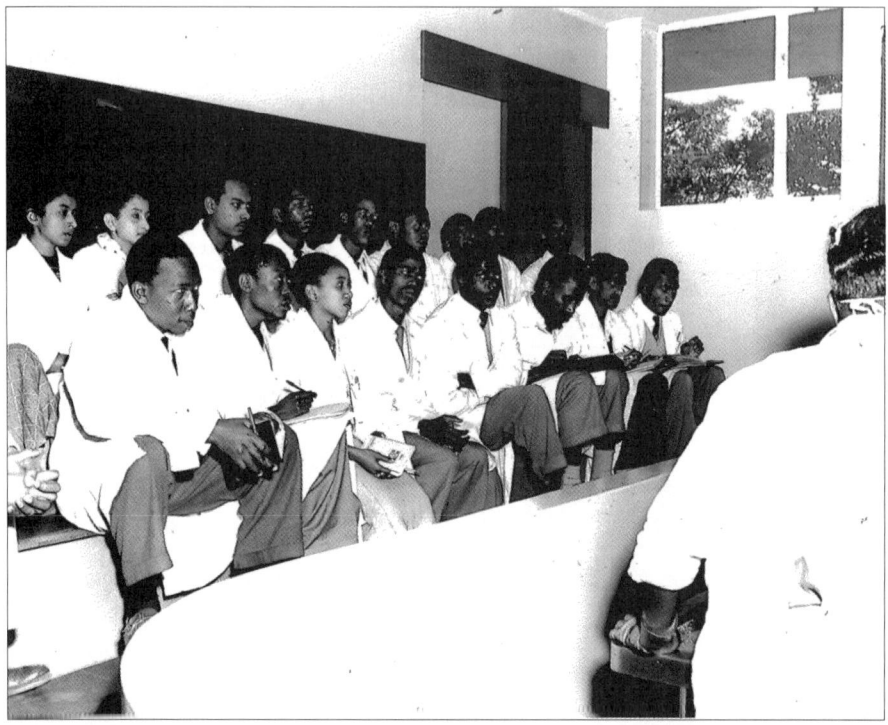

Photo 4.11 Third-year students in a post-mortem examination. (*UKZN Archives*)

As mentioned in chapter 2, a main point of contention amongst students stemmed from the school's racially skewed admissions quotas. Many African students sought admission each year with weaker individual subject passes and weaker overall matriculation-level passes than those of Indian and coloured students. For example, in 1960, only 26 African candidates, compared to 130 Indian candidates, obtained the minimum qualification needed for admission to the faculty – that is, matriculation with passes in mathematics and English.[45] As discussed in the last chapter, this stemmed from a number of factors. What was influential, however, was the later takeover of coloured and Indian schools by the apartheid government, and additionally, once this takeover was completed, Indian and coloured schools came to fare better compared to their African counterparts because of higher state-spending ratios on these schools. In an influential article on medical education and apartheid, Phillip Tobias has argued that a 'lower per capita expenditure on the education of African pupils (average R48.55 [$46.17]) than on "coloured" (R159.59 [$151.61]), Indian (R219.96 [$208.96]), or white (R645 [$621.30]) pupils . . .' produced major inequalities for different school-leaving students.[46]

Despite these factors, during the apartheid years the medical school's selection committee, under pressure from the government to train more Africans to meet the severe doctor shortage in African communities, accepted larger numbers of African students per year (at least 50%), with Indian and coloured students making up the difference.[47] Thus, many Indian and coloured applicants with higher passes in their matriculation subjects were denied acceptance at the medical school, despite having a better chance of graduating. This issue produced much dissatisfaction amongst Indian and coloured students who felt discriminated against, particularly after the passing of the 1959 Extension of University Education Act, which severely limited their available study options.[48] Some Indian and coloured students also felt frustration at being bypassed for government bursary-loans, which were given out mostly to African students on a racially skewed basis, doing nothing to alleviate the financial hardships experienced by many Indian and coloured students.[49]

Furthermore, academic competition and the stress to perform well placed enormous pressure on the school's students. While the desire to succeed would have been felt by all students, arguably the pressure would have been greatest on African students, especially those who came from the most disadvantaged Bantu Education backgrounds. In his book *Year of Fire, Year of Ash*, Baruch Hirson illustrates this point starkly. In 1966 it was reported that in four Soweto schools that consisted of 3 080 pupils, and in which 80 per cent of the pupils were supposedly being taught science, 'the total scientific equipment consisted of 13 Bunsen Burners, 6 balances, and 3 microscopes!'[50] Because the study of subjects like science in high school would have been a largely abstract experience for many students, who were often required to imagine what doing experiments would have been like, some Africans felt that they were unfairly placed to compete with their better-educated Indian and coloured colleagues. This became a point of contention amongst some students, as S.B. Pitsoe highlighted in an interview:

[W]e were disadvantaged in a sense that in our high schools we didn't have any laboratories . . . you know, [at the medical school] it was the first time some of our people saw a Bunsen burner or a beaker . . . So now we were competing with . . . Indians and coloureds who came from better schools. So with them it was more of a revision, whereas [with] us it was learning.[51]

The fact that many Africans were also second- or third-language English-speakers produced further difficulties. This was noted by a graduate who studied in Durban between 1973 and 1977:

[T]here was [a lot of pressure]. I mean, you would not deny that if you are being taught in a third or fourth language, which is English, firstly, it's not like being taught in mother tongue. And if you look at most Indian students, I mean, they were taught in English throughout [school]. We were taught through our vernacular African languages . . . until about . . . four years before you got to university . . . Then you go to Natal, the lecturers are . . . English and it's another culture.[52]

Recalling their medical school days, some African graduates also felt purposely excluded from study groups created by some Indian students, and felt discriminated against by certain Indian lecturers whom they felt favoured Indian students.[53] At times, this caused ill feeling in the student body.

Finally, despite the tendency to gloss over gender divisions amongst students in memories constructed about the medical school, a careful consideration of a variety of sources also highlights how tensions surfaced around inequalities and discriminations between men and women, in a profession dominated by men.[54] For example, in terms of numbers, Watts found that of 690 students admitted between 1951 and 1969, only 18 per cent were women.[55] In addition to being outnumbered by their male colleagues, women students found few women on the school's academic teaching staff to emulate.[56] The medical school environment reflected a masculine culture and one with blatantly sexist values that worked sometimes overtly, at other times covertly, to discomfort and marginalise women. Deena Padayachee, who studied medicine in Durban in the 1970s, provides an example of a common Indian male student's view about the 'proper' place of Indian women in South Africa at the time. In his book *What's Love Got to Do with It? And Other Stories,* Padayachee, who tries to portray everyday life for Indian South Africans in the apartheid era, writes of a heated debate that took place amongst a number of male and female students in the canteen on the Durban medical campus, where one student stoked the flames of controversy with his sexist attitudes:

> ... [W]e need doctors desperately ... These women ... most of them anyway, will simply get hitched ... Very few of them will contribute effectively to health care in our country once they're married. South Africa cannot afford it – and they occupy precious medical school seats here ... Those places could have been occupied by bread-winners who would have had medicine as their only career ... The concept of female doctors goes against every aspect of the Indian cultural outlook as we know it. Our society believes that the lady ought to devote herself to her family and home. Work, if it is to be considered at all, ought to be a part-time business. How will a female doctor cope with all the demands that her Indian husband will make on her?[57]

Discriminations varied from sexist jokes and remarks made by students about women students' supposed inferior intellectual abilities and socially prescribed roles in the home,[58] to the use of masculine 'norms' and universalising 'he/him' language in publications.[59] Sexist comments were also made by some lecturers in class, which served to ignore or undermine women's needs and experiences. Malegapuru Makgoba provides an example of this. In his autobiography, he discusses how one of his chemistry lecturers 'would often advise the young women in the class at least to grab a final year boyfriend, just in case they themselves failed to make it; [then] they would still be married to a doctor'.[60] During the earlier apartheid decades, women were also forced to endure stricter regulation of their movements through curfew restrictions and monitoring at ATR. B.T. Naidoo, who graduated in 1957, remembered this well:

> [There was] a small residence for ... women and they lived together ... and that was right next to the warden's quarters. So that was fenced off ... [It was separate] ... And there was curfew ... The girls couldn't come out after nine ... We could go out but the girls, after nine or ten o'clock, you know, although we used to study together, at the then appointed hour, they had to go into their quarters ... [and] there was a security officer that guarded ... [their] gate.[61]

Although this was aimed, in a more conservative time period, at 'protecting' the virtue of women students from possible sexual indiscretions whilst they were away from their families, it did not stop determined students from fraternising with one another.[62] Veronica Wilson remembers how, during the early 1970s, 'the guys devised ways of putting up a ladder there where you would climb over the wall and things like that'.[63]

Moreover, discriminatory social practices were a common feature of the student landscape, causing unease amongst some students. One graduate remembered how women students were sometimes treated as sexual objects by their male colleagues. For example, during her orientation week, students held a 'Miss Freshette Ball', where 'basically we were paraded like cows, you know, with our dresses walking up and down . . . [I]t was [intimidating] as new students, and, you know, see[ing] all these guys . . . the senior students already trying to, you know, looking for their next victim . . .'[64] Regular parties were also held at ATR on weekends, especially from the late 1960s onwards, where medical students socialised with one another, and invited guests in from outside the medical school. Nurses and nurse-trainees from King Edward VIII Hospital were commonly invited to these parties, and many medical students developed relationships and some even married nurses from this institution.[65] Makgoba recalled how these parties 'were just out of this world', fuelled by the musical inspirations of Curtis Mayfield, Roberta Flack, Nina Simone and James Brown, as well as 'the beer, and of course, the ladies from the surrounding metropolis', and 'many of my generation will remember romantic affairs, friendships and marriage proposals that were inspired by the record of Marvin Gaye entitled "Let's get it on"'.[66]

Steve Biko was a student who was well known for his 'womanising' activities at ATR.[67] As both a black consciousness political activist and medical student in Durban in the early 1970s, Mamphela Ramphele, who developed a romantic relationship with Biko, argued that his 'political sexuality' made him particularly susceptible to what she called 'the folly of admiring available women at every turn'. She discusses how Biko continued having affairs both within and outside the activist community, despite marrying a nurse from King Edward, who bore his children. Ramphele wrote in her autobiography that '. . . all three of us were constantly hurt by the tensions inherent in this triangular relationship', which continued right up to his death in police detention in September 1977.[68]

Sometimes, weekend parties at the medical school, or '*gumbas*' as they were called, developed into 'kinds of orgies' that were 'very wild'.[69] Women were used for sex and then discarded, as one African woman graduate who studied during the 1970s described in detail:

> I remember Alan Taylor [Residence]. If anybody was to dare go and do a sperm count in that swimming pool, it would have been a disaster! . . . [T]he culture of womanising was horrible . . . The parties would be going on and the guys would just be grabbing women from [the] parties and sleeping [with them] . . . I remember there was one guy . . . people said he wasn't so good at grabbing for himself . . . So he would get drunk and jive like everybody but [at] around 4 a.m. when the guys are kicking out what they've grabbed . . . he would go like an octopus and gather what has been kicked out and then he can get whoever [he wants] . . . [O]h . . . they loved . . . womanising! But not all of them by the way, but it was a [sub]culture that was there . . . I always think . . . if AIDS was during our years . . . half of that res. would have died from AIDS.[70]

A male graduate who was involved with the Christian Student Fellowship and did not embrace this subculture felt that it sometimes caused dissension in the student body: '. . . [I]t was very derogatory. I mean, these girls were being used. I mean, you could see it and you knew it was being done and those who perpetuated it were conscious of it.'[71] In 2006, Frank Mdlalose, who came from a rural Zulu background, explained in his autobiography that until marrying his wife and becoming 'very religious', as a medical student in Durban in the 1950s he had many girlfriends: 'To me girlfriends were friends and a good way to pass the time . . . My background was of course of a culture of boys having many girlfriends, of men being free to marry many women. My great-grandfather Thondolozi, I am told, had forty (40) wives!'[72] Other than having cultural meaning, in an apartheid context that denied black men power, sexual prowess could be regarded too as a central marker of 'being a man' and a way of maintaining power over women.

Not all students participated in these activities, however. Students who lived off-campus, as well as those who considered themselves religiously devout or did not consume alcohol, tended to avoid such parties.[73] But it was a powerful subculture that had a telling influence on many students' lives, sometimes resulting in close relationships, but often having detrimental effects on them, leading to womanising practices and drunken stupors. Alcohol abuse, resulting in the failure of some students who were overwhelmed by the experience of freedom from parental control for the first time, was another pivotal outcome.[74]

The fact that only a few – mostly female – alumni mentioned these diverse forms of gender discrimination in recent oral and written memory narratives does not undermine their significance. Instead, it highlights the constructed nature of memories and a selective bias in the way people remember things that were regarded as essential to them. In addition to a masculine bias in the collective memory narratives commonly produced about the medical school, it also captures once again the power of a recent celebratory and unifying, collective, nation-building memory narrative at work in structuring how individuals remembered things. This includes subsuming the complexity of gender divisions in a diverse student body to bring the school's and its graduates' achievements into line with the government's post-1994 triumphant collective memory agendas. Gender inequalities, together with divergences in the experiences of different 'racial' or ethnic groups, resulted in qualitatively diverse experiences for black students studying in Durban. As one Indian woman doctor said, reflecting on gender inequalities: 'I think it was just as important . . . [but] maybe the other problems were overwhelming, you know. Maybe the other problems were so much that people didn't even see . . . but it [was] there . . .'[75]

Staff-student relationships

In addition to tensions and schisms that emerged amongst students, staff-student relations could at times be strained, producing difficulties for students too. Partly an outcome of the challenges that emerged from the school's unusual set-up as a black faculty within the white University of Natal, these tensions can also be explained by the teaching staff's desire to maintain what they regarded as the highest standards, no matter the consequences. This was the view of Breminand Maharaj, who studied in Durban in the 1970s. He argued that many students felt that their lecturers were 'really being difficult, discriminating, trying to keep too high a standard and people were falling by the wayside'.[76] Although the academic staff worked within the state's framework of racial segregation at the medical school, largely because they had little choice, many worked hard to ensure that separate meant equal. This meant pushing educationally disadvantaged students, some to their breaking points, in an attempt to maintain the highest academic standards, comparable to those of their white medical colleagues being trained at other institutions. In fact, the attainment of the highest standards was not just to produce well-trained graduates; the quality of graduates trained also directly reflected on the reputation of the teaching staff. This produced deep contradictions for their black students as many could not meet the rigorous standards set.

During the early decades of the apartheid era, most of the academics on the staff in Durban were white, English-speaking men. In 1959 Alan Taylor wrote to inform a colleague overseas that 'the teaching staff are all young and enthusiastic'.[77] Whilst some received their training overseas, such as in the United Kingdom and Ireland, many received their training locally from more liberal university institutions such as at the UCT and Wits medical schools.[78] One of the early lecturers appointed in Durban, Y.K. Seedat, who had himself trained in Dublin before coming to work in the Department of Medicine, asserted that Durban 'had very good staff', many of whom were 'very liberal people'.[79] For him, their greater broad-mindedness in social and political affairs, which included encouraging improved race relations through gradualist reforms, was linked to the fact that some of the teaching staff came across from Wits and UCT to take up promotions at the Durban Medical School. Comparatively, many of MEDUNSA's predominantly white medical staff, especially those employed in the 1970s and 1980s, were state employees (certainly until MEDUNSA was granted its autonomy in 1985), and were drawn from the exclusively white, more segregationist and politically conservative Afrikaans-medium medical schools, such as Pretoria, Bloemfontein and Stellenbosch, which had opened since the late 1940s.[80] As the next chapter will show, this more liberal perspective would also have key effects on the overall political atmosphere on the campus, which was very different to MEDUNSA with its 'largely Afrikaner academic and administrative staff', and where 'all whites in the top structure were suspected of being Broederbond appointees'.[81]

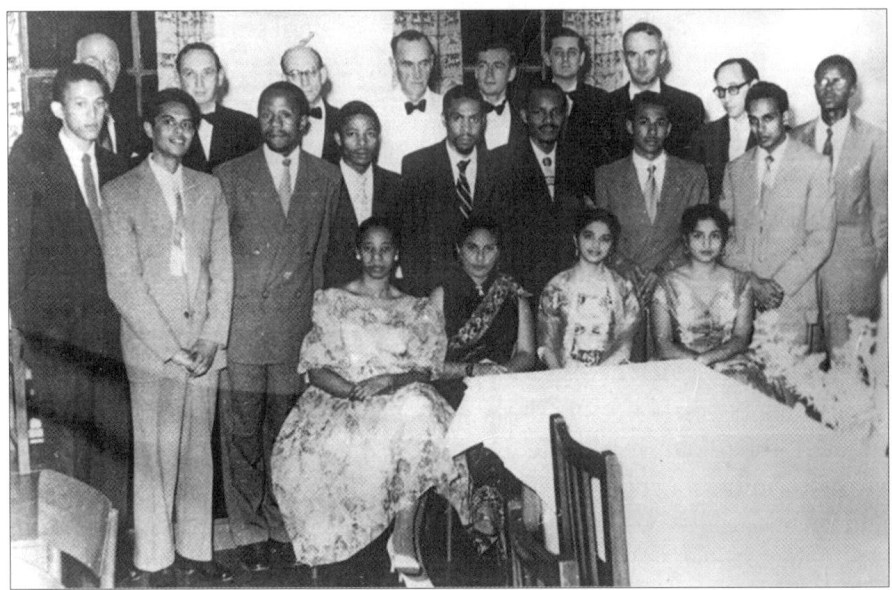

Photo 4.12   Pre-examination final-year dinner, 1957.
Back row: A.B. Taylor, S.L. Kark, I. Gordon, E.N. Keen, D. Crichton,
A. Kark, E.B. Adams and T. Culliman.
Middle row: N.E.G. Foster, B.T. Naidoo, A.M.S. Makunyane, H.M. Mogadime,
P.S. Ngakane, M.B. Zondi, C.H. Davidson, A.K. Thambiran and C.D. Marivate.
Front row: M.S. Mbambo, K. Naidoo, F.G.H Mayet and S. Kallichurum.
(*UKZN Archives*)

Slowly over time, black doctors, especially those of Indian descent, joined
the ranks of Durban's medical faculty as they graduated and specialised
from the 1960s onwards.[82] While Watts's 1970 survey of 26 faculty members
(some of whom had been there since the early 1950s) found that a small
number had no choice but to accept a position in Durban for the sake of a
job, or had felt a sense of frustration teaching academically disadvantaged
black students, and would have left given the opportunity to work at a
white institution, most were more positive about working in Durban.[83]
Sixteen of his respondents – most of whom were white – claimed they were
attracted to the challenges of an academic life and teaching in general,
regardless of the 'race' of the students, while a few mentioned that they
wished to teach black students specifically.[84] In fact, Taylor wrote in a 1954
letter to someone interested in applying for a post at the new school that the
early faculty board was very concerned to choose teachers who were more

than merely scientists but had humanitarian motives too, so that helping black students would be their priority.[85] The opportunity to work in a stimulating and 'multicultural' educational environment was also an imperative for some, while others thrived on being pioneers in the development of a new medical school project.[86] In addition, the wealth of clinical and research material available was an essential drawcard.[87] The chance of working close to where family members were settled was a further strong motivating factor.[88]

The desire to promote the highest scientific biomedical standards, however, was keenly felt by most. Head of physiology and former dean J.V.O. Reid commented:

> [T]he whole time from 1960 to 1980 I was there . . . my idea [was] . . . to produce a science-based black medical education. It had to not be some . . . indigenous healer's [school] . . . [T]hey had to base it on . . . science . . . [And] they had to be good. They had to think the way that we did. And that's what happened. At the end of 20 years we were producing very good doctors.[89]

Soromini Kallichurum, an early graduate and one of the first black employees at this institution, felt that being a pioneer black medical school in the country meant its staff felt the need to 'set a high standard . . . [and] if those students were around now, they'd have passed . . . The staff at this faculty had to prove that the end product would be good, that it's better than anywhere else . . . there was no leeway.'[90] Their reputations, after all, depended closely on the quality of their graduates.

Nevertheless, one cannot simply dismiss as poor the development of staff-student relationships at the Durban Medical School during the apartheid years. While relationships could be difficult and strained, we must avoid the trap of simply vilifying the teachers. The teaching staff was not simply a homogeneous enemy engaged in a drawn-out battle with their students. Staff-student relationships and interactions were much more complex.

While some graduates recall interactions as being very formal and focused exclusively on academic work,[91] others highlighted the supportive nature of relationships they established with some of their teachers. Kallichurum, for instance, remembered with fondness the caring attitude adopted by particular individuals. On an occasion in 1957, when Kallichurum was sick with viral pneumonia and had missed a few days of classes in her final year, her clinical lecturer in the Department of Medicine, A.J. Wilmott, actively sought her out in her off-campus flat. Finding her very ill, Wilmott arranged to take her to King Edward VIII Hospital for treatment. According to Kallichurum, 'the relationship between [some] staff and students was different' from what students have with their lecturers today.[92]

Some graduates also felt that certain lecturers worked to inspire them as students. Fatima Mayet said that Sidney Kark spent a lot of extra time motivating them. Mayet had taken Kark's innovative Social, Preventive and Family Medicine classes in the latter 1950s and saw that he showed a great deal of care for his students and patients in their home and community settings. *When* students attended the medical school was significant too, with regard to the development of staff-student relationships. This is particularly evident amongst the pioneering class of graduates, as their classes were very small. Mayet remembered how many of her lecturers, who taught her graduating class of twelve students in 1957, demonstrated great concern for their students, saying, 'if you showed interest and took initiative, they went out of their way to assist you and took an interest in you, a personal interest'.[93] Kallichurum agreed:

> You know that white staff spent more time with its students, much, much more time . . . than the staff presently does . . . I don't think any student today has . . . anywhere near the hours of contact we had with these people. It was a different era.[94]

In later years, some lecturers were regarded in a positive light for the interests they shared with some of their students. This was particularly the case with those who were involved in the Student Christian Fellowship (SCF) in the 1970s and 1980s. One African doctor who studied during the late 1970s said that 'deliberate efforts' and 'intentional partnerships' were made to 'cross the racial line'. He named two of his professors, Sam Ross and Hugh Philpott, who worked actively with students to do this, describing them as his personal 'mentors'.[95] Both were fondly remembered for their progressive attitudes and encouraging friendships and social intermingling in a context that could have got them arrested for their beliefs and actions. Students were often invited to spend weekends and holidays to socialise around the pool at Sam Ross's house. Ross, who taught alongside Hugh Philpott in the Department of Obstetrics and Gynaecology during the late

1970s and through the 1980s, was also affectionately remembered by May Mashego, who was a member of the SCF group too during her student days:

> We actually overwhelmed them [the Ross family]. We would go there in great numbers and . . . [even] sleep there . . . I mean really, we would spend time there, they would open up [their home] . . . He used to live in 12 Kilder Road . . . and his [phone] number was 212-642. I mean, that was how much [he meant to us], I cannot forget this number . . . They supported us . . . [They] went the extra mile.[96]

Of course, not all relationships with the academic staff invoked positive memories for graduates. Some felt certain lecturers evinced paternalistic and even patronising attitudes towards students, making their studies harder.[97] This particularly applied to students' intellectual abilities in class, and if students were having a hard time with something, statements such as 'If the cream of the nation is so bad, what about the scum?' were recalled.[98] Others felt intimidated by some of their lecturers, as B.T. Naidoo asserted:

> You were at their mercy because you were a student and . . . you know at the end of the year you would probably be hammered . . . so you just accepted whatever was coming . . . So here your grades depended on what you said or didn't say. The less you said the better.[99]

Blatant racist attitudes were also committed to memory. A number of graduates felt that certain lecturers who taught in the preliminary year were particularly racist. One former student asserted that it was an abusive year that pushed a lot of students out of medicine:

> It was an insulting year; it was not just a difficult year. I mean . . . the most racist utterances that we have a memory of were in those classes . . . I mean, it was completely insensitive for white guys, who were seeing black youngsters, teenagers coming in and, you know, be[ing] so abusive . . . I don't know anybody who thinks that they were helped by that course.[100]

A chemistry lecturer from the preliminary year was remembered by many graduates as having been particularly difficult and even ridiculing students. In a commemorative booklet published by the University of Natal in 1995, Koleka Mlisana publicly recorded her memories of one such lecturer:

Who could ever forget a certain Mr P. (God forgive him) who did not find it difficult to force a first year student in a strange and overwhelming environment to shout, 'I'm a monkey' to the whole class for having made a trivial mistake in a practical. Some unlucky students were threatened with expulsion on the first day.[101]

Mamphela Ramphele also described at length the politically conservative opinions of the white head of the Department of Medicine during her student days, which she found difficult to handle. She recalls how during tutorials, the professor thrived on pushing his students' buttons, especially her own. Although knowing that she was a student activist, he would tell her and her classmates his opinions on various politically contentious issues, such as the situation of Ian Smith's oppressive colonial government in Rhodesia in the 1970s. She also took umbrage at what she regarded as his patronising treatment of African patients, whom he commonly referred to as '"the old boy" or "old John" or whatever was the first name of the patient' during their clinical rounds.[102] Their relationship deteriorated so much that Ramphele stopped attending his tutorials, confronted him for his political insensitivity and was threatened with dismissal if she continued to defy him. Although he never reported her for her 'bad behaviour', she wrote: 'When I completed my final exams at the end of that year, he made it known to his colleagues that he would not have me in his firm in Ward D at King Edward VIII Hospital.' Instead, she had to work with other clinical lecturers in the Department of Medicine as she rotated through the various departments in her internship year.[103]

Another point of contention was the inconsiderateness displayed by some lecturers, who assumed, incorrectly, a common starting point when explaining medical issues or problems to their students. An African graduate recalled one such occasion, when a lecturer described bone changes that occurred in patients suffering from syphilis. These patients were described as being 'celery-stalk' in appearance, which confused and frustrated this student and many of his colleagues.

Now you come from the townships . . . [and] you didn't know what this celery was. You had to go to the dictionary and try to find out what it is. But it doesn't say what it looks like when it's cut across, so it's meaningless. And so you find that things are described from the cultural perspective of white people, which means nothing to you and you . . . just have to memorise the term, but you don't know what it means . . . So I think . . . there was limitation of how much knowledge we could generate . . . [Much] was falling . . . between the cracks because the concepts were not clear.[104]

As already mentioned, many of Durban's lecturers, including people in positions of leadership, such as deans of the medical school, focused on what they regarded as the positive and highest values that European scientific orientations and approaches could offer their black students. However, this example demonstrates that their general mode of communication and interaction took a lot of cultural background for granted. This made a number of students feel inadequate or 'other' rather than included, and added further stresses to their learning experiences in Durban. Some African graduates felt that they had to work much harder just to be recognised on a par with their colleagues, while others failed as a result.

Sam Fehrsen, now a retired family medicine professor who went to work at MEDUNSA in the 1970s, maintained that cultural misunderstandings played a large role in the high failure rate in Durban. He was told by many students who had come to study at MEDUNSA after having failed in Durban that lecturers there moved on too quickly with their scientific explanations, leaving many students behind. At MEDUNSA, where English was the medium of instruction even though most of the lecturers were Afrikaans-speakers, and most students spoke English as a second or third language, language difficulties would also have been an issue. However, Fehrsen expressed the view that having only a few who came to teach and learn at MEDUNSA with English as their mother tongue was actually 'a blessing because they all had to speak until everybody understood'.[105] In contrast to Durban, lecturers at MEDUNSA were forced to slow down and adapt their teaching to help students to understand the content. Having worked with many Zulu and Xhosa patients from his missionary hospital days (first at McCord Hospital and then in the Transkei), Fehrsen could speak their native languages. This enabled him to 'work with examples and idioms from an African perspective' and it enabled 'the guys [to] blossom . . .', he said. Despite these efforts, it would be naive to assume that 'othering' problems suffered by students in Natal simply evaporated once they arrived at MEDUNSA. Eurocentric perspectives, as well as cultural and linguistic misunderstandings, would have remained a challenge at this initially

Afrikaner-led, state-created institution too, where rigid segregation between its students and staff, race discrimination and language barriers, continued to prevail throughout the apartheid years.[106]

These examples all suggest that medical students had much to contend with once arriving at the Durban Medical School. Indeed, many of the students' hardships often extended beyond the purely academic. They included surviving distant, polluted and cramped living arrangements; scrambling to make up for deficits in inadequate secondary educations; and developing skills to navigate the choppy waters of shifting dynamics in student-student and staff-student relationships. And different race, class and gender experiences did much to muddy the waters, despite being purposefully ignored in recent glossy publications commemorating the history of the medical school. For the few students who successfully passed their studies each year, the challenges were not over. Those entering the latter clinical years of their medical degrees faced a daunting task. Now they had to work in underfunded and overburdened black public hospitals and were forced to deal with sick patients. Many contradictions and ambiguities would plague them at this level of study too.

Notes

1. UKZN EGML, 'Medical school – Durban's other campus', *Dome* 3 (April 1989).
2. Speech given by Soromini Kallichurum, *University of Natal, Nelson R. Mandela School of Medicine, Fiftieth Anniversary Banquet* (University of Natal, Durban: Audio-Visual Centre, 29 July 2000). For more on Kallichurum's background, see 'No stopping this doc of a "different" gender', *Mercury* (16 November 1995).
3. Patricia Anne Esselaar, '"Idealism tempered by realism": Dr E.G. Malherbe and issues of segregation and apartheid at the University of Natal, 1945–65' (Master's diss., University of the Witwatersrand, 1998), 40, 190–1.
4. Interview with Y.K. Seedat, Durban, 14 July 2003.
5. Speech given by Zweli Mkhize, *Fiftieth Anniversary Banquet*. For more on Zweli Mkhize's biography, see http://www.whoswhosa.co.za/zweli-mkhize-2310.
6. CC MH Mouldy Box Scans, Dr Taylor up to Dec 1958, page 70, Letter from Dr A.B. Taylor to Dr and Mrs E.A. Thompson, Grand Rapids, Michigan, 27 March 1951.
7. E.G. Malherbe, *Never a Dull Moment* (Southern and Eastern Africa and the UK: Timmins Publishers, 1981), 297.
8. E.H. Brookes, *A History of the University of Natal* (Pietermaritzburg: University of Natal Press, 1966), 87; and UKZNA H6/1/1, Medical School – History, G.W. Gale, 'The story of the Durban Medical School', 25 January 1976, 18.

9. NAR UOD 56, U3/26/4/5, University of Natal Building Grants and Loans for Medical School Non-Europeans Durban, 1949–53, 'Letter from Dr E.G. Malherbe to the Secretary for Public Works, Pretoria re. Wentworth Camp: Proposed Non-European University College', 14 August 1947, 2; and Brookes, *A History of the University of Natal*, 86.

10. I. Gordon, *Report on the Government's Intended Action to Remove the Faculty of Medicine from the University of Natal* (Durban: Hayne and Gibson, 4 March 1957), 11; and CC GP File 23, KCM 25915, W.R.G. Branford and A.W. Rees, 'Pre-medical courses in arts and science and the non-European hostel', addressed to all members of the Faculty of Arts, n/d [probably late 1950s].

11. Interview with ZM, Durban, 6 October 2003.

12. H.L. Watts. 'Black doctors: An investigation into aspects of the training and career of students and graduates from the medical school of the University of Natal. Part I: The Students' (University of Natal, Durban: Institute for Social Research, 1975), 27.

13. K.P. Mlisana, 'UND Black Section – Personal reflections', in *University of Natal Medical School Reconciliation Graduation Booklet 1995* (Durban: Indicator Press, December 1995), 11.

14. CC GP File 13, KCM 25735, 'Letter from Dr E.G. Malherbe to the Secretary for Education, Arts and Science re. Extension of hostel accommodation at Wentworth', 11 May 1953.

15. 'Reminiscences: The early days. Dr Thaven "BT" Naidoo's story', in *University of Natal Nelson R. Mandela School of Medicine: 50 Years of Achievement in Teaching, Service and Research*, eds Jack Moodley and Smita Maharaj (University of Natal Nelson R. Mandela School of Medicine: Connunications Office, 2001), 13.

16. NAR K296 E5/49 Medical Training, 1968–9, Komitee van Ondersoek oor Mediese Opleiding, Letter from G.A.H. Chapman (Warden, ATR) to I. Gordon (Dean Faculty of Medicine), 23 October 1968; UKZNA C10/6/1-2, 'Memorandum on the need to increase the accommodation available for medical students at the Alan Taylor Residence, 1972'; and UKZNA C10/7/1, 'Alan Taylor Residence', UN Council minutes, 18 March 1977, 215.

17. Interview with Hugh Philpott, Kloof, 14 July 2003.

18. UKZNA MQ 1/1/1-5, 'Facts you should know . . .', *The Amoeba* 2, no. 6 (1 September 1954), 3.

19. Interview with Mfanyana J. Ndlovu, Durban, 14 August 2003; Mamphela Ramphele, *Across Boundaries: The Journey of a South African Woman Leader* (New York: Feminist Press, 1995), 58; and UKZNA MQ 1/1/1-5, 'A response to gas smell from oil-refinery', *The Amoeba* 2, no. 4 (10 May 1954), 8.

20. CC GP File 23, KCM 25915, Branford and Rees, 'Pre-medical courses in arts and science'.

21. Interview with Maila J. Matjila, Durban, 11 July 2003.

22. Interview with Hugh Philpott, Kloof, 14 July 2003; and UKZN Board of the Faculty of Medicine minutes, 11, 13 and 15 May 1981.

23. Interview with Veronica Wilson, Durban, 6 November 2003. Also see see Padraig O'Malley Interview with Albertina Luthuli, 10 January 1993, http://www.nelson mandela.org/omalley/index.php/site/q/03lv00017.htm.

24. UKZNA MQ 1/1/1-5, 'The transport problem', *The Amoeba* 1, no. 5 (16 April 1953), 6; and UKZNA C10/7/1, 'Transport for black students', UN Council minutes, 15 June 1979, 204.

25. Interviews with Breminand Maharaj, Durban, 10 June 2003; Veronica Wilson, Durban, 6 November 2003; and MM, Durban, 28 July 2003.

26. Breminand Maharaj, 'University of Natal Medical School submission to the Truth and Reconciliation Commission', 23 June 1997, 2.

27. See CC GP File 6, KCM 25708, Appendix CC, 'Some comments by the organiser on pass and curfew laws that affect our African students', 24 April 1956.

28. Interview with B.T. Naidoo, Durban, 15 September 2003; Interview with S.B. Pitsoe, Durban, 17 June 2003.

29. UKZNA MQ 1/1/1-5, 'The transport problem', *The Amoeba* 1, no. 5 (16 April 1953), 6; and UKZNA C10/7/1, 'Transport for black students', UN Council minutes, 15 June 1979, 204.

30. Watts, 'Black doctors. Part I: The students', 5, 24.

31. Interview with Fatima Mayet, Durban, 4 June 1999.

32. See Muriel Horrell, *Bantu Education to 1968* (Johannesburg: South African Institute of Race Relations, 1968), 153; Surendra Bhana, 'University education', in *South Africa's Indians: The Evolution of a Minority*, ed. Bridglal Pachai (Washington, DC: University Press of America, 1979), 400; and Adam Starz, *Between Laughter and Tears* (Ladysmith, RSA: Sinclair Publishing, 1986), 9, 13.

33. Although an attempt was made to accommodate a few African medical students in a building near to Wits called Douglas Smit House in the late 1940s, under pressure from the apartheid government, this building was forced to close in the early 1960s. University accommodation was not made available for Indian students at Wits. See Wits CRO Box No. Reg. 00885, File no. 3, B19/2, Blacks – Training of Black Medical and Dental Students, June 1944 – July 1962, 'Admission of non-European students: The special case of medical education', 11 March 1954.

34. Wits FHSR M3/40 Internal Reconciliation Commission, 1998, Jules Browde, Patrick Mokhoba and Essop Jassat, 'University of the Witwatersrand Faculty of Health Sciences Internal Reconciliation Commission Report' (November 1998). For a discussion of the TRC health sector hearings, also see *Truth and Reconciliation Commission of South Africa Report*, Vol. 4 (Cape Town: Juta, 1998).

35. I. Gordon, 'Experience in the establishment of a medical school for non-white undergraduate students in South Africa', in *Medical Education in South Africa: Proceedings of the Conference on Medical Education held at the University of Natal Durban in July 1964*, eds J.V.O. Reid and A.J. Wilcot (Pietermaritzburg: Natal University Press, 1965), 296.

36. Haroon R. Elias, *Short Story Kaleidoscope* (Northmead, RSA: Prestige Publications, 1995), 22–31; Interview with MA, Durban, 6 November 2003; and Starz, *Between Laughter and Tears*, 21.

37. Interview with KM, Durban, 14 November 2003.
38. Interview with B.T. Naidoo, Durban, 10 November 2003.
39. Interview with May Mashego, Ashburton, 18 October 2003.
40. Also see, for example, Interview with May Mashego, Durban, 14 October 2003; M.W. Makgoba, *Mokoko: The Makgoba Affair: A Reflection on Transformation* (Florida Hills, RSA: Vivlia Publishers, 1997), 33-4; and Deena Padayachee, 'Whites and Indians opposed apartheid of the medical school', *Natal Witness* (7 September 2000).
41. Interviews with KM, Durban, 14 November 2003; and B.T. Naidoo, Durban, 10 November 2003.
42. Interview with TM, Pretoria, 21 August 2003. Similar perspectives were also expressed in Interview with May Mashego, Durban, 14 October 2003, and Pooba Govender, Questionnaire, 2003.
43. Watts, 'Black doctors. Part I: The students', 24, 41; and H.L. Watts, 'Black Doctors: An investigation into aspects of the training and career of students and graduates from the medical school of the University of Natal. Part II: The Graduates' (University of Natal, Durban: Institute for Social Research, 1976), 13.
44. Interviews with B.T. Naidoo, Durban, 15 September 2003, and Veronica Wilson, Durban, 6 November 2003. Also see UCT M&A, 'Apartheid education divides', *Varsity* (February 1984).
45. W.R.G. Branford, 'Examination systems and selection: The experiences of the admissions committee of the Board of the Faculty of Medicine, University of Natal', in *Medical Education in South Africa: Proceedings of the Conference on Medical Education held at the University of Natal Durban in July 1964*, eds J.V.O. Reid and A.J. Wilcot (Pietermaritzburg: Natal University Press, 1965), 195.
46. Phillip V. Tobias, 'Apartheid and medical education: The training of black doctors in South Africa', *The Leech* 60, no. 1 (March 1991), 97.
47. CC EGM File 463/5/2, KCM 56990 (59) f, W.R.G. Branford, 'Interim report on applicants of admission to pre-medical courses at UN 1951-60', 4–5; and Branford, 'Examination systems and selection', 193–4.
48. 'Indian accusations against medical school refuted', *Natal Mercury* (13 November 1964).
49. Interviews with Soromini Kallichurum, Durban, 29 May 1999, and B.T. Naidoo, Durban, 15 September 2003.
50. Baruch Hirson, *Year of Fire, Year of Ash: The Soweto Revolt: Roots of a Revolution?* (London: Zed Press, 1979), 60. Also see Tobias, 'Apartheid and medical education', 97.
51. Interview with S.B. Pitsoe, Durban, 17 July 2003. A similar comment was made in the interview with Mfanyana J. Ndlovu, Durban, 14 August 2003.
52. Interview with TM, Pretoria, 21 August 2003.
53. Interviews with KM, Durban, 14 November 2003, TM, Pretoria, 21 August 2003, and MM, Durban, 28 July 2003; and Speech given by Kgotsi Letslape, *Fiftieth Anniversary Banquet.*

54. Beryl Unterhalter, 'Discrimination against women in the South African medical profession', *Social Science and Medicine* 20 (1985), and 'Shattering the male monopoly: The history and struggle of female doctors', *The Leech* 62, no. 3 (November 1993). In 1963, 11 per cent of registered doctors in South Africa were women. This increased to 14 per cent in 1984 and to 20 per cent in 1994. See Chris P. Hudson, Jocelyne Kane-Berman and Rosemary Hickman, 'Women in medicine: A literature review – 1985–96', *South African Medical Journal* 87, no. 11 (November 1997), 1512.

55. This figure was made up of roughly equal proportions of female students amongst African (16 per cent) and Indian (19 per cent) students, while coloured women made up a slightly higher figure of 30 per cent during this period. Watts, 'Black doctors. Part I: The students', 37–8.

56. UKZNA MF3/1/1-8, J. Moodley, 'Inaugural lecture: Women, health and research development', *MedNews: Faculty of Medicine Newsletter* (November–December 1995).

57. Deena Padayachee, *What's Love Got to Do with It? And Other Stories* (Johannesburg: COSAW Publishing, 1992), 153–5.

58. See, for example, UKZNA MQ 1/1/1-5, V.K.G. Pillay, 'The university student', *The Amoeba* 1, no. 6 (27 May 1953); 'Analysis of woman', *The Amoeba* 1, no. 2 (12 October 1953), 5; 'My apologies to "cats"', *The Amoeba* 3, no. 1 (October 1954), 5.

59. See UKZN MQ 1/1/1-5, 'The ideal doctor', *The Amoeba* 2, no. 7 (September 1954), 7; G.W. Gale, 'The Durban Medical School: A progress report', *South African Medical Journal* (7 May 1955), 437; UKZNA CF 8/1/1 University of Natal, Hippocratic Oath Ceremony, 1975. 'Address by the Principal Prof. Francis E. Stock', 2; UKZN Board of the Faculty of Medicine minutes, 'Memorandum from the MSRC to Faculty of Medicine Board re. Other student problems', 2 February 1987, 5.

60. Makgoba, *Mokoko*, 34. Interviews with Veronica Wilson, Durban, 6 November 2003, and May Mashego, Durban, 14 October 2003.

61. Interview with B.T. Naidoo, Durban, 15 September 2003.

62. For more on the preoccupation of missionaries, school and university administrators and Christian Africans with protecting young African women's virginity whilst they were away from parental control studying in educational institutions, such as nursing school, see Shula Marks, *Divided Sisterhood: Race, Class and Gender in the South African Nursing Profession* (London: Macmillan Press and New York: St. Martin's Press, 1994), 103–4, 210.

63. Interview with Veronica Wilson, Durban, 6 November 2003.

64. Interview with Veronica Wilson, Durban, 6 November 2003. Also see Starz, *Between Laughter and Tears*, 23.

65. Frank T. Mdlalose, *My Life: The Autobiography of Dr Frank T. Mdlalose* (Wierda Park: Action Publishers, 2006), 21–2.

66. Makgoba, *Mokoko*, 32–3.

67. For more on this issue, see, for example, Aelred Stubbs, 'Martyr of hope: A personal memoir', in *I Write What I Like*, Steve Biko (New York: HarperSan-

Francisco, 1978), 171–4; Donald Woods, *Biko* (New York: Henry Holt and Company, 1978, 1987), 82; Lindy Wilson, 'Bantu Stephen Biko: A life', and Mamphela Ramphele, 'The dynamics of gender within black consciousness organisations: A personal view', both in *Bounds of Possibility: The Legacy of Steve Biko and Black Consciousness,* eds Barney Pityana, Mamphela Ramphele, Malusi Mpumlwana and Lindy Wilson (Cape Town: David Philip; London and Atlantic Highlands, NJ: Zed Books, 1991), 16, 36–40, 226.

68. Ramphele, *Across Boundaries*, 110, 117.

69. Makgoba, *Mokoko*, 35.

70. This interviewee did not want her name used.

71. Interview with ZM, Durban, 6 October 2003. Similar views were expressed in Interviews with Veronica Wilson, Durban, 6 November 2003; May Mashego, Durban, 7 October 2003; and KM, Durban, 14 November 2003.

72. Mdlalose, *My Life*, 21–2.

73. Watts, 'Black doctors. Part II: The graduates', 4. In this study, Watts found that sexual promiscuity was seen as 'occurring to a significant extent' by one-fifth of the 80 medical graduates surveyed.

74. Interviews with Veronica Wilson, Durban, 6 November 2003; ZM, Durban, 11 September 2003; and KM, Durban, 14 November 2003; and Watts, 'Black doctors. Part I. The students', 16, 22, 32.

75. Interview with MA, Durban, 6 November 2003.

76. Interview with Breminand Maharaj, Durban, 10 June 2003.

77. CC MH Mouldy Box Scans, Tied Together, Dr Taylor Personal 1959–60, page 130, Letter from Dr A.B. Taylor to Professor Clifford Herman, University of Vermont College of Medicine, Burlington, Vermont, 5 April 1959.

78. See UKZNA *UN Calendars*, Faculty of Medicine handbooks, 1950s–1970s.

79. Interview with Prof. Y.K. Seedat, Durban, 14 July 2003. Also see G.C. Moodie, 'The state and the liberal universities in South Africa: 1948–90', *Higher Education* 27 (1994).

80. Ina van der Linde, 'MEDUNSA at twenty', *South African Medical Journal* (December 1996), 1507–8; MA, MEDUNSA General, Periodicals with Substantial Information, 'Medical frontier', *Leadership* 8, no. 2 (April 1989), 94; Wits CRO, Taffy Adler, 'University of Natal, Black Medical School', *Wits Student* 23, no. 9 (30 April 1971), 9.

81. Van der Linde, 'MEDUNSA at twenty', 1507–8. The Afrikaner Broederbond was a cultural and political organisation formed in the early twentieth century with its main aim to further Afrikaner nationalism in South Africa. The foci on maintaining Afrikaner culture, developing a strong Afrikaner economy and gaining control of the South African government were major objectives. According to *South African History Online*, every prime minister and state president in South Africa from 1948 to the end of apartheid in 1994, not to mention most members of the National Party's changing cabinets, were members of the Broederbond. For more on this, see http://www.sahistory.org.za/organisations/afrikaner-broederbond.

82. Speech given by Kgotsi Letslape, *Fiftieth Anniversary Banquet*, and Maharaj, 'University of Natal Medical School submission to the Truth and Reconciliation Commission'.

83. H.L. Watts, 'Black doctors: An investigation into aspects of the training and career of students and graduates from the medical school of the University of Natal. Part III: The attitudes and opinions of staff' (University of Natal, Durban: Institute for Social Research, 1976), 1–2.

84. Interviews with Dennis J. Pudifin, Durban, 2 July 2003, and J.V.O. Reid, Plettenberg Bay, 16 June 2002; and Gordon, 'Experience in the establishment of a medical school for non-white undergraduate students', 296.

85. CC MH Mouldy Box Scans Dr Taylor up to Dec 1958, pages 109–10, Letter from Dr A.B. Taylor to Dr W.B.D. Evans, Bridgman Memorial Hospital, High Street, Mayfair, Johannesburg, 18 May 1954.

86. UKZN MSA, 'Address to be delivered by Professor I. Gordon, Dean of the Faculty of Medicine, to an extraordinary general meeting of medical students of the University of the Witwatersrand', 22 August 1958, 5; and Interview with Hugh Philpott, Kloof, 14 July 2003.

87. NAR UOD 1546, U3/40/4, Natal University College for Establishment of Medical School for Natives, 1945–48, 'Memorandum on the urgent need of establishing a fourth medical school in Durban', 22 July 1947.

88. Interview with Jerry Coovadia, Durban, 24 June 2003.

89. Interview with J.V.O. Reid, Plettenberg Bay, 16 June 2002.

90. Interview with Soromini Kallichurum, Durban, 29 May 1999.

91. Interview with Jerry Coovadia, Durban, 24 June 2003. Coovadia completed his postgraduate training in Durban.

92. Interview with Soromini Kallichurum, Durban, 29 May 1999.

93. B.T. Naidoo, 'A history of the Durban Medical School', *South African Medical Journal* 50, no. 41 (25 September 1976), 1627.

94. Interview with Soromini Kallichurum, Durban, 29 May 1999.

95. Interview with ZM, Durban, 11 September 2003.

96. Interview with May Mashego, Ashburton, 18 October 2003.

97. Watts also found that many black students also felt discriminated against by some of the school's white administrative staff. See Watts, 'Black doctors. Part I: The students', 12–3, 25.

98. Makgoba, *Mokoko*, 34; Questionnaire, HA, 2003; and Interview with Fatima Mayet, Durban, 4 June 1999.

99. Interview with B.T. Naidoo, Durban, 15 September 2003; and Interview with Veronica Wilson, Durban, 6 November 2003.

100. Interview with ZM, Durban, 11 September 2003. Others raised similar points: Interviews with Maila J. Matjila, Durban, 22 September 2003, and Mfanyana J. Ndlovu, Durban, 14 August 2003.

101. K.P. Mlisana, 'UND Black Section – Personal reflections', 11. Interview with Maila J. Matjila, Durban, 11 July 2003; and Starz, *Between Laughter and Tears*, 2–5, 25–6.

102. Ramphele, *Across Boundaries*, 69–70.
103. Interview with Y.K. Seedat, Durban, 14 July 2003.
104. Interview with ZM, Durban, 11 September 2003.
105. Interview with Sam Fehrsen, Pretoria, 22 August 2003.
106. In 1985, the entire MEDUNSA student body boycotted and demanded the dismissal of the Department of Anatomy head, Prof. G.G.J. le Roux, for physical and verbal abuse of students. 'Kick out Le Roux', *City Press* (24 February 1985); 'MEDUNSA offers pay to Le Roux to resign', *Pretoria News* (17 July 1985); 'Jubilation as professor quits', *Sowetan*, 20 July 1985. Also see Nimrod Mkele, 'Tragedy of the education system', *Star* (18 April 1983); MA, MEDUNSA General, Periodicals with Substantial Information, 'Medical frontier', *Leadership* 8, no. 2 (April 1989), 92, 94; and Van der Linde, 'MEDUNSA at twenty', 1507–8.

CHAPTER 5

King Edward VIII Hospital
and clinical training difficulties

'One's memories of the medical school are full of ambivalence and contradictions.'

— Taole Mokoena

The large, state-funded, 'non-European', public hospital – King Edward VIII – located immediately adjacent to the medical school's academic buildings on Umbilo Road provided Durban's aspiring black doctors with most of their hands-on clinical training.[1] This hospital provided a home for students completing the final three years of their undergraduate training, and for many others (including students who had trained at other medical school facilities) a practical base to complete a further mandatory one-year, post-graduation, internship training. Its location also served to provide easy access for black patients coming from the city centre and from the growing industrial area around Durban's busy harbour, and for African and Indian residents living in areas surrounding the city. Although coloured patients were not denied treatment at this facility, most coloured patients received hospital care at the white Addington Hospital on the Durban beachfront, which had a separate coloured section.

In 1954, a year before King Edward VIII hosted the medical school's first clinical training year, the hospital provided about 1 300 beds for inpatients (this increased to over 2 000 by 1976). It had a thriving casualty section, as well as an outpatients' department, and treated many patients for a variety of illnesses in its large medical and surgical wards. By the early 1960s, the hospital was treating roughly 600 000 outpatients and over 70 000 inpatients each year. By 1980, this figure had increased to over 830 000 outpatients and over 106 000 inpatients each year.[2] During the apartheid years, the hospital also had one of the largest maternity sections in the country, delivering close to 14 000 babies in 1960 and over 21 000 in 1980. However, as a state-subsidised hospital, its development during the apartheid years had pivotal effects – both positive and negative – on medical students' clinical training experiences.

Some graduates felt that they received an excellent training at King Edward VIII. Jerry Coovadia, for example, said that it was 'a good place to learn'.

> There w[ere] a lot of clinical problems to solve so we were exposed to a very wide range of diseases and issues. And . . . the teachers were very good . . . I've been in all parts of the world . . . [and] our kids are far superior clinically . . . [C]linical medicine has been their strength.[3]

Frank Mdlalose, a 1958 graduate, agreed that King Edward VIII's training prepared him and his colleagues well to practise medicine in South Africa. During a plaque-unveiling ceremony at the medical school in December 1995, Mdlalose noted that one of his most 'uplifting experiences' was during his fifth year when he attended a ward round at the black Baragwanath Hospital in Johannesburg. On this occasion, which brought together senior students from the UCT, Wits, Pretoria and Natal medical schools, Mdlalose emphasised that after just that one hour of ward rounds together, in comparison, 'I knew we were being taught medicine at our University of Natal!'[4]

However, as was the case with the varied opinions about students' early medical school training years, not all black doctors trained in Durban recalled their clinical experiences in so positive a light. A negative factor, one shared by black students at Wits and UCT, was that black medical students were restricted to examining and treating black patients only, whereas their white colleagues could learn from and work with both black and white patients. Many graduates felt that this limited their clinical training, especially when they continued to be taught about certain diseases that mainly affected white patients. Though their theoretical training might have been on a par with those of their contemporaries in other medical schools in the country, they received a limited practical understanding of the full spectrum of diseases affecting different population groups. This situation was captured in the memories of an African doctor, who argued that some diseases were known to him and his colleagues only in theory:

> I mean, in paediatrics for instance, I would mention the inherited disorders, you know, which you didn't find in us . . . But you had to learn about them . . . I mean, some . . . [diseases] because they are known from white patients, they're described in terms of white patients and you don't really know what the iris of a white person looks like. And then all of a sudden now you've got to remember what Kayser-Fleischer rings [are] . . . and you've got to try to imagine these things.[5]

As a black public institution in the apartheid era, the medical school's teaching hospital was also put under enormous pressure because of insufficient or outdated equipment, inadequate staff-to-patient ratios and a lack of space. The reasons for this were multiple. The post-Second World War period, bringing increased urbanisation and the improved efficacy of curative treatments, such as antibiotics, saw a marked increase in the number of black patients. During the years of apartheid, and the 1970s and 1980s particularly, several applications were made by the university to the state to upgrade the hospital and to establish a new, larger academic teaching hospital, but it was only many years later – in the post-apartheid period – that funds were actually made available for these purposes.[6] A key reason for the delay in obtaining permission to extend its buildings was the hospital's presence in what had, from the early 1950s, been zoned a white residential area. It was hoped by apartheid ideologues that this contradiction would be removed once alternative hospital facilities were made available for Indians in Chatsworth at the R.K. Khan Hospital (which was opened in the early 1970s), and for Africans in Umlazi township at the Prince Mshiyeni Hospital (which was opened in the late 1970s), to bring Durban hospitals more into line with the country's separate-development health policies.[7]

Despite these intentions, the eventual opening of these hospitals did not result in the closure of King Edward, because of growing black patient numbers across the province during the 1970s and 1980s. The state continued to provide limited funds for King Edward's daily operational costs, and by the 1980s it was a beleaguered hospital, literally 'begging for funds'.[8] Of course, King Edward was not the only hospital to suffer these vastly overcrowded, inadequately equipped, and short-staffed conditions that made proper instruction for black medical students, not to mention good patient care, extremely difficult. This dismal situation prevailed at many of the country's black hospitals, such as Baragwanath in Soweto, and even at Ga-Rankuwa Hospital – the teaching hospital used to train MEDUNSA's medical students – which, despite being built in the early 1970s, was much more recent than King Edward and Baragwanath.[9] The large 'Bantu' Ga-Rankuwa Hospital had been established in the Bophuthatswana homeland and, by the late 1980s and early 1990s, the report of MEDUNSA's vice-chancellor and principal noted that 'conditions at our teaching hospital have deteriorated to an appalling level', and its staff were also begging for additional funds to expand and improve their 'hopelessly inadequate' hospital.[10]

And, the situation became more dismal as the years continued. In 1990, it was reported that the per-day budget allocated by the state to King Edward was only 49 per cent of the budget given to white teaching hospitals.[11] As a result, patients literally overwhelmed the available facilities and personnel, with some wards operating at 200 per cent capacity, while hundreds of outpatients queued down Umbilo Road every day hoping to see a doctor or nurse who might assist them.[12] Janet Giddy, a family medicine specialist who studied at UCT's well-resourced and mostly white Groote Schuur teaching hospital, remembered well King Edward's dire state of affairs. Having come to Natal to do her internship training in 1984, she recalled the shock she felt when she first arrived at King Edward. In her opinion, Groote Schuur was well resourced, the hospital had 'enough of everything', including staff and supplies, and it tried to deliver a dignified service to its patients where privacy was protected. Comparatively, she exclaimed:

> King Edward was a total shock because . . . you couldn't find anything, [and] it was so ugly! I felt like I was in a third-world hospital in Africa . . . And if you wanted to put up a drip, well, you'd be lucky to find a drip stand in a whole ward of a hundred patients! And you'd sort of have to find a nail in the wall, or be near a window and hook it onto a window . . . [I]t was totally overcrowded and . . . patients would get lost in the wards, literally. You wouldn't find them for days! . . . [A]nd half the patients would be on what they called floor beds . . . [and] under the beds. There weren't enough nurses. The nurses were . . . a mixture of harassed, exhausted, run off their feet and totally indifferent.[13]

Dennis Pudifin, a long-serving specialist physician in the Department of Medicine, agreed. He asserted that working at King Edward during the apartheid period was 'very depressing at times', especially when the 'work pressures were really heavy . . . And you just struggle to manage with inadequate equipment, and equipment which is not working, inadequate support structures, help from the nurses, help from the porters . . .'[14] Thinking back to his time at this teaching hospital, Pudifin felt the problems were multilayered, which is why they were so difficult to solve. And they were exacerbated during times of political violence during the 1970s and 1980s, which resulted in increased numbers of gunshot and knife-wounded township patients being admitted to already overstretched casualty and surgical wards.[15] Many black patients died because they were denied treatment at the nearby state-sponsored Addington Hospital, which had beds and high-tech equipment available, while King Edward was almost crippled under its patient load.[16]

These overcrowded and substandard conditions were not conducive to teaching medical students and interns, as many of the hospital's doctors and nurses were inundated with work and had little time or patience left to teach students. In addition, many graduates felt exploited, unappreciated and exhausted as they often had to work 100-hour weeks doing many of the menial tasks of the hospital. One doctor who trained in the early 1970s described internship as 'no bed of roses'. 'The interns worked; and they worked some more. "Vampires", "bloodsuckers" and "slaves" they were called, and every one of their titles suited them aptly. The registrars used them, the consultants abused them.'[17] What is more, the lack of privacy in wards meant that students were taught in conditions that were dehumanising for the patients. In conditions where the number of patients overwhelmed the doctors and nurses, as well as the hospital's facilities, privacy screens were seldom used when patients were examined. With both regret and embarrassment, B.T. Naidoo recalled:

> We were [not] taught th[e proper] sort of set-up . . . and we examined the patients wherever and whenever, you know. We didn't worry about privacy . . . [The labour ward] was terrible . . . these ladies were exposed to the world, you know . . . And when you did your internal examination . . . everybody could see . . . and hear, you know.[18]

Graduates also remembered how doctors would discuss their patients with their colleagues or students without including or consulting with their patients about their medical problems. In these appalling working conditions, medical students were seldom taught about patients' rights, and slow improvements were only noted in the late 1980s when these issues were publicly discussed and later codified into patients' rights laws in the post-apartheid period.[19]

The grossly overcrowded conditions in King Edward's maternity wards were so bad for teaching purposes that professors in the Department of Obstetrics and Gynaecology at the medical school had to make other provisions. This included, as already mentioned, an alternative arrangement negotiated with the nearby McCord mission hospital which allowed some of the school's students to gain practical experience in its maternity wards once their clinical training years started.[20] Significantly, McCord Hospital also provided a valuable alternative site for black students to do their internship training in Durban. In its smaller, more intimate surroundings, McCord doctors and nurses took great pains to teach students and junior doctors in a variety of medical and surgical wards, as well as in their outpatients' department.[21] This hospital was also unique for policies of non-racialism, its strong service ethic, and promotion of a Christian 'family' ethos amongst its staff and students which encouraged close working relationships amongst different black doctors, but also between white and black doctors, as well as nurses.[22]

Furthermore, Mfanyana J. (Joe) Ndlovu, a Natal graduate and today a practising psychiatrist, chose to do his internship at McCord's because he saw that interns were not only allowed but actively encouraged to take on more work responsibility than they were in other hospitals. Furthermore, at McCord's, he said, working conditions were 'a lot better than King Edward' because it was a smaller hospital and therefore had a stronger morale.

> There was a sense of family, a sense of being very intimate and a lot of comradeship among the interns . . . There were Africans, there were whites and there were Indians at that time . . . My reason for choosing McCord's, yes, I did want to work in a Christian environment, but I think a more overwhelmingly important reason was the fact that I wanted to get more responsibility and a better training. There is absolutely no doubt that you

got better intern training at McCord's than at King Edward or any other place in this province . . . The best internship you would get at McCord's and it has been like that for years.[23]

Besides inferior working conditions at King Edward VIII Hospital, Durban medical graduates recalled experiencing hurtful forms of discrimination whilst in clinical training. This worsened relationships and caused resentment. Fatima Mayet relayed how she and her colleagues, as interns and, later, doctors working on the wards, had to endure the use of separate toilet facilities – a humiliating experience. This practice also extended to the theatres, where black students were not allowed to use the same facilities – such as change-rooms – as their white colleagues. Differences in food quality and quantity for staff based on race, as well as separate overnight sleeping facilities, and separate tea rooms and cafeterias were noted as well at this institution. During the 1950s and early 1960s, the petty nature of apartheid also extended to the requirement that black doctors wear blue name tags, while red ones were worn by whites, which Leo Kuper suggests might have marked a separate 'laundry arrangement, since the doctors live[d] in segregated quarters'.[24] Of course, these discriminatory learning and working conditions were not unique to King Edward and played out at other black teaching hospitals too.[25]

Even salaries were not the same for doctors in public service, which resulted in staff dissatisfaction, especially after the imposition of discriminatory pay increases in the late 1960s. In 1968, Indian and coloured doctors earned approximately 65 per cent of a white doctor's salary, while Africans earned only 55 per cent, despite having the same training and doing the same work. These unequal salaries and poor hospital working conditions led to black doctors' embarking on strike actions at King Edward in 1968 and 1969. Dramatic headlines ('Non-white doctors in big pay revolt: Whites get rise, they get nothing', 'Never same pay for doctors' and 'Pay gap angers doctors') were carried in the press for several months. The go-slow strikes almost crippled King Edward's services until improvements were negotiated with the Natal Provincial Administration (NPA).[26]

A number of medical graduates who had trained in Durban and were either working or doing their postgraduate studies at King Edward participated in the strike. The consequences were extreme for a few, such as B.T. Naidoo and Fatima Mayet, who were labelled as 'agitators' and forced by the NPA to resign. The result of the protest was that the salary structure was reduced from three tiers to two tiers – one for whites and one for blacks. However, it would not be until the early 1980s, after many years of struggle and negotiation, that parity in doctors' salaries was achieved in the public sector.[27] Yet, total compensation packages, including medical aid, pensions, housing subsidies, bonuses and travel allowances, etcetera, were still skewed in favour of white doctors for many years thereafter. King Edward VIII Hospital was truly a microcosm of racial inequalities that played out in South Africa's wider apartheid society, as Jerry Coovadia remembered with frustration about his postgraduate training and working experiences:

> Every level of normal existence was divided between black and white . . . [T]here was no social life that was common. So the only place where we interacted was in our work. We shared the labour of providing a health service, but that was the only interaction . . . And that was also fraught with tension given the fact that our colleagues who were white were earning a higher salary than us . . . There was a huge gulf between them and us.[28]

Students and doctors also had to endure interpersonal racism during the apartheid years whilst based at King Edward. One issue discussed repeatedly by graduates was the refusal of the hospital's white nurses to take orders from black interns and doctors. This point was made by B.T. Naidoo, who remembered that during the late 1950s, when most of the hospital's nurses, and certainly those in senior positions, were white, black doctors were treated as part of the 'lower echelons':

> They didn't give you the respect that a doctor deserves . . . [T]he white sisters . . . wouldn't join you in ward rounds, you know . . . They would always send black nursing sisters to join you on ward rounds or to accept orders from you and they would only come on the ward round when the white consultants or the white junior doctors were there.[29]

Some white matrons and nurses were remembered for being 'bossy' and for 'bullying' black doctors, producing 'huge barriers, psychological and others, between us and the senior white staff'.[30] This was particularly the case from the mid-1950s, when the medical school's first black doctors received their clinical training at King Edward, and then from the late 1950s, when the first black doctors started graduating to work as interns and later doctors at the hospital.

Obviously, these issues did not occur only at King Edward VIII Hospital. Historian Shula Marks has traced the long history of discontent between white nurses and black doctors at other institutions during South Africa's segregation and apartheid eras.[31] Unlike in European settings, where nurses usually occupied a professional position below doctors in the broader medical hierarchy, Marks showed how in South Africa's complex racial order this relationship was inverted in instances where the doctor was black and the nurses were white. Race took precedence over professional status. Increasingly through the 1960s, however, King Edward's nursing staff became African – in line with the apartheid state's separate-development policies – thus paving the way for improved working relationships between King Edward's nursing staff and the mostly black students and doctors who trained and worked on its wards. The transfer of white nurses to white hospitals during this period also helped clear the way up the promotional ladder for black nurses to make their mark.

Some white doctors also humiliated and intimidated black students and doctors on the teaching wards. Bongiwe Bolani vividly recalled one such professor whom she worked with on the obstetrics and gynaecology wards in the 1950s:

> He was a horrible man. He always shouted at the nurses and doctors – everybody . . . He was cruel. He put such terror in people. He screamed, he shouted, he humiliated us, made you feel like imbeciles. He had such a sense of his own importance . . . [H]e treated people badly. I was young then, so his effect on me was enormous. Other people, older white males, terrified me from that time for many years. It took a long time for me to get over it. Many people resigned and left because of him.[32]

Similar cases were also recorded by the Medical Students' Representative Council in 2004. A report documenting alumni's experiences of racism whilst training at the medical school and King Edward Hospital told of how students were shouted at or ignored by consultants 'as if they were children'.[33]

A number of international scholars have argued that medical training often had built into it a difficult 'rite of passage' process which involved the embarrassment and belittlement of students by their superiors. This process supposedly worked to teach students the medical knowledge they required, as well as respect for those senior to them. Furthermore, it was also supposed to help advance individuals from the student status of 'medical boys' to the full adult status upon graduation of 'medical men'.[34] However, this training placed adult student doctors, some of whom were older, already married and had children, in subordinate positions in a hierarchical medical environment. In the apartheid South Africa context, it also infantilised them.[35] Although this humiliating rite of passage in medicine was not unique to South Africa, extra layers of insult were added because of racial hierarchies and inequalities.

What is more, gender discriminations also played out at the clinical training level. As in the earlier years of medical school, women students who reached the latter clinical years were always outnumbered by male colleagues. They found few women consultants to emulate and continued to face sexist attitudes and opinions about their capabilities and roles. Some felt brushed aside or ignored by their clinical instructors on the wards.[36] Others faced greater obstruction in their professional advancement, which included exclusion from supportive male networking groups and channelling of their careers into less prestigious and lower-paying specialities. Women doctors also received lower salaries and reduced benefits once in practice.[37] One woman felt that her professional identity as a doctor on the wards was sometimes questioned by patients because of her gender:

> Some people don't believe . . . that I am a doctor. . . . They would think I'm a nurse . . . I mean, I would be sitting there working with a doctor and maybe he's a junior doctor, but because he's white and I'm there, the patient would say to me, 'Nurse, please tell him what my problem is'.[38]

Indeed, reflecting on their clinical training experiences, some women doctors felt that their skills and knowledge were not taken seriously by many of their male colleagues, even if they were more senior in status. An Indian woman doctor commented:

[M]en, whether they were white, Indian or black [African], were disparaging towards me . . . I had interns [and] medical officers that refused to do investigations because they didn't think it was appropriate even though I was the registrar and said they had to do it . . . We had a hard and long battle.[39]

This questioning of their expertise sometimes extended to black nurses too. While some nurses felt threatened by women doctors, whom they saw as undermining their supportive roles to male doctors, the existence of broad social prejudices which held that men made better doctors, also assisted. In addition, feelings of jealousy in institutional situations where many nurses found spouses amongst male doctors were essential to understanding tensions between female doctors and nurses.[40] In his study of black doctors, Watts found that more than half of the spouses of male medical graduates were from white-collar backgrounds, with medicine and nursing being the most dominant professions.[41]

Though the numbers of women entering medicine were small, the presence of women served to unsettle socially constructed understandings of the profession as a traditionally male preserve. Their achievements also disturbed the stereotypical view that women should be demure and subservient to men. Mamphela Ramphele stood out for her assertiveness, for example. One of her lecturers, Y.K. Seedat, remembered her as a 'very articulate and very fiery' student who was also 'very conscientious as a worker'.[42] She stood up for what she believed in, including opposing male students and professors if she thought they were out of line. Her lecturer in obstetrics and gynaecology, S.B. Pitsoe, agreed that she was 'quite a fighter'. She was 'fiery', 'outspoken' and 'strong' – 'you couldn't do anything to her', he said.[43] Soromini Kallichurum ruffled feathers as one of the first black female professors and the first female dean of the medical school. Reflecting on his long-time colleague, Seedat regarded her 'as more manly than female', as in these powerful positions 'she used to bully people around, especially the males!' To succeed in medicine, many black women felt the need to be assertive and determined, and had to work harder to prove themselves as equals to their male peers. This point was emphasised by Kallichurum, who said she had no difficulty succeeding because she made sure that her male colleagues did not cause her any difficulty: 'Really, that [was] very important . . . you had to be one step ahead of them at all times . . . I always said, "If anybody does the trampling, it's going to be me" . . . You ha[d] to, you know, to survive.'[44]

These women paved the way for larger numbers of women to follow them into the profession of medicine, though the costs could be steep for these early generations, especially for those who decided to go into demanding specialities. In addition to professional glass ceilings that continually had to be smashed along the way, sometimes leading to friction and tensions with their male colleagues, many of these women often felt the need to work extra, long hours to prove themselves in a male world.[45] It was an uphill struggle for them. Besides causing burn-out and relationship difficulties, such as marital problems and other family estrangements, such as with their children, psychologically it would have been a lonely road to travel with few women doctors around to provide them with support. What is more, in an attempt to regulate the profession and justify their success, these early generations of medical women were often regarded by their male peers as having almost 'left the fold of women', as exceptions to the rule and even as 'honorary men'.[46] As Seedat's and Pitsoe's quotations above suggest, it was easier for their male colleagues to accept this view which portrayed women as being changed by their association with a masculine profession, rather than consider the possibility that the profession was being feminised by the presence of women. Therefore, clinical medical experiences were not simply a result of racial discrimination under apartheid, but were also determined by differentials in power between men and women. In the largely white, male-dominated medical profession, interlocking racial and gendered discriminations thus affected the clinical experiences of black doctors in different ways.

'Patients can relate to me': Doctor-patient interactions

Another issue producing ambivalence and contradictions for black student doctors was the experience of working with patients. This was especially the case when patients arrived at hospital having exhausted other popular healing avenues, including self-medication and consultations with 'traditional healers'.[47] During the nineteenth and twentieth centuries, individuals and families living in Durban, as well as in the rest of Africa, sought remedies for a variety of ailments in many places, with hospitals usually being a last resort. A number of historians have provided invaluable research on the long and intricate history of medical pluralism that existed in South Africa both before and after the arrival of Europeans.[48] However, despite being aware of this complex history, the Durban Medical School's lecturers and clinical teachers, with much to prove in an apartheid context, were determined to teach their students using the latest western or scientific medicine approaches in line with those taught at the country's internationally recognised white medical schools. Additionally, they worked hard to steer their students away from what they regarded as the 'dangers' and 'backwardness' of the philosophies and practices of indigenous healers. They wanted to enthuse in their students a firm commitment to what they regarded as the superiority of biomedicine.[49]

Over the years, Durban medical students certainly learnt much in the way of content from their lecturers, but their lecturers' perspectives also rubbed off on them, leading to the internalisation of the biomedical paradigm as the paramount healing approach. In fact, for some students, this perspective was already firmly entrenched before starting their studies. Fatima Mayet, who had attended Wits before studying medicine in Durban in the early 1950s, recalled her 'reluctance to come to this medical school' because of concern for the 'perception' that it was going to be a 'tribal medical school and we would be sort of second grade' when it first opened.[50] It was only once she had been there for a few months that she could see the emphasis her lecturers placed on maintaining the highest biomedical standards, and she could settle into her studies.

For some students, the internalisation of biomedical perspectives and approaches dovetailed with moralising religious beliefs. This promoted, amongst some religiously devout Christian students, for example, uneasiness as well as contemptuous attitudes towards traditional healers and their therapies, which actively led to their discouragement when dealing with patients, as one African graduate highlighted adamantly in an interview:

> [W]ith my religious . . . Christian background, I mean, there are certain things which I just don't believe in. And so, I mean, if patients would come with whatever stories that they come with, I would just discard those and tell them straight that, you know, 'there's nothing like that' and just carry on with . . . what one is trained for . . . [O]ne might . . . say I may have been unfair to patients but . . . I believe in it because I think it's the right way . . . I would just tell the patient, 'You know what? You're just wasting your time. This is what you should be doing.'[51]

Like the devout European missionary doctors who came before them, some student doctors who professed to be Christians placed themselves in the vanguard of the battle against what they regarded as superstitious and 'witchcraft'-based healing practices. On the other hand, their condescending attitudes towards indigenous healers and their non-Christian patients could lead to social distancing in their doctor-patient relationships. Indeed, many factors might have worked against a close doctor-patient relationship for these student doctors. While divergent religious and healing perspectives were key, so were differences that stemmed from educational and gender differences, as we have already seen, as well as personality and maturity. What is more, depending on the case, on occasion Indian and coloured student doctors at King Edward might have had a hard time communicating with their African patients because they came from different sociocultural backgrounds, or because they spoke a different language, thus reducing their levels of empathy. The same would have applied to African student doctors working with Indian or coloured patients, or for that matter, Africans from different ethnic backgrounds too.

Of course, the situation was often more complex in practice during one-on-one interactions. Although some students might not have identified with their patients, and might not have agreed with their healing perspectives, coming from the same or similar sociocultural background could and often did help to improve doctor-patient relationships. So too did being able to speak a patient's language. Because of linguistic similarities between the Nguni languages spoken in South Africa, as well as the propensity of Africans to speak more than one local language, many African students and doctors (as well as nurses) provided vital translation services for their patients on the wards, and for colleagues and even professors who did not speak African languages. This was essential over the years as the majority of patients who used King Edward's services during the apartheid era were African. Many patients, coming to town from rural areas, spoke little English, or none at all. An African doctor provided an example of being able to understand her patients culturally:

> If, for instance, a mother brings a child in who is dehydrated . . . the questions I'm going to ask that mother, I'm asking them because I've got background information. I know . . . where this mother's coming from, I know the environment, I know what generally the communities are using

and therefore I'll be able to ask the relevant questions. And even, you know, assisting the mother [or] educating the mother, I'm in a better position to do so ... And the mother is not going to feel ... you're just talking about something you don't know ... At least he or she can relate to what I'm saying. So I think it helps ... I mean, even now ... I always feel I've got a better standing ... dealing with patients and understanding [them] ... and patients can relate to me.[52]

On the opposite side of the spectrum, other student doctors identified strongly with their patients and were accommodating of their traditional beliefs and practices. Some of these people even came from families where individuals practised as indigenous healers, or whose family members consulted with such healers on a regular basis.[53] Many of these individuals were aware of the psychological value that traditional healing approaches held for easing tensions between individuals within their wider family and community structures. They also appreciated the value of understanding their patients holistically, which indigenous approaches stressed. As a result, some graduates thought it counterproductive to simply brush aside a patient's beliefs. For these students and doctors, the ability to listen carefully to a patient's perspective and provide a firm attempt to accommodate their beliefs was essential to a successful doctor-patient consultation.

May Mashego explained that if patients asked her if they could go home because they needed to perform particular rituals to complete their healing processes, she always considered their requests, and often let them go:

If it's not going to be dangerous for the person to go and that person is taking oral medication, I see no harm in giving a person a pass-out and let them go and do their rituals, because in treating diseases ... [it is also] mental. So if I haven't done what I think should be done, I will not get better.[54]

As this African doctor implied, some traditional healing beliefs and practices gave their patients a psychological sense of security and so a holistic and pragmatic approach was beneficial. Thus, while indigenous healing beliefs and approaches were not actively encouraged at the medical school, some student doctors turned a blind eye to what they considered as 'harmless ritualistic practices' that did not interfere with their biomedical treatment protocols.[55]

Black medical students and doctors were not merely the ideological and practical instruments of a growing biomedical empire in South Africa. They were not simply trained to work in clinical settings to replace indigenous beliefs and practices with western ones. Instead, it could be argued that many of them were positioned both inside and outside the biomedical world: although they had been schooled and worked within the biomedical paradigm, some exhibited a willingness to draw eclectically upon indigenous healing explanatory devices as needed. The internalisation of biomedicine approaches was a complex process which varied from individual to individual and often built upon earlier foundations where belief in the value of indigenous healing approaches was already long established.

The experience of black student doctors offers many interesting insights into the history of biomedicine's operation and impact in South Africa. While in one sense it would be correct to see them as agents of biomedicine, a deeper analysis of their activities helps us to see past any rigid, simplistic and dichotomous healing encounter with supposedly 'modern' and 'progressive' western-trained doctors on the one side, and supposedly 'traditional' and 'backward' patients on the other.[56] Though Durban's black student doctors were trained and worked within the biomedical field, and certainly could and did reinforce situations of asymmetry in the power relationships with their patients, they could and did also act as brokers.[57] These were individuals who straddled and mediated interactions between the different social and medical worlds of those who worked at their teaching hospital and those coming in for treatment. As Mashego tried to explain, using meningitis as an example:

> You've got to explain meningitis in their terms whilst you understand there could be a bacterium here . . . If they explain it in a different term, try and understand what terms they're using and then try and bridge the two . . . negotiate between the two . . . But you have to understand where people are [coming] from [and] how they analyse disease.[58]

The history of South African biomedicine was shaped in complex ways by hybrid interpretations and translations by black students and doctors in practice. Analysis of their training and work in clinical settings therefore highlights how biomedical, clinical, healing spaces were sites of translation, negotiation and debate. These aspiring doctors built on a long history of pluralistic paths to healing in Africa that saw both healers and patients draw on different healing traditions based on their efficacy. Though some of their activities might be viewed by a few as compromised forms of medicine, by taking the middle ground these students and doctors helped overcome patients' scepticism about western forms of medicine and its culturally alien and sanitised clinical environments, and ultimately helped facilitate the spread of western medicine as a popular and effective healing option for black populations.[59] In addition to helping their colleagues and teachers as cultural and linguistic translators, they assisted their patients to better understand unfamiliar scientific diagnostic explanations and treatments in a language and idiom in which they were more familiar.[60] However, while being vital intermediaries in clinical spaces, in the South African medical hierarchy black medical students and doctors were subordinate members who continued to remain racial and professional 'others'.

During the apartheid years, messy uncertainties and hurtful discriminations greatly influenced black students' and doctors' experiences in Durban. The medical school and its main training hospital were contradictory institutions that produced both positive and negative outcomes for those studying and working there. Graduates' oral and written memory narratives about these institutional spaces have provided important information about the hardships they faced, highlighting the many obstacles that had to be overcome if students wanted to graduate. However, not all students graduated. Some obstacles were just too high, and many attempting to complete this long and difficult journey fell by the wayside. Until now, the story of the Durban Medical School has largely been one focused on the stories of those who succeeded. While memories promoting students' successes in line with the nation's triumphant 'struggle' narratives provide uplifting reading in the post-apartheid period, these stylised public memory narratives also conceal a great deal.

Many black students who were granted admission to the medical school did not succeed. This was yet another contradiction of an institution designed for this very purpose. Those students who progressed each year to experience the many discriminations and inequalities discussed so far were the lucky few. Studying the history of the Durban Medical School requires a consideration of its multifarious sides, as well as the selective biases in the way memories are constructed about this place. The many failures that have been airbrushed out of recent celebratory publications should not be forgotten. They are a significant part of the medical school's history too.

'Whole groups of students would be failing . . . and being excluded.'
— Breminand Maharaj

After the Durban Medical School opened its doors in 1951, the years of study that produced the most anxiety in terms of failures were the preliminary and second years. As already established, the preliminary year was introduced as a bridging year to help students who came from disadvantaged educational backgrounds, especially those with inadequate science and English-language preparations needed for medical school. Many students, however, felt that this year was not useful to them. They viewed it as a punishment for coming from Bantu Education schools and saw it as serving to push students out of, not into, medicine.[61] A good example of this was the English I course requirement which, at the University of Natal, was a course in literature. It proved too difficult for many second- or third-language English speakers and accounted for 'more failures than any other premedical subject'.[62] Thus paradoxically, many weaker students, which the preliminary year was designed to help, regularly failed this introductory year of the medical school's teaching programme.[63]

If students managed to pass the preliminary year, the second year of study, with its high volume of work, especially in physiology and anatomy, proved exceedingly difficult too. In her autobiography, Mamphela Ramphele discusses how hard she found dissecting animals, especially 'slimy creatures' like frogs in her physiology class, despite her lecturer's attempts to desensitise her to them by encouraging her to play around with her hand in a bucket full of frogs. One of the compulsory experiments that caused her much distress was the 'pithing of a live frog'. This required destroying its spinal cord by puncturing it with a needle, then dissecting out its calf muscle and conducting tests to measure its muscle function under different conditions. 'There were various stories at Medical School,' she recalled, 'of people whose careers had been frustrated by this particular experiment.'[64] One such student, Matsapola, after whom the experiment became nicknamed, walked away never to be seen again, while the requirement to handle and dissect cadavers in the anatomy class proved too much for some students also.

In fact, the second year of study, with its voluminous course content, was viewed by some professors as 'the sieve with the finest mesh', and produced the highest annual failure rate at the school, with an average of about 40 per cent during the 1950s and 1960s.[65] This caused much apprehension amongst students, as one graduate highlighted: 'I mean, whole groups of students would be failing second year and being excluded . . .'[66] This anxiety was particularly acute amongst African students who had been accepted in larger numbers into the school to meet the 50 per cent admissions quota, but who failed and were excluded in higher numbers over the years. This is reflected in the school's graduation statistics. For the sixteen years from 1957 until 1972 inclusive, on average, fewer than eleven African students graduated per year. Moreover, of 2 413 students who graduated between 1957 and 1994 inclusive, only 804 Africans (about 33%) graduated, with the remaining 67 per cent made up of mostly Indian (1 489, or about 62%) and coloured (120, or about 5%) graduates.[67]

In addition to ill feelings that built up amongst students over the school's skewed admissions quota system (which ultimately failed to produce larger numbers of African graduates as intended), some African students felt that their Indian colleagues were being favoured in some way, and this worsened relations between these two groups. Negative racial stereotypes against Indian students were also prevalent. Bongiwe Bolani, who married a student – Themba Bolani – who attended the medical school during the 1950s, foregrounded these issues. She argued that her husband would discuss these matters exhaustively with his friends, as well as herself. In her opinion, African medical students seemed to think it was mostly Africans who failed at the medical school. Furthermore, she knew of some students 'who did not feel good about Indians'. She said:

> Africans thought Indians were favoured somehow, when Indians passed so well and Africans failed. They were angry and bitter and felt that some mischief was going on. [The issue] of Indian bribery always surfaced – that Indians were bribing the professors in order to pass . . . My husband . . . did not visit with Indians, nor did the others. There was no friendship as such between the students, just a working relationship only.[68]

Far fewer women students finished their studies. Although not an uncommon trend in other medical schools around the country, the lower number of women students graduating did represent a serious problem at Durban's medical school.[69] For example, of the 2 413 students who graduated between 1957 and 1994, only 552 (or 22.88%) women, compared to 1 861 (77.12%) men, successfully completed their degrees. While similar academic problems would have obstructed men's and women's study progress, some women left medical school, or failed to complete their degrees on schedule, because of additional domestic burdens they were forced to bear living off-campus or through early marriage (which sometimes occurred during their studies).[70] For students who practised unprotected sex, this sometimes meant dealing with the extra burdens of unplanned pregnancies too.

This came up for discussion in a special issue on women in medicine published in 1997 in the *South African Medical Journal* recording the experiences of a variety of women doctors who studied and worked in South Africa during the apartheid era. One African doctor, who graduated from the University of the Witwatersrand, poignantly described how her difficulties started when she got married in 1953, the same year she started her medical studies. 'That was when the drama started,' she said. About nine months later, she bore her first son. After returning to medical school to resume her studies in 1955, she fell pregnant again. She spoke of her daughter being born on the morning she was supposed to write her final-year exams. She wrote of her exasperation, the inadequate contraception available to women at the time and the delays in her progress to attain a medical degree:

> [T]here were tears of frustration in my eyes. I had to lose that year as well ... Oh it was so difficult in those days. To put in one of those vaginal rubbers ... they were like condoms, but circular and so hard, and you could not get them in without struggling! You must remember, there were no pills and no injections and there was a husband ... My husband was also a medical doctor, busy with his private practice. Traditionally men are not supposed to care and did not feel obliged to help.[71]

May Mashego also spoke of her experiences of falling pregnant whilst studying in Durban a couple of decades later. With her mother's support, which included taking over childcare responsibilities until she graduated, Mashego was able to complete her medical degree. Although it is impossible to determine to what extent pregnancy influenced the drop-out rate of students, when other issues such as financial and academic difficulties might have been the determining factors, Watts found that of the 690 students admitted to the medical school between 1951 and 1970, there was a higher drop-out rate amongst women students; only 42 per cent of women students, compared to 55 per cent of male students, completed their degrees on schedule.[72] While extra domestic responsibilities really depended on the personal circumstances of the individuals concerned, including how much child-care support they could draw upon, dealing with pregnancies and child-care duties was usually viewed as a woman's responsibility. Coping with the ramifications of an early pregnancy mostly fell on women students and their extended female kin and not on their male partners, especially if pregnant students were not married. For a woman this meant facing the need to drop out of her studies if extended child-care support was not available.[73]

Whatever the causes of the high failure rate and exclusions from the Natal Medical School, large financial debts had to be paid back by students.[74] Students who failed often had little to show for their efforts and had to find low-paying jobs to pay back their loans. This was the case with Themba Bolani, who was excluded from the medical school at the end of 1957 for failing to pass his physiology exam after his second attempt. Once excluded, he gained employment as a clerk in a Durban-area high school, and later became a health inspector for the Durban municipality. He and his wife, who was employed as a nurse at King Edward VIII Hospital at the time, had to struggle for many years to pay back his government bursary-loan.[75] Bongiwe Bolani remembered how for her husband and his colleagues, the pressure to succeed at the medical school was immense, and how his failure nearly destroyed him. 'It was important for him to make something of his life,' she argued, so when he failed

[h]e was very bitter about it. He didn't believe he should have failed. It was very important for his family and people back home in Johannesburg for him to come back a doctor . . . He blamed the professors at the Medical School . . . The medical students used to talk angrily about it when they got together. Many others failed. Some of them went and took up teaching.[76]

Others who failed went on to work in family businesses, or in other white-collar jobs. Some went overseas to study. Once MEDUNSA opened in 1978, some African students even went there to complete their degrees. A number of African students who had failed their medical courses in Durban were accepted into MEDUNSA to try again. Sam Fehrsen argued that many passed at MEDUNSA because of a more supportive study environment that was created to assist disadvantaged African students.[77] This included, for example, increased contact time with their lecturers and the provision of academic bridging or remedial programmes to help students better understand a number of problem subjects such as maths and science. The provision of more generous bursaries, improved student counselling services and better-quality residential facilities also, in his opinion, helped students to cope better with their studies and ultimately succeed. In his position as head of the Department of Family Medicine at MEDUNSA, Fehrsen was able to monitor his students' progress as well as discuss their educational advancement with them. In addition, he felt strongly that African students advanced because they did not experience the added stress of trying to compete with their better-educated Indian and coloured colleagues. In 1982, MEDUNSA graduated its first 34 doctors, and by 1986, 225 students had graduated with an MB ChB degree; in 1987 alone, more than 50 African doctors graduated.[78] Comparatively, as late as 1987, Durban produced only twenty African doctors from its 100 graduates that same year.

For Themba Bolani, just one of the many to be excluded from the medical school over the years, his failure was not merely a personal or private matter. It represented a crushing blow for his family, who had sacrificed so much to get him through. It was a blow also for his wider community, who would have carefully followed his progress with the hope that he would have made something of his life. For these students, having been placed on pedestals and lauded by their communities for their extraordinary achievements to get into medical school, their fall from grace would have been devastating.[79] Bongiwe Bolani captured this aptly in her memories of her husband, who struggled to be positive again after what he regarded as one of his biggest failures:

> I think he got over it in the end. But it did affect him. The sense of failing was great, failing the thing he desired so much . . . It affected him a lot. But he was a good father and his family meant a lot to him and if we were not there he probably would have crumbled and been destroyed in the end . . . [M]edicine was his life-long dream.[80]

The anomalous set-up of Durban's medical school as a state-funded 'non-European' faculty within a white university produced much uncertainty and many inequalities, as well as numerous contradictions for its students. By studying at this school, a small number of black students were given the rare opportunity, though through years of hard work, to enter one of the most esteemed and highest-paying professions in apartheid South Africa. Once they graduated, their clinical work would provide invaluable health-care services for their black communities too. However, arrival at the school, despite the enormous odds of disadvantaged socio-economic and education backgrounds, did not automatically secure their professional success. Instead, it exposed them to further hardships, and forced them to struggle against many obstacles that would thwart the aspirations of many. While there were positive experiences that served to motivate and inspire some, its racially segregated and unequal teaching arrangements, including those at the school's King Edward VIII teaching hospital, saw its students suffer deeply hurtful racial indignities to achieve their goals. They learnt to practise medicine in apartheid conditions that perpetuated racial divisions and inequalities for their patients.

Moving beyond the everyday social and educational issues facing students, the story of the Durban Medical School now shifts to focus on the unique set of circumstances which came together to mould the political outlooks and activities of students at the school on the Durban campus. At the centre of this story was the Alan Taylor Residence. As already discussed, this unusual residence environment forced students coming from different backgrounds to live and study together, and the outcomes were contradictory. Many tensions and deep divisions emerged academically and socially among African, Indian and coloured medical students, who had not interacted with, let alone lived with, people of different races before. However, the discriminatory educational experiences students were forced to endure also resulted in much frustration and dissatisfaction amongst many of the school's students.

Contrary to the government's intentions, this led to the politicisation of many medical students from the late 1960s onwards. They would turn to anti-apartheid political activities as a way to try to address their numerous grievances. Student activism would make the Durban Medical School a vital crucible in the 1970s and 1980s. Of course, in a context of apartheid-induced racial tensions and divisions, discussing this part of the school's history is not a simple matter either. As with students' social and educational experiences, their activities in the political arena were rarely unified, as the next chapter will demonstrate.

Notes

1. For more on the history of King Edward VIII Hospital, see, for example, Isidor Gordon, 'King Edward VIII Hospital: The teaching hospital of the Durban Medical School', *South African Medical Journal* (2 December 1961); and C. Dyer, E.B. Adams, A.M. Seedat and J. Morfopoulos, 'Fifty years at King Edward VIII Hospital, Durban', *South African Medical Journal* (22 November 1986).
2. For more on the history of this hospital, in addition to the above sources, see *The University of Natal Durban Medical School: A Response to the Challenge of Africa* (Durban: Hayne and Gibson, 1954), 23; 'Hospital serves non-whites', *South African Panorama* (February 1962); and UKZNA H6/1/1, Medical School – History, 'University of Natal Medical School twenty-fifth anniversary/Silver Jubilee', 1976.
3. Interview with Jerry Coovadia, Durban, 24 June 2003.
4. UKZN MSA, 'Address by Premier Dr F.T. Mdlalose', Unveiling of plaque, University of Natal Medical School, Durban, 6 December 1995, 2–3. http://www.whoswhosa.co.za/frank-mdlalose-4125.
5. Interview with ZM, Durban, 11 September 2003. Kayser-Fleischer rings are a common symptom of Wilson's disease, a rare inherited disease that occurs mostly in European population groups, where too much copper accumulates in the body's tissues. The excess copper damages the liver and nervous system, and often causes a brown ring to form around the edge of the iris. http://www.nlm.nih.gov/medline plus/ency/article/000785.htm.
6. UKZN MSA, File: Hospitals, Natal, King Edward Hospital, 'It's no go on hospital expansion', *Natal Mercury* (29 July 1971); UKZNA C10/8/1, 'Medical school, teaching hospital and Alan Taylor Residence', UN Council minutes, 16 April 1981, 185; UKZN EGML, 'Crisis at King Edward', *NU Partners* 1, no. 2 (September 1990), 8; and 'Inkosi Albert Luthuli Central Hospital', *Sunday Tribune* (17 December 2000).
7. UKZN MSA, 'Extracts from memorandum for Executive Committee: Hospital facilities for Bantu: State policy', prepared by J. Parker, Natal Director of Hospital Services, attached to Board of the Faculty of Medicine minutes, 26 March 1963.
8. 'King of hospitals is begging for funds', *Natal Mercury* (25 November 1986).
9. For more on the history of Baragwanath, see Simonne J. Horwitz, '"A phoenix rising": A social history of Baragwanath Hospital, Soweto, South Africa, 1942–90' (DPhil. diss., Oxford University, 2006).
10. 'History of MEDUNSA', http://www.medunsa.ac.za/faculties/nsph/nsph_about/about_medunsa1.htm; MA, Principal – Annual Report, MEDUNSA 1989, Report of the Vice-Chancellor and Principal, 3, and MEDUNSA 1990, Report of the Vice-Chancellor and Principal, 12. For more on Ga-Rankuwa's inadequacies, also see MA, MEDUNSA General, Various Publications and Documents, 'The National Assembly Portfolio Committee on Health. Report on Visit to MEDUNSA/Ga-Rankuwa Complex', July 1995, 2–5.
11. UKZN EGML, 'Crisis at King Edward', *NU Partners* 1, no. 2 (September 1990), 8. Also see Y.K. Seedat, 'The health crisis in Natal – A personal view', *South African Medical Journal* (7 July 1990).

12. 'King Edward's daily nightmare', *Daily News* (25 June 1974); and 'The war zone that is King Edward: If you're critically ill the service is excellent', *Sunday Tribune* (16 August 1987).

13. Interview with Janet Giddy, Hillcrest, 24 May 2003. A similar perspective is mentioned in Interview with Y.K. Seedat, Durban, 7 July 2003; and Isobel Shepherd Smith, 'This social disgrace: New-born babies, mothers and pregnant women are forced to sleep on the floor', *Sunday Tribune* (28 July 1985).

14. Interview with Dennis J. Pudifin, Durban, 2 July 2003.

15. Y.K. Seedat, 'The health crisis in Natal – A personal view', *South African Medical Journal* (7 July 1990), 3.

16. Breminand Maharaj, 'University of Natal Medical School submission to the Truth and Reconciliation Commission', 23 June 1997, 5.

17. See Adam Starz, *Between Laughter and Tears* (Ladysmith, RSA: Sinclair Publishing, 1986), 129. For more on the exploitative work conditions of interns in South Africa, see S.F. Oosthuizen, 'The intern year', in *Medical Education in South Africa: Proceedings of the Conference on Medical Education held at the University of Natal Durban in July 1964*, eds John V.O. Reid and Alexander J. Wilcot (Pietermaritzburg: Natal University Press, 1965), 379; V.K.G. Pillay, 'Some thoughts on intern training', *South African Medical Journal* (2 December 1961), 1026–7; and Wits SAHA NAMDA – *Critical Health* Publications, 1980–1992, 'The internship year in South Africa', *Critical Health* 23 (August 1988), 49–52.

18. Interview with B.T. Naidoo, Durban, 10 November 2003. May Mashego, who attended the medical school as a student two decades later, during the late 1970s and early 1980s, and who gave birth to her first child in this labour ward, concurred with Naidoo's assessment that there was no privacy for its patients. Interview with May Mashego, Durban, 14 October 2003.

19. Interviews with B.T. Naidoo, Durban, 15 September 2003; May Mashego, Durban, 14 October 2003; Jerry Coovadia, Durban, 24 June 2003; and 'Institutional hearing: The health sector', in *Truth and Reconciliation Commission of South Africa Report*, Vol. 4 (Cape Town: Juta, 1998).

20. Derk Crichton, 'The clinical work of the Department of Gynaecology and Obstetrics of the University of Natal during 1957: A brief review', reprinted from *Medical Proceedings* 4, no. 19 (20 September 1958).

21. CC MH Box 7 Series II Medical Superintendent Reports 1956 to 1962, Annual Reports of McCord Hospital, 1957, 1960 and 1962.

22. Leo Kuper, *An African Bourgeoisie: Race, Class, and Politics in South Africa* (New Haven, CT, and London: Yale University Press, 1965), 239, 243. Similar arguments were raised in Interviews with ZM, Durban, 11 September 2003; Steve Reid, Hillcrest, 24 May 2003; and Sam Fehrsen, Pretoria, 22 August 2003. Steve Reid and Sam Fehrsen did their internships at McCord's in 1985 and 1963 respectively.

23. Interview with Mfanyana J. Ndlovu, Durban, 14 August 2003.

24. Kuper, *An African Bourgeoisie*, 239–240.

25. Wits, FHSR M3/40 Internal Reconciliation Commission, 1998, Jules Browde, Patrick Mokhoba and Essop Jassat, 'University of the Witwatersrand Faculty of Health Sciences Internal Reconciliation Commission Report' (November 1998), 13–4.

26. UKZN MSA, 'Non-white doctors in big pay revolt: Whites get rise, they get nothing', *Natal Mercury* (11 July 1968); '"Never" same pay for doctors: Professor called "agitator"', *Daily News* (23 April 1969); 'Pay gap angers doctors', *Daily News* (2 December 1970). For more on this issue, also see UKZNA C10/1/1, 'Differential salary scales for non-whites: Faculty of Medicine', UN Council minutes, 15 March 1968; UKZNA C10/2/1, 'Revision of non-white salary scales: Medical school', UN Council minutes, 23 March 1972; M. Horrell, *The African Homelands of South Africa*, (Johannesburg: South African Institute of Race Relations, 1973), 165; UKZN MSRC, Meeting of the Executive Committee, 28 July 1997, Committee Room, Mpala House, Medical School, 'University of Natal Medical School Submission to the Truth and Reconciliation Commission', 23 June 1997; and Browde, Mokhobo and Jassat, 'University of Witwatersrand Faculty of Health Sciences, Internal Reconciliation Commission Report', 14–5.

27. 'Elimination of salary discrimination on the basis of race', *South African Medical Journal* (18 July 1981), 82; and Wits FHSR M3/40 Internal Reconciliation Commission, 1998, 'Preliminary Submission to the Truth and Reconciliation Commission from the Faculty of Health Sciences, University of the Witwatersrand', submitted by Max Price (Dean) on behalf of the faculty, 23 May 1997, 9, 13.

28. Interview with Jerry Coovadia, Durban, 24 June 2003.

29. Interview with B.T. Naidoo, Durban, 15 September 2003. Similar views were expressed in an Interview with S.B. Pitsoe, Durban, 17 June 2003. Also see Hilda Kuper, 'Nurses', in *An African Bourgeoisie: Race, Class, and Politics in South Africa*, Leo Kuper (New Haven, CT, and London: Yale University Press, 1965), 240–1; and Padraig O'Malley Interview with Albertina Luthuli, 10 January 1993, http://www.nelsonmandela.org/omalley/index.php/site/q/03lv00017.htm.

30. Interview with Jerry Coovadia, Durban, 24 June 2003; Watts, 'Black doctors. Part II: The graduates', 19, 34.

31. Shula Marks, *Divided Sisterhood: Race, Class and Gender in the South African Nursing Profession* (Johannesburg: Witwatersrand University Press, 1994), 59–60, 140. Also see Helen Sweet and Anne Digby, 'Race, identity and the nursing profession in South Africa, c. 1850–8', in *New Directions in the History of Nursing: International Perspectives*, eds S. McGann and B. Mortimer (London: Routledge, 2004).

32. Interview with Bongiwe Bolani, Durban, 1 May 1999.

33. See Ali Modiba, 'MSRC Racism Report presented to the faculty and students of the University of Natal, Nelson R. Mandela School of Medicine', 26 September 2004, 3–4, Interviews with TM, Pretoria, 21 August 2003, and B.T. Naidoo, Durban, 15 September 2003; and Watts, 'Black doctors. Part I: The students', 40.

34. For more on the medical doctor socialisation process, see, for example, Howard S. Becker, Blanche Geer, Everett C. Hughes and Anselm L. Strauss, *Boys in White: Student Culture in Medical School* (Chicago and London: University of Chicago

Press, 1961); Eileen C. Shapiro and Leah M. Lowenstein, eds, *Becoming a Physician: Development of Values and Attitudes in Medicine* (Cambridge, MA: Ballinger Publishing, 1979).

35. See Robert Morrell, 'Of boys and men: Masculinity and gender in southern African Studies', *Journal of Southern African Studies* no. 4 (December 1998).

36. Interviews with May Mashego, Ashburton, 18 October 2003, and Veronica Wilson, Durban, 6 November 2003.

37. Elizabeth Walker, 'The South African Society of Medical Women, 1951–92: Its origins, nature and impact on white women doctors' (PhD diss., University of the Witwatersrand, 1999); Beryl Unterhalter, 'Discrimination against women in the South African medical profession', *Social Science and Medicine* 20 (1985), and 'Shattering the male monopoly: The history and struggle of female doctors', *The Leech* 62, no. 3 (November 1993).

38. Interview with May Mashego, Durban, 7 October 2003.

39. Interview with MA, Durban, 23 September 2003.

40. Interviews with May Mashego, Ashburton, 18 October 2003, and Bongiwe Bolani, Durban, 1 May 1999.

41. Watts, 'Black doctors. Part II: The graduates', 5.

42. Interview with Y.K. Seedat, Durban, 14 July 2003.

43. Interview with S.B. Pitsoe, Durban, 17 June 2003.

44. Interview with Soromini Kallichurum, Durban, 29 May 1999. Also see Mamphela Ramphele, *Across Boundaries: The Journey of a South African Woman Leader* (New York: Feminist Press, 1995), 71, 175–7; Mamphela Ramphele, 'The dynamics of gender within black consciousness organisations: A personal view', in *Bounds of Possibility: The Legacy of Steve Biko and Black Consciousness*, eds Barney Pityana, Mamphela Ramphele, Malusi Mpumlwana and Lindy Wilson (Cape Town: David Philip; London and Atlantic Highlands, NJ: Zed Books, 1991), 219–20; Interviews with K. Goonam, Durban, 13 October 1997, and May Mashego, Durban, 7 October 2003.

45. Interviews with Fatima Mayet, Durban, 4 June 1999, and Veronica Wilson, Durban, 6 November 2003.

46. Interview with May Mashego, Durban, 7 October 2003. Also see Lucy M. Candib, 'How medicine tried to make a man out of me', in *Women in Medical Education: An Anthology of Experience,* ed. Delese Wear (Albany, NY: State University of New York Press, 1996); and Regina Morantz-Sanchez, *Conduct Unbecoming a Woman: Medicine on Trial in Turn-of-the-Century Brooklyn* (New York and Oxford: Oxford University Press, 1999), 8.

47. I am keenly aware of the problematic, ahistorical and static usage of terms such as 'traditional healer', which have often been used simplistically and in oppositional ways – 'western' being more scientific, modern and superior, and 'traditional' being more superstitious, backward and inferior – to examine different healing traditions. Many scholars have shown how both these healing systems are cultural artefacts that have evolved in specific historical contexts, have actually involved much ideological and practical overlap and borrowings, are both dynamic and

changing healing traditions, and are not homogeneous entities but made up of diverse healing approaches. Tracy J. Luedke and Harry G. West, eds, *Borders and Healers: Brokering Therapeutic Resources in Southeast Africa* (Bloomington and Indianapolis: Indiana University Press, 2006).

48. See, for example, Anne Digby, *Diversity and Division in Medicine*, especially chapters eight and nine; Julie Parle, *States of Mind: Searching for Mental Health in Natal and Zululand, 1868–1918* (Pietermaritzburg: University of KwaZulu-Natal Press, 2007); and Karen Flint, *Healing Traditions: African Medicine, Cultural Exchange, and Competition in South Africa, 1820–1948* (Athens, OH: Ohio University Press; Pietermaritzburg: University of KwaZulu-Natal Press, 2008).

49. Unlike the western paradigm that focuses on science-based 'germ theory' as the underlying cause of diseases, African 'traditional' healing approaches explain illnesses using both natural and supernatural (spiritual) causes. For a useful summary and comparative analysis of the work of indigenous healers, western doctors and their healing beliefs and practices, see Digby, *Diversity and Division in Medicine*, chapter 7.

50. Interview with Fatima Mayet, Durban, 4 June 1999.

51. Interview with KM, Durban, 14 November 2003.

52. Interview with KM, Durban, 14 November 2003.

53. See, for example, M.W. Makgoba, *Mokoko: The Makgoba Affair: A Reflection on Transformation* (Florida Hills, RSA: Vivlia Publishers, 1997).

54. Interview with May Mashego, Ashburton, 18 October 2003.

55. For more on this, also see Watts, 'Black doctors. Part II: The graduates', 42–3.

56. Frederick Cooper, 'Conflict and connection: Rethinking colonial African history', *American Historical Review* 99, no. 5 (December 1994); and Frederick Cooper and Ann Laura Stoler, eds, *Tensions of Empire: Colonial Cultures in a Bourgeois World* (Berkeley, Los Angeles and London: University of California Press, 1997).

57. For more on African health workers as cultural brokers, see, for example, Nancy Rose Hunt, *A Colonial Lexicon: Of Birth Ritual, Medicalization, and Mobility in the Congo* (Durham and London: Duke University Press, 1999); Anne Digby and Helen Sweet, 'Nurses as culture brokers in twentieth-century South Africa', in *Plural Medicine, Tradition and Modernity, 1800–2000*, ed. Waltraud Ernst (London and New York: Routledge, 2001); and Luedke and West, eds, *Borders and Healers*.

58. Interview with May Mashego, Ashburton, 18 October 2003.

59. Megan Vaughan, *Curing their Ills: Colonial Power and African Illness* (Cambridge: Polity Press, 1991), 25; and Digby and Sweet, 'Nurses as cultural brokers', 113–4.

60. Interview with TM, Pretoria, 21 August 2003.

61. Interviews with ZM, Durban, 11 September 2003, and S.B. Pitsoe, Durban, 17 July 2003.

62. W.R.G. Branford, 'Examination systems and selection: The experiences of the admissions committee of the Board of the Faculty of Medicine, University of Natal', in *Medical Education in South Africa: Proceedings of the Conference on Medical Education held at the University of Natal Durban in July 1964*, eds John V.O. Reid

and Alexander J. Wilcot (Pietermaritzburg: University of Natal Press, 1965), 191, 194, 196.

63. I. Gordon, 'Experience in the establishment of a medical school for non-white undergraduate students in South Africa', in *Medical Education in South Africa: Proceedings of the Conference on Medical Education held at the University of Natal Durban in July 1964*, eds John V.O. Reid and Alexander J. Wilcot, (Pietermaritzburg: University of Natal Press, 1965), 295.

64. Ramphele, *Across Boundaries*, 51–2.

65. See J.V.O. Reid, 'A study of second-year examination', in *Medical Education in South Africa: Proceedings of the Conference on Medical Education held at the University of Natal Durban in July 1964*, eds John V.O. Reid and Alexander J. Wilcot (Pietermaritzburg: University of Natal Press, 1965), 184.

66. Interview with Breminand Maharaj, Durban, 10 June 2003.

67. See graph in appendix based on the Faculty of Medicine's 1957–94 statistics.

68. Interview with Bongiwe Bolani, Durban, 1 May 1999.

69. For more on this issue, see Unterhalter, 'Discrimination against women in the South African medical profession' and 'Shattering the male monopoly: The history and struggle of female doctors'; and Liz Walker, 'The colour white: Racial and gendered closure in the South African medical profession', *Ethnic and Racial Studies* 28, no. 2 (March 2005).

70. Some students married whilst still studying or doing their internship year, producing extra domestic responsibilities for them. Interviews with Soromini Kallichurum, Durban, 29 May 1999, and Fatima Mayet, Durban, 4 June 1999. See also Nophasika Maforah, 'Black, married, professional and a woman: Role conflicts?' *Agenda* 18 (1993), 5–7.

71. 'Interviews: South African women doctors speak', Special Issue on Women in Medicine, *South African Medical Journal* (November 1997), 1565.

72. Watts, 'Black doctors: Part I. The students', 37–8.

73. See research conducted by Rowena Martineau, 'Women and education in South Africa: Factors influencing women's educational progress and their entry into traditionally male-dominated fields', *The Journal of Negro Education* 66, no. 4 (Autumn, 1997), 391–3; and Ann Perry, *A Study of the Employment Experiences and Attitudes to Employment among African Secondary School Leavers in Durban* (Johannesburg: South African Institute of Race Relations, September 1974), 18–9.

74. Reid, 'A study of second-year examinations', 184; and Watts, 'Black doctors. Part I: The students', 12, 40.

75. For more on Bongiwe Bolani's life story, see Janet Lea Twine, '"I'm just an ordinary nurse": A life history of Matron Bongiwe Bolani' (Honours thesis, University of Natal, 1997).

76. Interview with Bongiwe Bolani, Durban, 1 May 1999.

77. MA, MEDUNSA Yearbook, 1994/95, 'MEDUNSA – the background', 11; Interview with Sam Fehrsen, Pretoria, 22 August 2003; and Interview with ZM, Durban, 11 September 2003.

78. L. Taljaard, 'An historical overview: MEDUNSA and black medical education', *Journal of the Dental Association of South Africa* 42, no. 10 (October 1987), 585 and UWC MAC; MEDUNSA, 1989, 'Prof. rides the "white elephant" to glory', *Pace* (April 1988), 62.
79. Interviews with KM, Durban, 14 November 2003; ZM, Durban, 6 October 2003; and Veronica Wilson, Durban, 6 November 2003.
80. Interview with Bongiwe Bolani, Durban, 1 May 1999.

CHAPTER 6

The 1950s and 1960s
Medical students and the anti-apartheid struggle in Durban

'I learnt to be an activist at medical school.'

— May Mashego

Claims have been made in numerous post-apartheid commemorative publications that the students of the Durban Medical School were a united entity that successfully overcame the adversities of apartheid and produced 'leaders who were in the forefront of the struggle for political freedom in South Africa'.[1] Analysed more carefully, the history of the medical students' involvement in politics was much less certain. While it is clear that a number of students did get involved in extracurricular political activities to tackle their many grievances, which will form the subject of the next chapter, others tried actively to keep their heads down and remain out of politics. An exclusive focus on memories that promote 'unity-in-adversity' struggle narratives for graduates of the school are only one side of a much messier, though interesting, history.

So far, the story has touched on the many racial, class and gender tensions and divisions that played out in this school's changing student body during apartheid. Attention in this chapter focuses on how students responded to the numerous forms of discrimination they faced whilst studying at the medical school, starting with an examination of some of the reasons for the lower level of political activism in the 1950s and early 1960s, and moving on to consider the factors propelling greater numbers of students to get involved in politics by the late 1960s. As will become clear, within the realm of politics too, student activities were ambiguous and could both reflect and oppose apartheid influences.

Students' involvement in anti-apartheid organisations

'Apathy and indifference ... makes for a disunited ... body of individuals.'

— V.R. Makgalomele

Over the years, medical students in Durban have been involved in a variety of extracurricular activities. Depending on the year and level of interest, a quick perusal of student publications reveals how students either led or participated in different organised activities, including, for example, drama, dancing and debating clubs, a students' clinic, a medical women's cultural group, a science society, a Students' Christian Association (SCA), a choir, a film society and numerous sports clubs, such as rugby, soccer, tennis and athletics.[2] However, when turning to the issue of their involvement in political activities during the 1950s and early-1960s period, things were less clear-cut.

Although some medical students might have been members of or sympathised with the aims and activities of anti-apartheid political organisations, few publicly involved themselves in activities of the major political organisations in operation at the time. This was despite a long history of black doctors who had in earlier times actively involved themselves in anti-apartheid politics, such as A.B. Xuma and James S. Moroka, succeeding presidents of the African National Congress (ANC) through the 1940s and early 1950s, or G.M. Naicker and Yusuf Dadoo, leaders of the Natal and Transvaal branches of the South African Indian Congress, to mention but a few.[3]

Two examples of students who were involved in political activities at this time included Albertina Luthuli, the daughter of Chief Albert Luthuli who was elected president of the ANC in 1952. Albertina Luthuli remembered how her father's election coincided with her first year at the medical school, as well as with the Defiance Campaign, a political campaign organised by the ANC which sought to build alliances with different race groups to fight apartheid. The campaign was a coordinated and mass defiance effort, involving protest rallies, demonstrations, stay-at-home strikes and voluntary arrests. It was an opportunity for many thousands of South Africans to publicly voice their opposition to apartheid laws and regulations.[4] Though little political action was actually made by medical students at this time, she recalled how most tried at least to stay informed of events going on around them:

> As medical students we often followed a lot of my father's meetings, especially those he addressed in Durban Square, off what was then Grey Street. He would tell people about the situation in our country and the need to do something about it. Those years were spent mainly growing the ANC.[5]

The Defiance Campaign ended in a wave of arrests by the government and the promulgation of a number of new security laws intended to suppress resistance to apartheid.

Another medical student who involved himself actively in party politics at this time, despite the many risks, was Dan Ncayiyana, who studied at the medical school during the late 1950s. He was arrested in the early 1960s for his association with the Pan-Africanist Congress (PAC).[6] This organisation, which had been formed in 1959, over four decades after the formation of the ANC, was banned by the state, as was the ANC, in 1960, following a period of heightened opposition to the apartheid state and the state's vicious containment of Sharpeville anti-pass demonstrations that resulted in the deaths of 69 people by police shooting. Sam Fehrsen, a UCT-trained doctor who was working as an intern at McCord Hospital in Durban during the early 1960s, and knew Ncayiyana, spoke of the stresses of the time for black political activists:

> People were being locked up all around us ... And so we were involved with the people in jail, taking them parcels and things like that ... [I]t was a very tense time. Whenever there was trouble, they just locked up all the leaders, you know, the student leaders in the university, whether they were involved or not ... Dan Ncayiyana was boarding with us ... [at] McCord's. So there would be like lunchtime off to the cells to go and deliver some food to the guys and we would come back.[7]

Eventually, after a Durban judge granted him bail, Ncayiyana left South Africa and made his way to the Congo, where he was stationed for a while as a PAC representative. He then resumed his studies at a medical school in the Netherlands, later settling in the United States with his family, where he pursued an advanced medical degree and opened a private practice. In 1988, he returned to the Transkei, where he helped develop a medical school at the University of the Transkei, becoming its first dean.[8]

The late 1950s and early 1960s was a period of intense state repression which saw nationwide imprisonment or exile of a whole generation of prominent anti-apartheid leaders in political organisations like the ANC and PAC, whose organisations were banned and forcibly pushed underground.[9] These repressive measures left a noticeable above-ground political void, except within the framework of government-sanctioned structures such as the Bantustan homeland authorities. Even discussing politics was a high-risk activity for black South Africans, as a barrage of oppressive state legislation, including the Riotous Assemblies Act (1956), the Unlawful Organisations Act (1960), the Sabotage Act (1962), the General Law Amendment Act (1966) and the Terrorism Act (1967), for example, silenced many. During the 1960s, the police were granted almost unlimited powers of arrest and detention, and insidiously recruited an army of black informers with pay-offs or threats. Many people even suspected of political activities were harassed or detained (often without trial and for lengthy periods of time), while others were served with banning orders, placed under house arrest or banished to remote areas. Many individuals also lost their lives in detention.

The state's overt and covert activities promoted a climate of fear and mistrust in black communities, which effectively paralysed above-ground political activities.[10] B.T. Naidoo, who completed his undergraduate medical degree in Durban in 1957 and stayed on into the early 1960s to do postgraduate studies, remembered that medical students were negatively affected by this repressive political climate. For the most part, students were not directly involved in politics. He said:

> You must remember at that time . . . the state was very powerful and as soon as you uttered something they just swatted you down or they marked you. So people were very circumspect at that stage . . . [Many political organisations] were quietened and they went underground . . . [T]here was a regular [police] visit to campus and we were all suspicious that there were plants on the campus . . . [W]e were very much aware of certain people who might have been informers . . . And this of course quietened us down.[11]

In a context where political obstacles and state repression seemed formidable, fear was a strong motivator influencing many students to keep the focus on their medical studies. Minding their own business and remaining out of politics seemed the safest option when involvement produced such severe consequences.

Lack of student involvement in political matters is also evident in comments made in students' publications from the time, comments that contrast starkly with student writings and activities in the 1970s and 1980s. A strong concern with organisational indifference and detachment was noted repeatedly in the student newsletter, *The Amoeba*, published in the 1950s. In one edition it was recorded: 'The story of student organisation at our school is as uninspiring as it is challenging. It is a chapter of inevitable failures and frustrations.'[12] In another edition a student editor asserted: 'We are of the opinion that we ourselves are more often at fault than not. In our characters, in our very personalities, in our everyday dealings with one another, there is that apathy and indifference that makes for a disunited, opinionless, spineless body of individuals.'[13] Leo Kuper, a professor of sociology who conducted research on African professionals in the 1950s and 1960s, maintained that Durban 'medical students seem fairly content with the academic situation, or at any rate their dissatisfactions have not yet developed into protracted strikes and demonstrations'.[14]

Other factors also reduced student political involvement at this time. Recording the history of the University of Natal, Edgar Brookes argued that 'amazed gratitude' amongst early students might have mitigated protests, as many medical students did not want to jeopardise a unique opportunity that was being offered to them on their newly built Umbilo Road campus.[15] Student numbers were small in the early years too, weakening any strong oppositional stance based on the numbers game. The fact that students came to the medical school with different socio-economic backgrounds and interests might also explain some students' apathy. Some students' families were not politically inclined and encouraged their children to stay out of politics.[16] The gruelling nature of their schedule, which saw most hours in a student's day occupied with lectures, laboratory work or clinical work, also left little time for involvement in extracurricular activities.[17]

Furthermore, the first generations of medical students were under enormous pressure to succeed academically. Many families had struggled a great deal to find the money to send them to medical school. This gave many students a strong sense of familial duty to get on with their medical training. Others feared losing hard-won scholarships and bursaries if they got involved in politics, as B.T. Naidoo pointed out: 'You must remember we were on scholarships or bursaries and the threat was that if you were involved in any of these things, you know, you'd lose them and you'd be kicked out. So . . . [in] that way they silenced quite a lot of activities.'[18] Medical students' career prospects were also more favourable than those of black students studying in the humanities or social sciences. During these early years, most of these university students trained as teachers, an occupation that offered meagre financial rewards and declining prestige after the introduction of the Bantu Education system.[19] If medical students managed to avoid distractions and passed each year, an elevated social status and comparatively higher financial rewards awaited them after graduation, especially for those who entered private practice. Graduates could then, in turn, help to improve the quality of life of their families who had helped to support them through medical school for so many years.

For those students who did get involved in politics, the choice was often a difficult one between balancing the altruistic interests of helping their wider communities – which involvement in anti-apartheid political activities sought to advance – and obtaining potential success as an individual in what could be a profitable profession.[20] Of course, the high drop-out rate of students who were politically active introduced a further ambiguity for those making this choice, as failure – for whatever reason – served to undermine their future ability to provide desperately needed health-care services to 'their own communities' too.

Medical students and the students' representative council

While the above factors help to explain the tendency for most medical students to steer away from involvement in politics (at least publicly anyway), it is essential to note that a couple of issues did rally students into action during this early period. One entailed the struggle during the 1950s to get the university to recognise officially the existence of a separate students' representative council (SRC) from the other SRCs that existed at the University of Natal at the time. These included two white SRCs (which represented the Howard College and Pietermaritzburg campuses), and the University of Natal's 'Non-European' SRC (UNNE SRC), which was created in 1948.[21] Although medical students had been encouraged to join the UNNE SRC, arguments were made that it did not adequately represent their interests.[22] Its student leaders were based in other locations – either the Marian Buildings or Sastri College buildings – far from the Umbilo Road medical campus, which made it difficult to attend meetings. What is more, it tended to be dominated by students studying in the humanities and social sciences.[23] Although little progress was made by medical students for many years, B.T. Naidoo remembered how a medical students' representative council, which fell under the general umbrella of the UNNE SRC, was eventually formed towards the end of his undergraduate studies to try to deal specifically with medical students' issues.[24]

The issue that eventually brought forward momentum on this matter and engaged the school's students in protests was the state's attempts to pass through Parliament the contentious Separate University Education Bill in 1957. The bill, in addition to calling for the closure of white universities to black students and the creation of new black university colleges to accommodate them, advocated the removal of the black medical school from the white University of Natal and the closure of the university's 'non-European' section. A variety of individuals and organisations protested loudly and very publicly, including black medical students who came out to support the declaration of their white lecturers to resign en masse. Soromini Kallichurum, a final-year student at the time, recalled how hard 'the staff fought to keep this place' and how students protested by 'walk[ing] around the streets [and] making a noise' with placards, as well as writing letters to gain support for their cause.[25] However, while the many protest actions ultimately helped save the medical school, the passage of this Act through Parliament in 1959 led to the closure of the university's 'non-European' section. The numbers of black students studying at Natal dwindled and those registered were allowed to finish off their degrees. However, what this action did lead to was that black medical students finally gained a stronger voice on the 'non-European' SRC, which from the early 1960s onwards effectively became the representative council of medical students.

During the 1950s and 1960s, black SRC students tended to focus their attention on the university's role in perpetuating racial inequalities. Complaints about and boycotts against the poor quality and insufficient quantity of food served to students at the Alan Taylor Residence (ATR) and at the medical school's canteen were good examples of this.[26] Annual graduation boycotts provided another occasion of student opposition. The boycotting of graduation ceremonies had been initiated some years earlier by non-medical black students who objected to the segregated and inferior conditions they were required to study in at the University of Natal. Now it became a form of protest for medical students also. From the late 1950s onwards, when the first medical students started graduating, some students chose to boycott this celebratory occasion.[27] The aim was to protest against the practice of racial separation and discrimination in education, which included segregated seating arrangements at the earlier graduation ceremonies.[28] The graduation boycott, which often included picketing by graduates, was an embarrassment to the University of Natal. It also represented a great sacrifice for students (and their parents) as it was a significant milestone in their lives, particularly for black students who had succeeded despite years of struggle to achieve their educational goals.

The Natal Medical School was the 'home of black consciousness'

During the 1960s, medical student representatives on the 'non-European' SRC in Durban came to play a more prominent role as members of the National Union of South African Students (NUSAS).[29] Formed initially in 1924 as a university student organisation open to white students nationally through their SRCs, and with its headquarters at UCT and Wits, over time NUSAS opened its membership to all university students from across the country.[30] Since students would become the country's future leaders, NUSAS encouraged students to be informed about broader political and social issues in South Africa, and promoted amongst students, especially at their national conferences, the 'free discussion of the vital questions of the day'.[31] By the 1940s, its development as a multiracial student organisation that promoted racial tolerance and cooperation, and its attempts to represent the interests and fight for the educational rights of university students attracted growing numbers of black students. A crucial moment for NUSAS was the role it played in galvanising student support and encouraging student protests against the Separate University Education Bill in 1957.

Nevertheless, despite its noble aims and strident oppositional voice, which saw many of its leaders harassed, beaten up and even arrested by the security police in the late 1950s, by the 1960s NUSAS had effectively become a national organisation of English-speaking white students, with only a few black SRC representatives.[32] This occurred for a number of reasons. Firstly, as a form of protest against the lack of academic freedom at their black institutions, students at the universities of Fort Hare and Durban-Westville refused to form SRCs. This effectively removed their presence through elected SRC representatives at NUSAS events. Secondly, other black campuses, which were allowed to have SRCs, were forbidden by their universities from sending delegations to NUSAS conferences or to partake in NUSAS activities. The University of Natal was one of the few campuses that allowed its black students to participate in NUSAS activities.

By the late 1960s, however, black students represented at NUSAS felt increasingly frustrated and disillusioned by what they considered the organisation's white-dominated liberal and reformist politics. For these students, NUSAS essentially helped to maintain the status quo, and did not go far enough in promoting the interests and needs of black students in apartheid South Africa.[33] Moreover, they objected vociferously to the indignities they were forced to endure in segregated housing arrangements at the annual NUSAS conferences. In March 1967, for example, in a letter addressed to John Sprack (a white NUSAS leader), Steve Biko, who introduced himself as the 'Wentworth chairman of NUSAS', wrote that his Durban medical campus was 'a very uncompromising campus' and that students felt a growing 'hostility to NUSAS' because of unequal treatment they continued to receive at the hands of this organisation.[34]

In December 1968, after many months had passed and nothing substantial had been done to address their grievances, black student leaders from across the country organised and met separately at a conference held in Mariannhill, near Durban. At this conference, they agreed to form a breakaway student organisation. This new organisation, the South African Students' Organisation (SASO), was formally inaugurated the following year at another conference held at the University of the North (or Turfloop), in July 1969. Medical students from Durban who attended and played a pivotal role at this 1969 conference included Steve Biko, who was elected SASO's first president, Aubrey Mokoape, Keith Mokoape, Vuyelwa Mashalaba and J. Goolam (who, like Biko, had been a NUSAS branch chairman at the medical school).[35] In addition, this organisation's first general students' council was hosted by Natal medical students at their ATR in Wentworth a year later.

A large amount of research has been done on the history of SASO, the Black Consciousness Movement (BCM) and the broader collection of pro-black organisations (including the Black People's Convention [BPC], the

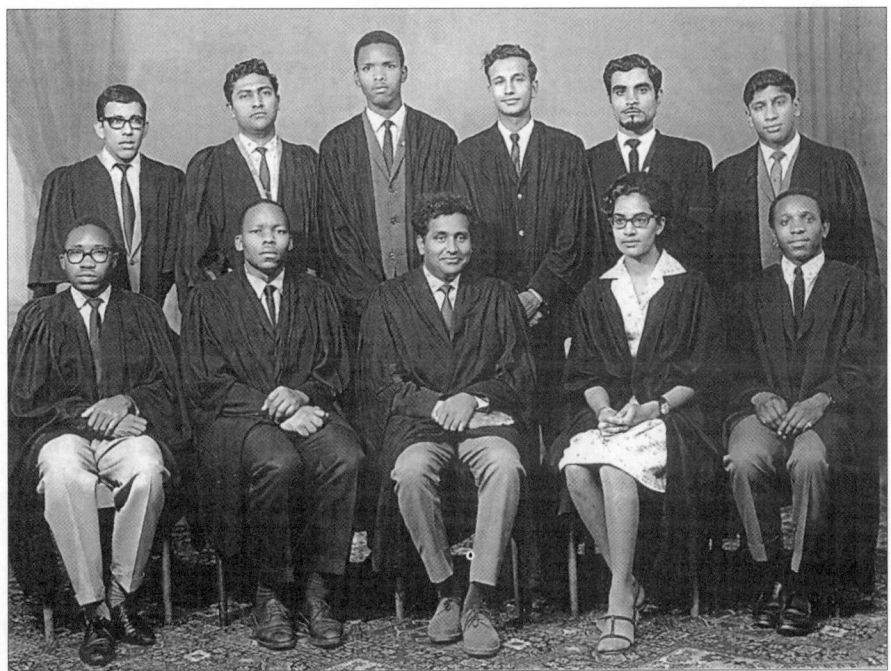

Photo 6.1   Members of the 1966 Medical School SRC.
Back row: N. Soni, D.P. David, B.S. Biko, S.M. Naidoo, R.P. Juggatt,
K.S. Govender
Front row: V.S. Ramasuola, B. Ngubane (Vice President), R. Pillay (General
Secretary), J. Mosendane (Treasurer).
(*UKZN Medical School Archives*)

Black Community Programmes [BCP] and the Black Women's Federation)
that grew out of this.[36] Here the focus is on SASO's early emergence from
and central connection to medical students studying in Durban. For these
students, the ATR became a fulcrum of student anti-apartheid politics
during the late 1960s and through the 1970s. In fact, in 1971, a student
writing for the *Wits Student* newsletter recorded that Durban's 'UNB
[University of Natal Black Section] is the centre of SASO, whose aim is the
consolidation of blacks into a power group which will be able to negotiate
with the white power bloc'.[37] Steve Reid, a graduate of UCT Medical
School and now the Director and Glaxo-Wellcome Chair of primary health
care at UCT's Faculty of Health Sciences, concurred: 'Some of the leading
lights in the Black Consciousness Movement were medical students in
Durban.'[38]

SASO emerged in the late-1960s period for a variety of reasons that extended beyond the specific conditions that existed at the Durban Medical School. Many of the SASO generation of students, who surfaced as the key challengers to the state, had been too young to have witnessed the harsh repressions of the late 1950s and early 1960s. As a result, unlike their parents' generation, they were not completely intimidated by the power of the apartheid state. Scholars like Saleem Badat argue that these students thus felt heightened anger towards the inequalities and discriminations they experienced, and frustrated and impatient with what they viewed as the general apathy and acquiescence of their parents' generation.[39] Maila J. Matjila, who studied medicine during the early 1970s, also felt that generally, as a group, students had fewer social responsibilities, such as wives and children, to support. They thus had much less to lose and this enabled them to be less restrained in their thoughts and actions.[40]

On the other hand, while it is true that many students might have had fewer social responsibilities, one could argue that black students were in many ways more emotionally mature than their privileged white counterparts. This may have inclined them to greater social awareness as they had been forced to grow up quickly under the harsh realities of apartheid. Mamphela Ramphele, whose student days in Durban overlapped with Matjila's, made this point strongly in her autobiography: 'I believe that growing up under apartheid promoted premature ageing. One's childhood, adolescence and young adulthood were knocked out of one very rudely. One either grew up and survived, or was destroyed along the way.'[41]

In a highly repressive political climate, education was viewed by many black families as one of the few chances for their children to escape the ever-widening cycle of poverty and hardship into which so many black South Africans were trapped. This is reflected in educational statistics collected from the time as, despite the apartheid state's creation of separate and unequal facilities for different black population groups after 1959, there was a considerable increase in enrolments at black tertiary institutions. For example, between 1960 and 1965, enrolments at black tertiary institutions increased by almost 400 per cent, doubled between 1965 and 1970, and increased more than 100 per cent between 1970 and 1976.[42] Also, by 1970, 92 per cent of black students were studying at their specific racially or ethnically designated black university campuses. As already mentioned, growing access to these universities was facilitated by increased numbers of

212

black students who obtained the necessary matriculation passes for entrance to university, by the lower fees charged to students at black universities and by the provision of state bursaries and loans.

What is interesting, however, is that this apparent compliance of black students with the state's segregated higher-education policies also created the ideal conditions for large groups of black students to draw together in resistance against their shared racial oppression under apartheid. At universities, students had time to think, read and discuss issues, ask questions and criticise the established order of things. As a result, in a manner contradictory to the state's original aims, university spaces provided fertile breeding grounds for the expression of student opposition to apartheid inequalities. For Matjila, who studied during this period of heightened political ferment, students did not have much to lose. Instead, they had 'every reason to think for the future', and if the future seemed bleak because of the conditions they lived and studied in, 'they have got every reason to focus on that. It is not surprising that many . . . revolutionary ideas, revolutionary discussions, start from the students.'[43]

While many of these broader issues influenced the development of student politics at the medical school from the late 1960s onwards, there were three additional reasons that help explain SASO's early origins on this campus. Firstly, Barry Kistnasamy, a community health specialist who did his undergraduate medical degree in Durban in the 1970s and later became dean of the medical school in the post-apartheid period, felt that medical students were 'high achievers' by nature. Being high achievers was a noteworthy factor as it ensured the existence of 'a certain element of innate arrogance' amongst medical students. This made these particular students more confident in themselves and their abilities and, as a result, less easily 'broken down by racism or whatever it is'. This attitude, according to Kistnasamy, would have made medical students as a group more prepared to take a stand when their rights were being violated.[44]

Secondly, the Natal Medical School most likely captured the pool of the very best-educated black students in the country.[45] Since studying medicine was often regarded as the first choice for the brightest black students, and since the state's 1959 university legislation effectively removed Wits and UCT as institutional choices, during the 1960s it was on the Durban medical campus that the largest number of such students would have congregated. This created the opportunity for critical discussions. While just a handful of Indian and coloured students did manage to get ministerial permission to study at Wits and UCT after 1959, they were so few in number on these campuses that they largely bore their difficulties and discriminations in silence for the sake of obtaining their degrees. Janet Giddy, a white doctor who studied at UCT during the late 1970s and early 1980s, recalled how quiet these students were, how they tended not to be vocal in student politics, and instead worked to 'lie low . . . minding their ps and qs and didn't want to cause any ripples'.[46] They would have felt overwhelmed or sidelined, compared to the situation in Durban, where black students felt a greater sense of solidarity in numbers. At Wits and Cape Town, black students would have been 'like a speck in a sea of white faces', Jerry Coovadia asserted, and 'many blacks would have preferred to have been here [Durban] because at least in the student body they felt at home'.[47]

The third reason, and arguably one of the most important, had to do with the University of Natal's more liberal approach, and its continued acceptance of a diverse mix of black students into its medical student body after 1959.[48] While the Natal Medical School was originally established as an apartheid institution, and was certainly caught up in and perpetuated many discriminatory policies in the name of the state, the campus also, arguably, provided a more protected educational space which gave its students the opportunity to explore political issues. In this manner, it once again reflected, but also paradoxically opposed, apartheid influences.

During the apartheid years, like Wits and UCT, the University of Natal was a 'fully fledged' university that was *state-aided* through financial subsidies, not *state-controlled* in all facets of its operation.[49] It stood in stark contrast, therefore, to the situation at other black universities created by the state after 1959. Although not completely free to do as it pleased, since it continued to rely on state subsidies, the University of Natal had more academic freedom and autonomy over its staff and student affairs compared to the black 'ethnic' campuses, which would be granted autonomous status only in later years.[50] In Durban, black students were thus allowed more political freedom too, which included the operation of a functioning SRC, which enabled its students to affiliate to NUSAS. In a 1988 interview conducted whilst she was in exile in London, Nkosazana Dlamini Zuma told her interviewer why she thought SASO thrived as an organisation at the University of Natal:

SASO took advantage of other existing structures; because SASO could just become one of the subcommittees of the SRC . . . [And] in Natal, it automatically got a budget from the SRC. That's why in Natal it was much more active initially compared to other places. Because [at] other places they had to try and raise funds from the students, and they had to struggle for everything.[51]

At the black universities, where the state had direct control over the appointment and dismissal of the academic staff, as well as over what courses they taught, and was able to intervene directly in the admission and expulsion of students, there was far less academic freedom. Here, students were often summarily expelled or criminally charged if found to be involved in political activities. In fact, the state often retained a standing and very visible armed police or army presence within or just outside these institutions, to maintain the strictest possible control.[52] Students were often baton-charged and tear-gassed by police at the slightest sign of student opposition, while strict curfews were imposed to restrict their movements. By the late 1960s, student politics of any kind, including the existence of SRCs and membership of NUSAS on most of these black campuses, were forbidden.

An African medical graduate, who studied at Turfloop (the University of the North) before being accepted to study medicine in Durban in the early 1970s, argued emphatically that the University of Natal was much more liberal in its policies with regards to student politics than Turfloop, which was 'actively pro-state at that time'.[53] During his time at Turfloop, he remembered how the administration was 'really actively involved' and 'would pass information to the security police', including student residence room numbers, so that those involved in anti-apartheid politics could be raided and detained.

Comparatively, MEDUNSA too was administered as a 'state university without the same autonomy and rights as other [white] universities'.[54] In addition to the big decisions, such as policies and procedures affecting finances, staff appointments, conditions of service and student selection, 'even day-to-day decisions were dictated by the then Dept of Education and Training', until it was granted its autonomy in the mid-1980s. Academic freedom and university autonomy were therefore virtually non-existent. Journalist Nimrod Mkele wrote the following about MEDUNSA in a newspaper article in April 1983:

The first thing one notes about the MEDUNSA campus is the security that permeates this institution of higher learning. It is surrounded by a high security fence and can be entered only from two closed gates manned by armed security guards who search cars as they enter and demand passes from the inmates.[55]

Furthermore, although students at MEDUNSA were allowed to have an SRC, its impact was limited as attempts to take a stand on political issues were usually quickly suppressed.[56] In fact, most protest activities that occurred on this and other black university campuses, especially during the 1960s and 1970s, were usually ruthlessly dealt with by the authorities.[57]

Two other medical graduates, whose time at the medical school collectively spanned the 1970s to early-1980s period, also highlighted that the University of Natal gave students comparatively more space to manoeuvre politically, although it was certainly not completely sympathetic or accommodating. In fact, support could and did vary depending on the political perspectives of the leaders in power at the university at a particular time. For instance, during his time as a student, Matjila remembered how the dean and a few other University of Natal upper-level managers made determined efforts to keep the security police off the medical campus, in an effort to protect its students. For him, this was a big deal because 'the police were the almighty force. I mean, they could get anywhere, anytime.'[58] According to Matjila, these efforts 'allowed the students an opportunity to have gatherings and meetings and discussions' because without that, the formation of SASO would not have been possible.

Joe Ndlovu, who studied in Durban between 1979 and 1984, a few years after Matjila, agreed. While he felt that the University of Natal was not actively supportive of students engaged in anti-apartheid political activities, it did help to create a protective environment for this to occur. According to Ndlovu, although many students studying at the University of Zululand or Turfloop, for example, were politically active,

I think in fairness one must acknowledge that those universities in the homelands were limited in what they could do by the brutality of the homeland forces that operated in those areas. And Natal Medical School was more or less free. I mean, the governors of the University were old liberal white people who really, in a sense, you know, allowed or tolerated a lot of political activity. And sometimes they themselves actually got into trouble from the government . . . for allowing student protests.[59]

In his opinion, as long as students were 'protesting what was happening in the country in general' and not specifically engaged in critiquing aspects of the University of Natal, 'it was fine. Not that you were . . . encouraged as such or assisted, but . . . a kind of a blind eye was turned to those issues.' Furthermore, by the 1970s and 1980s, as more black doctors qualified and some were appointed as staff members at the Durban Medical School, a greater level of empathy and support developed amongst the staff for students too.[60]

The person who instigated and led the black student breakaway movement from NUSAS in 1968, and who spearheaded the formation of SASO in 1969 as its president, was Bantu Stephen Biko. Steve Biko, as he was popularly known, was an African student who came to Durban from the Eastern Cape, having had a taste of state repression in his home area when his older brother was arrested in 1963 for his PAC political activities. He had been sent to Mariannhill's Catholic missionary school to complete his matriculation subjects and his good grades secured him a place at the medical school at the start of 1966. Here he studied for a number of years until he was expelled in June 1972 because of poor grades obtained as a result of distractions caused by his extracurricular political activities.[61]

Whilst at the medical school Biko, together with Barney Pityana (a Fort Hare student, who became the first general secretary of SASO and its second president), spent much time travelling around the country, such as during their varsity holidays and on other occasions including inter-varsity sports events and for conferences, to establish early contacts and build up SASO's network of support amongst black students around South Africa.[62] In fact, for a time, the state encouraged these activities and supported the formation of SASO as it seemed to fit within the separate-development scheme. It quickly spread to all black university campuses with Biko and Pityana captivating members with their ideas and leadership. SASO's ideas were also disseminated through the publication of the *SASO Newsletter*. After Pityana took over the organisation's presidency in July 1970, Biko became the director of SASO publications, and wrote many articles for this newsletter from his dormitory room at ATR. His column was called 'I Write What I Like', under the byline 'Frank Talk'. He used the platform to expound on many of the basic tenets of SASO and the BCM more broadly.[63]

Matjila, whose own study time in Durban overlapped with Biko's, recalled clearly the inspirational speaking abilities and personal charisma of his contemporary, who had first played a leadership role on his university's 'non-European' SRC before being elected as president of SASO:

> Biko was very, very articulate . . . He was one of the most eloquent speakers I have yet ever seen . . . [H]e had a major influence . . . on student politics in this country and certainly on this campus. I think the concept of black consciousness would not have flown on this campus had it not been for the type of person that he was at that time . . . [H]e was able to communicate his convictions and back it up with evidence.[64]

Additionally, what he really marvelled at about Biko was that under very difficult circumstances, especially the oppressive apartheid era of the time, 'he had the guts' to stand up and 'to call a spade a spade'. Others shared Matjila's admiration: Y.K. Seedat, who was a senior lecturer in the Department of Medicine at the time, spoke in awe of Biko's public speaking skills and his abilities to spellbind an audience.

According to Malegapuru Makgoba, who was also a medical student during the early 1970s when SASO was in its formative years, Steve Biko and his colleagues campaigned hard to establish the organisation, as well as to educate the students and inspire them into action. For Makgoba, they always seemed to be at meetings and campaigning amongst different students to try to conscientise them:

> They were very articulate and convincing in their arguments and most of us identified with their cause . . . We joined as members in droves . . . They read poetry, sang liberation songs, showed banned movies and discussed liberation politics. Even the most virgin of us began to understand the serious nature of our political problems. These guys were dead serious, dedicated and hardworking.[65]

What is more, he felt that involvement in SASO was 'exciting, stimulating and unifying' for students, and 'these leaders gave us pride, hope and things to aspire towards'.

From 1969 and through most of the 1970s, SASO became a key sub-culture at the medical school, and Biko's room at ATR at first doubled up as the SASO head office until he was able to negotiate with university authorities to use a separate room at the residence for this purpose.[66] Abba Omar, who was a student leader at the Indian University of Durban-Westville during the 1970s, remembered how Biko and other medical student activists served as a magnet, attracting many student leaders and activists from around the province and from around the country to the medical students' residence. According to Omar, 'You could come from anywhere in the country. If you were in Durban on political business, you went to Alan Taylor Residence. Here you had a ready group of students to do the work and people could meet here and work out national political campaigns.'[67]

This campus's leadership would also prove essential as growing government crackdowns took place on SRC and SASO branches on the country's black university campuses. This point was stressed by Breminand Maharaj. As a graduate of the medical school in 1977, he argued that the Natal Medical School 'was the home of black consciousness'. For Maharaj, the BCM started off in Durban:

> I mean, all the other institutions . . . were pretty pressed down, they couldn't [organise] . . . I mean, they would be beaten up, you know, to a pulp literally. So this was the hotbed . . . And people would come in, and feed in and feed out. It was really, as I told you, a lot of other people coming here and taking part in the activity and kind of like disappear[ing] into the community and do[ing] their work . . . So SASO had to be born here because that was the strongest point.[68]

It was thus in this small and cramped office at the ATR that black consciousness ideas were vigorously debated amongst its diverse student body. It was to this office that other, more politically oppressed black university students around South Africa looked for leadership and direction in this era of growing student political mobilisation.

The black consciousness ideology that emerged from the mouths and pens of SASO leaders was inspired by several international as well as local organisational and individual precedents, such as the 1950s and 1960s Civil Rights and Black Power movements in the United States; revolutionaries from South American countries, such as Che Guevara and Paulo Freire;

early independence leaders in Africa, such as Kwame Nkrumah and Julius Nyerere; African intellectuals, such as Frantz Fanon and Aimé Césaire; and banned local ANC and PAC leaders, whom their parents would have told them about. It also emerged as a response to the harsh experiences of apartheid racial discrimination and inequalities black South Africans endured on a daily basis.[69] Additionally, Dlamini Zuma felt that events in the southern African region, including the independence of Mozambique and Angola in 1975, had a 'very important part to play'. During an interview recorded whilst in exile in London in 1988, she reminisced about how as a medical student in the mid-1970s, and just after television had been introduced into South Africa, someone had donated a TV set for students to use at ATR. Students would 'scramble for space' whenever a news programme about their northern neighbour came on. 'You see, people were seeing liberation as a very distant thing, an impossible thing. But if they realised that five hundred years of Portuguese rule has just been crushed by people just like them . . . then all that gives an impetus in the struggle.'[70]

For SASO leaders, the aim was to fill the political vacuum left by the outlawed organisations. In a nutshell, the major concerns of these activists included the liberation of black South Africans from the psychological oppression caused by apartheid that had incapacitated them from political action, and the promotion of a positive dignity and pride in themselves and their cultural backgrounds.[71] They were also centrally concerned with building a strong, defiant, anti-apartheid consciousness and oppositional politics. Recent scholars, including one of Biko's sons, have argued that for Biko and his colleagues, 'meaningful integration would only come about once the whites had been stripped of their paternalistic tendency and the blacks their arsenal of inferiority complexes'.[72]

One of SASO's most visible innovations was its promotion of the term 'Black' with a capital 'B' as a positive affirmation of self-worth for all black South Africans oppressed by apartheid laws. The reclamation of this term was done in direct opposition to derogatory terms like 'non-European' or 'non-white' in use at the time – terms which negated their being. It was also a challenge to the racist nomenclature of apartheid that worked to separate people of colour.[73] Its early origins amongst Durban medical students ensured that SASO developed an inclusive definition of 'Black', actively working to incorporate African, Indian and coloured students in its leadership and membership. Instead of differences and fragmentation, it stressed the shared suffering among black students to build a resistance movement.

Moreover, the organisation was open to both men and women. Durban's SASO leaders worked hard to cultivate a broader sense of unity amongst black South Africans. The aim was to encourage them to become common allies in opposition to the apartheid state's policies, which aimed to divide and weaken them, such as the Bantustan or 'homelands' policy that was created to accommodate the different African ethnic groups separately from whites and each other.[74] Those leaders who worked within the Bantustan authorities, who accepted ethnic politics and worked within the apartheid system, were viewed by SASO leaders as sell-outs.

However, despite the Durban Medical School being considered by some to be 'the home' of the BCM in South Africa, it is imperative to stress that SASO ideologies did not appeal to all students at the medical school or elsewhere for that matter. Celebratory narratives, while inspiring to many, also hide a great deal in their attempts to bring the medical school's political history into line with the post-apartheid state's 'unity-in-adversity', nation-building narratives. Furthermore, it is impossible to gauge accurately how many black students in Durban, or across the country, were active SASO members. During the 1970s, the security police raided SASO's headquarters in Durban and its branches around the country, leading to the confiscation and destruction of many SASO records. In addition, it was dangerous to keep careful membership records as the security police could obtain these records through raids and other means and then use them to identify and arrest students who were involved in SASO activities.[75] Before considering the experiences of those students in Durban who involved themselves in SASO political activities, the next section will first give some attention to the stories of those students who tried to stay out of politics.

'There were some . . . students who weren't interested in politics.'
— Y.K. Seedat

Despite SASO leaders' best efforts to mobilise all black students and to create an inclusive and unifying political ideology, not all students studying in Durban from the 1960s onwards wanted to get involved in its politics. Some students did not identify with its ideologies. Others did not feel that they 'belonged'. Despite the repeated rhetoric of 'belonging', they did not consider their interests adequately represented by this organisation. While opposition to apartheid inequalities provided common ground and did at times bring many medical students together in opposition to their general oppression as 'non-Europeans', the state's efforts to keep black 'race' groups apart had deep roots, and neither before, during or after SASO's time were students completely unified politically.

It is also essential to highlight that on occasions, some student support for political activities, such as boycotts, was coerced, as Y.K. Seedat highlighted in an interview:

> [T]here was intimidation too . . . by students towards other students [for]
> . . . not subscribing to [certain] viewpoints . . . pressuring people. And so
> one never knew what the student following really was . . . Meetings were
> well attended, particularly on controversial matters . . . [but some] students
> wouldn't subscribe to the view of boycotts, and then, of course, that's
> when the intimidation came through.[76]

Even as late as the 1980s, the University of Natal instituted a series of investigations into various charges of physical and verbal intimidation of certain students at ATR who refused to participate in boycott activities. These institutional records discuss how some students had their dormitory rooms forcibly entered by other students and possessions stolen when they refused to participate. Notices about student 'dissenters' were posted on noticeboards at ATR to shame errant 'offenders' and occasionally harassment became so severe that some students abandoned their studies altogether.[77]

Tensions and divisions fractured SASO's political mobilisation in a number of ways. One issue that emerged during SASO's development was the question of political cooperation with what some students considered to be more socially and economically privileged Indian and coloured minority groups.[78] Differences of race and social class inhibited easy political identification amongst all African, Indian and coloured students. Some Africans felt that students from minority groups saw their best interests served in maintaining their own separate identities as intermediate groups enjoying a few extra privileges and not in supporting the African majority in their fight against the apartheid state. This issue was made clear by Mosibudi Mangena, a student who attended the University of Zululand (or Ngoye) during SASO's period of operation:

During our debates at Ngoye, there were those who maintained that while they agreed with and supported the aims and policies of SASO, they could not accept the presence of Indians in its ranks . . . because they are privileged . . . No matter how much we argued, a few people . . . felt they could not identify their aspirations with those of Indians and thought Indians could not be allies.[79]

Concerns were also raised by some African students about their Indian colleagues' apparent lack of commitment to the struggle against apartheid, as fewer Indian students participated in political activities. This produced strained relations as it was felt that African students sacrificed more than Indian students, as one African graduate, who studied in the 1970s, remembered:

There were tensions between Indians and Africans, always tensions . . . I think part of it was the commitment to the struggle. I think African students were always committed to the struggle. Indian students, there were a few that were committed, but the majority were not committed to the struggle . . . Indian students were . . . more focused on academic things . . .[80]

Although involvement by Indian students in political activities would have varied year by year depending on the individuals concerned, the perceived lower overall participation of Indian students over the years can be explained by a variety of factors. As discussed earlier, a large number of Indian students who lived off-campus were somewhat shielded from the political activities that went on at ATR.[81] Some students did not want to risk jeopardising their careers by getting involved. Studying medicine was viewed as 'a ticket to freedom' for many students and their families, where improved earning power gained after qualifying would help elevate their socio-economic positions and soften the harsh consequences of racial inequalities under apartheid.[82]

What's more, very few Indian students received state bursary-loans, which meant that families had sacrificed much to finance their studies, placing enormous pressure on students to pass.[83] Others did not want to endanger private scholarships or bank loans. Some stayed out of politics as they felt that they could better serve their communities by completing their degrees and providing desperately needed health-care services for black patients.[84] Reflecting on the many reasons why students might not have participated in politics, Jerry Coovadia asserted:

> [T]here [was] never a period when all students would be involved in politics . . . [T]he ethos was for political freedom, and the disputes were the level [or] the tactics by which we attained [it]. So the question might be, students are going on boycott too often and the Indians, you know, complained that we want to write the exams and these people are preventing us. So there were numerous divisions like that . . . numerous disputes and disagreements.[85]

Furthermore, some Indian students did not identify with SASO's inclusive definition of 'Black' which they felt worked to undermine their cultural heritage. This was the view of Kogila Moodley, who argued that from the beginning, SASO tried hard in their mobilising efforts to include Indian and coloured students and, despite having an appeal for some of these students, it 'failed to provide the psychological identity they needed'. Rather, Moodley believed that many experienced in the movement 'a certain denial of self at the grassroots level' and 'felt pressured to replace their cultural heritage'. In addition, she maintained that many felt that they 'were never accepted as authentically "black" enough'.[86]

This perspective was supported by Ben Ngubane, a medical student who had been an SRC representative in NUSAS before his constituents pressured him to resign in 1967. In July 1969, Ngubane wrote a letter expressing his concerns about SASO, whose policies he regarded as reactionary. In this letter, he also laid out the enormous amount of opposition that was initially raised against SASO when its policies were first discussed on the Durban medical campus. Referring to the SASO leaders as 'my local fascists', he wrote that they were

> . . . trying to rally support for their SASO but they will never win a straight fight on this issue – most of the people are fairly sceptical of the intentions and motivations behind this effort. To be brutally frank, the Indian and Coloured students are so anti SASO that I need only pack the hall with them to get a motion of centre affiliation to [have] SASO kicked out.[87]

Furthermore, although only a tiny number of coloured students studied medicine in Durban each year compared to their Indian colleagues, these students also experienced identity ambivalence when SASO was launched. Veronica Wilson, who studied in Durban during the early 1970s, said that as a student

> . . . you know, with the classification of coloureds . . . where did you fit? . . . you found that . . . the blacks [Africans] didn't really want you and the whites . . . and the Indians [neither] . . . [A]nd then, of course, you were supposed to be have been privileged.[88]

Involvement in extracurricular political activities was a 'dangerous game in those days' that could threaten students' academic work and their personal safety too.[89] The harsh consequences that resulted for students involved in anti-apartheid political activities, including police harassment, raids, assault and imprisonment, along with the presence of unknown police informers in the student body, dissuaded many Indian and coloured students, but also some African students, from actively participating in politics.

In addition to 'deep underlying issues' that divided Africans, Indians and coloureds, political tensions amongst Africans complicated the quest for a unified student body in Durban too.[90] One such tension emerged during SASO's formation years. During the late 1960s, a clear division surfaced between African students who wanted to remain members of NUSAS, which encouraged non-racialism, and those aligned with SASO, who wanted to exclude white students altogether.[91] Students who supported NUSAS were suspicious of SASO's aims and interpreted its endorsement of a blacks-only membership as support for apartheid separate-development plans. In her autobiography Mamphela Ramphele discussed how Ben Ngubane (the same person mentioned above) was Steve Biko's main opponent in the debates when she joined the medical school's student body in 1968. While Ngubane supported Biko's arguments that apartheid was oppressive and needed to be fought, he did not agree with Biko's suggestion that 'black politics be consolidated away from the white liberal fold'. According to Ramphele, 'Ben defended NUSAS on the Medical School campus to the very last, when the student body finally voted narrowly in favour of Steve's motion of central disaffiliation from NUSAS thus paving the way for [SASO] . . .'[92] Right until the end, when Ramphele claims he became 'more cynical and disillusioned, finally fading out of the political arena, only to re-emerge in the 1980s', he continued to argue that NUSAS had 'stood firm in the face of harassment by the apartheid state and thus deserved the loyalty of all freedom-loving students'.

Even through the 1970s, some African students felt uncomfortable with SASO's anti-white politics. One of these graduates said that his personal premise was to 'always watch carefully . . . [against] catching [him]self in an emotional reverse racism'.[93] For this doctor, a big concern was that 'extremists would find a home there' in the BCM. This included a number of his friends who were 'pushing it to being anti-white . . . [B]ut I had a different argument.' He felt that his strong Christian beliefs helped him in this regard. Some students continued to align themselves with non-racial political ideologies like that of the ANC, even if these organisations were banned at the time.[94]

Of course, on the other end of the spectrum, there were other African students who felt that SASO did not go far enough in its politics, and would have preferred the exclusion of Indian and coloured students too, more in line with PAC policies.[95] Additionally, as an organisation, SASO also experienced divisions between those students who supported armed struggle to achieve their aims, and those who did not, fearing that such a move would get the organisation banned. One crisis along such lines was raised at the 1972 conference by a group of delegates, led by medical student Keith Mokoape (and later a senior member of the ANC's armed wing, Umkhonto we Sizwe), who called for a policy supporting military struggle.[96] Although suppressed at this conference, growing calls within SASO and other BC organisations towards the engagement in military action would be made in the years after 1972, leading up to these organisations being banned in October 1977.

However, while the exclusion of whites but also the inclusion of Indians and coloureds caused ideological tensions and disagreements amongst African students on the Durban medical campus, it was ethnic differences which produced serious political divisions too. These schisms became particularly evident during the 1970s and 1980s. On the one side of this political divide was the larger grouping of medical students supporting organisations whose membership was open to a variety of ethnic groups, such as SASO, and after SASO was banned in October 1977,[97] non-racial political movements like the United Democratic Front (UDF), which adopted the ANC's Freedom

Charter and consulted with ANC leaders in exile.[98] On the other side were the few African students who supported the KwaZulu homeland government's cultural-cum-political organisation known as Inkatha, which was formed in 1975 and promoted Zulu ethnic interests.[99]

Since African medical students who came to study at the University of Natal over the years were an ethnically mixed group and had come to Durban from across the whole of South Africa, those who became involved in politics tended to belong to organisations with a broader membership base, and not to ethnically based organisations like Inkatha.[100] In addition, those who became involved in SASO and later UDF/ANC politics saw Inkatha supporters as traitors and sell-outs who undermined the anti-apartheid cause by working for conservative reforms for Africans within officially sanctioned Bantustan political structures.[101] Two African graduates, who did not want their names used, argued that during the late 1970s and through the 1980s, there was great hostility amongst students on the medical school campus towards Inkatha. In addition, student supporters had to keep their support for this organisation a secret:

> [Inkatha] ... was almost tabooed ... There were a few ... sympathisers, especially people who would come from across the Tugela River or the north coast of Natal, but they were in such a minority and they were completely, you know, unmentioned in political speak.

> [It] just didn't have support ... I think those who belonged to Inkatha, they must have done so privately ... but they were quiet about it because there was going to be no support. Remember, people who were at the Medical School came from all over the country, so we were not thinking provincially or [in terms of] Bantustans ... We were thinking nationally ... [so Inkatha] wouldn't have appealed to the masses ... [W]e had to have something that was very inclusive.[102]

One issue that sparked tensions in the student body involved a change in the conditions required of bursars accepting state bursary-loans. As already discussed, from the opening of the medical school, many African students were able to study medicine because of bursary-loans made available to them from the central government, which they were then required to pay back in service in approved 'non-European' areas for a number of years.

However, from the late 1970s, a shift in the management of the scheme to the different homeland governments that were created by this date, required bursars to agree to work, after graduating, in the public service of the particular Bantustan that had sponsored their studies.

Another issue made matters more contentious for those accepting money from the KwaZulu government – the homeland closest to the medical school where many black doctors went to work over the years. Chief Mangosutho Buthelezi, the leader of both the KwaZulu government and Inkatha, stipulated that African students accepting KwaZulu bursary-loans had to sign a pledge of allegiance to himself and Inkatha.[103] This pledge was a law passed by the KwaZulu legislature in the early 1980s as a condition of service for bursars. It required all KwaZulu public servants to sign an undertaking not to vilify or denigrate the KwaZulu government or its leaders. In effect, it was an oath of personal allegiance to Buthelezi and his Inkatha political party. It affected all civil servants including doctors, nurses, teachers and clerks who were required to sign the Inkatha pledge.

Although some medical students signed the pledge and thus, according to one African graduate, 'play[ed] this game of apartheid . . . and benefited from it' to advance their individual careers, many SASO and later UDF/ANC-aligned students refused to sign what amounted to a political pledge of loyalty to a leader and party that were anathema to many.[104] The outcomes were dire for students who refused to accept these conditions. These included having their bursary-loans revoked; having to pay back the entire amount with accumulated interest after graduating; or not getting jobs in KwaZulu health services near to their homes. In the 1970s SASO members and in the 1980s UDF/ANC-aligned activists in the medical student body often spoke out publicly against the pledge conditions and other Inkatha political activities. In addition, those who had accepted KwaZulu bursary-loans before the pledge condition came into effect felt that this government's retroactive requirement that they also sign the pledge was a breach of contract. In an interview one African doctor spoke passionately about his student experiences during the early 1980s. In his opinion:

> [Inkatha] hated the . . . medical school . . . [and] there were some very hot exchanges between [Inkatha] and the medical school . . . [The students] were very outspoken against [its] policies. Very, very outspoken . . . We

were meant to sign it [the pledge] in 1983 or '84 . . . just before graduating
. . . Well, we refused to sign it. Most of us refused. There were perhaps one
or two IFP supporters who actually signed it . . . [The school] was always a
hive of activity and those students were always known as hotheads
politically, very much, you know, ANC-affiliated.[105]

Though these exchanges were usually verbal, they also occasionally became
serious physical threats to students too.[106] For example, on 29 October
1983, four students were killed and scores more injured when Inkatha
supporters attacked students with assegais and clubs at the University of
Zululand (Ngoye) for refusing to participate in a Shaka Day celebration.[107]
This was vividly remembered by a professor who worked at the medical
school at the time and who travelled up to Empangeni that night with a
number of other doctors to help look after those who were injured. He said:
'All the theatres were opened all night and so we saw first-hand what had
happened, so nobody can deny that to us. We saw it, we saw them in the
mortuary, those who had died, and it was a terrible massacre.'[108] The
following week, he and four other colleagues drove up to Ulundi to speak
to Buthelezi about the Inkatha pledge issue. This was a very tense meeting.

> I remember the day we met in one of the board rooms in the Holiday Inn
> . . . and Gatsha [Buthelezi] was there and the five of us . . . And I had to say
> how our students felt about what had happened both in the massacre
> against the Zululand students and in the demand for signing the pledge.

He recalled how 'very angry' Buthelezi got and his parting threat. 'I'll never
forget . . . he pointed to me and he said, "You go back and tell young Diliza
Mji I'm out to get him".' Diliza Mji had made a name for himself as a SASO
activist at the medical school in the mid- to late-1970s. Furthermore, Durban
sociologist Fatima Meer discussed a specific example of how UDF/ANC-
aligned students living at ATR were forced to flee the residence during a
weekend in August 1985 following rumours that Inkatha vigilante groups
'were coming to deal with them' during a time of violence in the nearby
African townships of Umlazi and KwaMashu.[109]

Eventually, due to the large public outcry and lack of doctors prepared
to work in KwaZulu hospitals after graduating, Buthelezi and his health
ministry were forced to back down on the issue and remove the clause that

bursars were required to sign a pledge of allegiance in their contract agreements. The great anger the Inkatha pledge provoked in many people resulted in a severe shortage of African doctors in the KwaZulu homeland during the 1980s. According to Cedric de Beer, KwaZulu health institutions had vacancies for 70 doctors in the early-1980s period.[110] Many African doctors who had been forced to use the bursary-loan scheme to fund their medical studies found jobs in other provinces or started their own private practices. They chose to pay back every penny of their bursary-loans together with interest, under great personal strain on themselves, rather than work under these conditions.[111]

Finally, gender divisions also affected medical student politics in Durban. Over the years, male students dominated the leadership positions in organisations like SASO, while women were generally encouraged to play supportive roles.[112] Being outnumbered and socially conditioned to be subservient in their societies also meant that many women students did not challenge patriarchal gender roles themselves. Mamphela Ramphele, who was one of the few women to become active in a leadership position in SASO at the medical school in the early 1970s, remembered how responsibility for domestic chores, such as catering and cleaning up at SASO conferences, as well as at seminars and workshops, always fell on women members.[113] Some SASO male student activists, as discussed in an earlier chapter, also became involved in sexually exploitative, 'womanising' activities at ATR.

Other than being 'looked at as part of the entertainment',[114] Nkosazana Dlamini Zuma, reflecting back on her experience as a medical student and SASO activist in Durban during the early 1970s, succinctly captured the overall position of women in the organisation:

> [SASO was] a male organisation. There were very few females who were really involved in it. There were a lot who were associated with it, but it was the kind of association at the girlfriend level rather than at comrade [level] . . . But when I got involved in it I did not get involved to try to put my female element in it. It was just that I felt I wanted to participate in the struggle. I wasn't conscious of that aspect at the time. I don't think many people were, but women tended to be treated as just girlfriends or acquaintances but not equal.[115]

This highlights how the fight to end racial inequalities overshadowed gender issues.[116] The priority of SASO and other BCM organisations was the liberation of black South Africans from apartheid oppression, and women were involved in these organisations because they were black, not because they were women.[117] It is prudent to remember too that the category of gender was not politicised and theorised as an issue in South Africa during the late 1960s and early 1970s as it is today. The tiny number of women activists who participated in SASO activities injected little feminist influence into BC theory and praxis. It was only in the late 1980s, when black women became increasingly involved in leadership positions in anti-apartheid political bodies, such as the UDF and later the ANC, that a stronger women's rights agenda was developed.[118]

While, now and again, determined women such as Ramphele and Dlamini Zuma were recognised as 'honorary men' and occasionally placed in leadership positions in organisations like SASO, this was rare, and generally men were the empowered speakers and decision-makers, not women.[119] And, women who reached such positions had to be strongly outspoken to have their ideas heard, as Dlamini Zuma asserted, recalling her election to the position of vice-president of SASO in 1976: 'You had to be quite determined to put your views across for them to be seen.'[120] Ramphele concurred: 'I was one of a group of women within BC ranks who became assertive, to the point of arrogance. We learnt to be tough, insistent, [and] persistent and to hold our own in public and private debates.'[121]

Moreover, since SASO politics were dominated by male leadership, their political ideologies also reflected their masculine gender bias, which showed little concern for women's particular problems or interests. This even filtered down to the type of universalising masculine language used in SASO speeches and publications, as is evident in a pivotal September 1970 article by Steve Biko published in the *SASO Newsletter*. In this newsletter, Biko, who was the head of SASO publications at the time, asked a series of questions about the psychologically defeatist attitude that he regarded black South Africans as suffering. This was a key factor, according to Biko, which made them submissive and politically inactive. A section of this article is quoted at length here to highlight the biased language that was used to refer to problems that supposedly affected all black South Africans:

What makes the black *man* fail to tick? Is *he* convinced of *his* own accord of *his* inabilities? Does *he* lack in *his* genetic make-up that rare quality that makes a *man* willing to die for the realisation of *his* aspirations? Or is *he* simply a defeated person? The answer to this is . . . nearer to the last suggestion than anything else. The logic behind white domination is to prepare black *men* for the subservient role in this country . . . To a large extent the evil-doers have succeeded in producing at the output end of their machine a kind of black *man* who is *man* only in form. This is the extent to which the process of dehumanisation has advanced. Black people under the Smuts government were oppressed but they were still *men* . . . [T]he type of black *man* we have today has lost *his manhood*. Reduced to an obliging shell, *he* looks with awe at the white power structure and accepts what *he* regards as the 'inevitable position'. Deep inside *his* anger mounts at the accumulating insult . . . All in all the black *man* has become a shell, a shadow of a *man*, completely defeated, drowning in *his* own misery, a slave, an ox bearing the yoke of oppression with sheepish timidity. This is the first truth, bitter as it may seem, that we have to acknowledge before we can start on any programme designed to change the status quo.[122]

Gender-specific words such as 'castration', 'impotence' and 'emasculation' also appear in a number of other *SASO Newsletter* articles to describe the negative effects of apartheid on the experiences of black South Africans. For SASO's male leadership, only once the 'Black man's' sense of self-worth, pride and confidence was restored through an inward-looking process that enabled 'him' to overcome a feeling of inferiority, and to re-appreciate the positive value of 'his' identity, culture and history, that a powerful and defiant anti-apartheid opposition could emerge, which was strong enough to challenge the apartheid state.[123] Whether done consciously or not by SASO leaders, this language subordinated women and their concerns. SASO's anti-apartheid politics developed as a hyper-masculine endeavour that worked to enable black men involved in this organisation to regain their battered sense of manhood by participating in a defiant, proud and sometimes dangerous 'struggle politics' that bravely challenged their racial oppressors.[124] SASO's fight to end racial oppression did not include an attempt to eliminate gender oppression in a patriarchal society where black men traditionally exercised and fought to maintain their power and control over black women.

Thus, divisions plagued the student body in the political realm as much as in the social and educational arenas. SASO failed to grapple effectively with the simultaneity of different racial, ethnic, class and gender oppressions in South Africa's social structure, which meant that not all black South Africans were equally represented by it. For SASO, some subjective experiences – that is, those of Africans or men – were ranked higher than other subjective experiences. This fractured the medical student body and influenced the effectiveness of SASO's political mobilisation efforts.

'Natal Medical School ... offered an environment for ... a political education for me.' — Mamphela Ramphele

While SASO's political ideology did not appeal to everyone, did not represent all black students' interests equally and therefore limited the number of students who actually actively joined this organisation, its influence on the Durban medical campus was considerable before it was banned in the late 1970s. Indeed, its influence reached well past its own active membership. Just living in the same residence, studying in the same classes or eating together in the same cafeterias, where the 'hot issues of the poverty in the country, the harassing of people with pass laws, the homeland issues of dividing South Africa, the detentions which was ongoing [sic]' were discussed by SASO activists on a regular basis, would have awakened students to a variety of political discussions and issues.[125] This was the case for Veronica Wilson. Coming from what she described as a 'sheltered upbringing' in the small town where she grew up, it was only when she came to university that she felt really 'exposed to politics in the true sense and attended meetings'.[126]

This medical school campus provided a broader political education for its students. While the activist climate at the school helped to conscientise most students, it actively politicised some. According to Wilson, the medical school was an 'eye-opener' for her and exposed her to 'a totally different world!' It was in this environment that she became politically conscious with all the discussions going on around her when she arrived in 1969. As part of their orientation, May Mashego, who attended medical school a few years after Wilson, recalled how all new students were given a '*mlevo*' session (a Zulu word meaning 'to sit down and chat') upon entering the medical school, which changed some students' lives, including her own:

Alan Taylor Residence was a very good residence ... [Although] the buildings ... were barracks ... the life that was inside there was different ... People welcomed you, people supported you and people wanted to put you in the right perspective about life. You were young, you've just arrived ... [and] the people who were already there wanted us to know exactly who we were ... [So] they told you about the studies, but at the same time, they told you a lot about life. I mean, I learnt to be an activist ... a political activist at medical school. I learnt to actually understand what [was] happening in the country and what we should be doing to correct the ills at the medical school.[127]

The circulation of positive black consciousness ideas made students more politically aware if not always politically active. Whether they belonged to SASO or not, black consciousness ideas would have encouraged them to feel pride and confidence in themselves, and this gave many medical students in Durban a distinct psychological advantage. Joe Ndlovu, today a qualified psychiatrist who entered the medical school in 1979, felt that on this campus, 'things would have been better' compared to those black students studying at Wits and UCT, 'because, I mean, black consciousness would have had its best impact there among all these black students living and working and studying together'.[128] For Ndlovu, a Durban medical student would have felt more 'worthwhile as a person; you're not as inferior as the white people have told you. And this would translate into a degree of confidence, you know, which would permeate through to your performance at school ... your relationships ...'

Many other graduates described in interviews how lucky they felt to be exposed to SASO's black consciousness message for what it did for their lives. Breminand Maharaj, who graduated in 1977, felt that when he first arrived at the school, 'suddenly you were told you're an entity, not a non-entity, right. You're not a non-something, you're not a non-white, you're Black.' It was a deeply positive experience that made him 'feel ... worthy [and] proud'.[129] Wilson concurred. It taught students to like and respect themselves once again:

... the apartheid system did affect people in that you had that self-worth that sometimes you questioned ... and you actually felt inferior. But when the black consciousness came ... it was actually telling the people that, you know, you must be proud of who you are and of the way you look . . . and where you come from and your history.[130]

Other than offering medical students a boost in self-confidence and a political education, for those who stayed at ATR, their training in Durban helped create a greater sense of unity amongst some of its students too. Maila J. Matjila felt this keenly. Despite the inferior conditions students were expected to live in, 'it really built a spirit of unity . . . a spirit of oneness among the people.[131] And . . . I think it brought us closer together . . . people from all different backgrounds, different . . . parts of the country.' In his opinion, 'a very close-knit family' atmosphere was created amongst some students. This view was supported by Maharaj, whose time in Durban overlapped with Matjila's. Many students 'were allowed to bond at a level that was never known before . . . It [ATR] was a terrible arrangement but it allowed people to unite . . . and, I mean, we just really supported each other.'[132] Both Matjila and Maharaj asserted that many people got on well because 'we had a common enemy – apartheid . . . and of course people here . . . [also] felt discriminated against by the main campus'. And, when students did experience 'the hit' of apartheid oppression and inequalities, since in Durban black students lived and studied together as a large group, they could be there for each other and 'at least lick each other's wounds' during trying times, which helped them cope with their situations.[133]

Memories of Alan Taylor

Before moving on to discuss students who actively involved themselves in anti-apartheid politics, it is worth dwelling further on the medical school's ATR, particularly on what is silenced publicly when certain memories are commonly promoted. Interviews gathered for this review of the school's history suggested consistently that the production of knowledge about the residence – what students often just called 'Alan Taylor' – overlooked the contributions of Alan B. Taylor, the man, and, by extension, the long history of Christian missionaries on the development of black medical education in South Africa.[134] As discussed in chapter 1, Taylor, together with Dr James B. McCord, worked assiduously in the early twentieth century to provide a medical education for black students in Durban. And it was largely because of their efforts that the Durban Medical School was opened in 1951. Too often, when alumni discuss the ATR, the missionary connection is completely omitted. For example, not once 'on this Alan

Taylor occasion' – referring to the ATR reunion that was held in October 1989 shortly before the closure of this residence, and an explicit moment of public remembrance – was Dr Alan Taylor, the man, and his contributions remembered.[135] And, if mentioned at all, it is only done so in passing, and usually by early generations of students.[136]

Oral and written memories recorded about ATR have focused instead on its inferior conditions and its importance as a site of anti-apartheid conscientising and organising for students. For many alumni, despite its hardships, it was often portrayed as 'a very good residence' that moulded their characters and 'built a spirit of oneness' amongst its students, who together stood 'united' against their common apartheid enemy. However, while these celebratory narratives provide flesh to the bones of the medical school's history, and bring the contributions of the school's alumni firmly into line with the post-1994 collective memory framework of 'liberation struggles' waged against apartheid, in the process they conceal vital aspects that would help us understand better the history of this institution.

Historian David William Cohen has argued that the process of remembering is often closely linked to the process of 'forgetting'.[137] Once again, this issue helps point us to the constructed nature of memories. As readers, we need always to bear in mind the possible erosion of memories with the passage of time, and the sway a particular present can have in influencing how memories are constructed in a specific way. Memories are selective and involve not only processes of recovery, but also processes of silencing. Ironically, in the telling and writing of history, much can be forgotten in the act of actively remembering, and in repeatedly saying a name. Taking seriously what is remembered, but also what is supposedly 'forgotten', in narrative productions is essential in understanding any history, including that of the Durban Medical School.

In the next chapter, the focus of attention moves to consider medical students who participated in anti-apartheid political activism. Although SASO only occasionally drew all students together to oppose a particular issue, it did win many students over to their cause, which stimulated a defiant mood and gave those who became politically involved the confidence to question and challenge apartheid discriminations that affected them and their wider communities. Those students who became involved in SASO would strive to make friendships across age, gender and racial categories and 'b[ind themselves] together by the perception of apartheid and the need to fight it'.[138]

Notes

1. See, for example, 'Message from Dr U.G. Lalloo, President, Medical Graduates Association', in *The University of Natal Medical School 1951–1991: Meeting the Challenge of Change*, brochure to mark the fortieth anniversary of the Faculty of Medicine of the University of Natal, (University of Natal: Communication and Publicity, 1991); and 'History's hand in the shaping of the medical school', *University of Natal Nelson R. Mandela School of Medicine: 50 Years of Achievement in Teaching, Service and Research* eds Jack Moodley and Smita Maharaj (University of Natal Nelson R. Mandela School of Medicine: Communications Office, 2001), 9.

2. See, for example, UKZNA MQ 1/1/1-5, 'Student society round-up', *The Amoeba* II, no. 7 (September 1954), and 'Student activities', *The Amoeba* 1, no. 1 (September 1956).

3. For more on the early political contributions of black medical doctors, see Anne Digby, 'Early black doctors in South Africa', *Journal of African History*, 46, no. 3 (November 2005).

4. For more on the general history of anti-apartheid politics in South Africa in the 1950s and 1960s, see, for example, Tom Lodge, *Black Politics in South Africa since 1945* (London and New York: Longman, 1983); Ian Liebenberg, Fiona Lortan, Bobby Nel and Gert van der Westhuizen, eds, *The Long March: The Story of the Struggle for Liberation in South Africa* (Pretoria: HAUM, 1994); and Thomas G. Karis and Gail M. Gerhart, *From Protest to Challenge: A Documentary History of African Politics in South Africa, 1882–1990*, Volume 5 (Pretoria: UNISA Press, 1997).

5. Online article by Khululiwe Makhaye: http://www.northcoastcourier.co.za/2009/sep25/luthuli.htm. Albertina Luthuli and Pascal Ngakane (another Durban Medical School graduate, whom she married) continued with their anti-apartheid political work after graduating. However, they eventually went into exile because of continual police harassment and after her husband's detentions and imprisonment on Robben Island between 1964 and 1967. Also see Padraig O'Malley Interviews with Nomsa Ngakane, 26 August 1992, and Albertina Luthuli, 10 January 1993, http://www.nelsonmandela.org/omalley/index.php/site/q/03lv00017.htm.

6. In the post-apartheid period, Ncayiyana became deputy vice-chancellor of UCT and then vice-chancellor of the Durban Institute of Technology. UKZNA MF3/1/1-8, 'Homecoming for activist and scholar', *Mednews: Faculty of Medicine Newsletter* 3, no. 1 (January–December 2002).

7. Interview with Sam Fehrsen, Pretoria, 22 August 2003. Ncayiyana's arrest was also discussed by Alan B. Taylor in the CC MH Mouldy Box Scans, 56–63 Folder 2 Loose Papers[S], page 22, Letter 'To the Kids', 28 June 1963.

8. UKZNA MF3/1/1-8, 'Homecoming for activist and scholar', *Mednews: Faculty of Medicine Newsletter* 3, no. 1 (January–December 2002).

9. Other smaller political organisations were negatively affected by the state's repressive actions in during the 1950s and early 1960s. For example, the Communist Party of South Africa was forced to disband in 1950 ahead of the state's passing of the

Suppression of Communism Act, while the South African Indian Congress's momentum was greatly stifled by arrests and bannings of key leaders too.

10. For more on this subject, see, for example, Lodge, *Black Politics in South Africa since 1945*; and Karis and Gerhart, *From Protest to Challenge.*
11. Interview with B.T. Naidoo, Durban, 10 November 2003.
12. UKZNA MQ 1/1/1-5, A.B.T. Mohlomi, 'A review of student organisation', *The Amoeba* 1, no. 2 (16 September 1952).
13. UKZNA MQ 1/1/1-5, V.R. Makgalomele, 'Editorial: Wentworth aspect', *The Amoeba* 1, no. 3 (14 October 1952).
14. Leo Kuper, *An African Bourgeoisie: Race, Class, and Politics in South Africa* (New Haven, CT, and London: Yale University Press, 1965), 154.
15. Edgar Brookes, *A History of the University of Natal* (Pietermaritzburg: University of Natal Press, 1966), 165–6.
16. Wits SAHA South African Political Materials 1964–1990s, The Karis-Gerhart Collection, Part I: Interviews, Folder 8, Jerry Coovadia, 2 June 1988, 1.
17. UKZNA MQ 1/1/1-5, 'Editorial: 1953 – A new era', *The Amoeba* 1, no. 4 (11 March 1953).
18. Interview with B.T. Naidoo, Durban, 10 November 2003.
19. Kuper, *An African Bourgeoisie*, 154.
20. Digby, 'Early black doctors', 427, 444.
21. Brookes, *A History of the University of Natal*, especially chapter 23.
22. UKZNA MQ 1/1/1-5, 'A review of student organisation', *The Amoeba* 1, no. 2 (16 September 1952), and V R Makgalomele, 'Editorial: Wentworth aspect', *The Amoeba* 1, no. 3 (14 October 1952).
23. In addition to the above two *Amoeba* articles, also see A.B.T. Mohlomi, 'A review of student organisation', *The Amoeba* 1, no. 3 (14 October 1952); 'Editorial: 1953 – A new era', *The Amoeba* 1, no. 4 (11 March 1953); 'Why a medical students' representative council?' and 'Complexities of the University of Natal', *The Amoeba* 1, no. 6 (27 May 1953); 'The dilemma of the S.R.C.', *The Amoeba* 2, no. 5 (21 June 1954); C.D. Marivate, 'The UNNE SRC', *The Amoeba* 2, no. 7 (September 1954); 'Student politics after all', *The Amoeba* 3, no. 2 (May 1955).
24. Interview with B.T. Naidoo, Durban, 10 November 2003.
25. Interview with Soromini Kallichurum, Durban, 29 May 1999. Also see 'A student's view on the stand of our staff as regards the Separate University's Bill', *The Amoeba* 1, no. 4 (April 1958); 'Bill shocks med professors and lecturers: Public demonstrations by students; medical school staff to decide on future', *Daily News*, 14 March 1957; and 'Threat of medical staff boycott', *Natal Mercury*, 15 March 1957.
26. UKZNA C10/1/1, 'Alan Taylor Residence and the medical school canteen', UN Council minutes, 15 October 1965.
27. Kuper, *An African Bourgeoisie*, 154–61; and Brookes, *A History of the University of Natal*, 166.
28. 'Reminiscence: The early days: Dr Thaven "BT" Naidoo's story', in *University of Natal Nelson R. Mandela School of Medicine: 50 Years of Achievement in Teaching, Service and Research.*

29. Through involvement on the UNNE SRC, medical students became involved with NUSAS from the early 1950s. See N.G. Moodley (NUSAS Treasurer), 'What NUSAS does for you?' *The Amoeba* 1, no. 4 (11 March 1953), and 'Wentworth students decide to affiliate to NUSAS', *The Amoeba*, 1, no. 5 (16 April 1953).

30. Saleem Badat, *Black Student Politics, Higher Education and Apartheid from SASO to SANSCO, 1968–90* (Pretoria: HSRC, 1999), 79–83.

31. Bruce K. Murray, *Wits the Early Years* (Johannesburg: Witwatersrand University Press, 1982), 340–2. For more on the history of NUSAS, see, for example, Graeme C. Moodie, 'The state and the liberal universities in South Africa: 1948–90', in *Higher Education,* 27 (1994), and Murray, *Wits the 'Open' Years*, especially chapter 9.

32. Murray, *Wits the Early Years*, 339–45. Afrikaans students also formed their own separate organisations.

33. See 'Black souls in white skins?' in Steve Biko *I Write What I Like* (New York: Harper-SanFrancisco, 1986), 19–26; and Badat, *Black Student Politics*, 81–3.

34. Quoted in Mbulelo Vizikhungo Mzamane, Bavusile Maaba and Nkosinathi Biko, 'The Black Consciousness Movement', in South African Democracy Education Trust (SADET), *The Road to Democracy in South Africa. Volume 2, 1970–80* (Pretoria: UNISA Press, 2006), 118.

35. Mzamane, Maaba and Biko, 'The Black Consciousness Movement', in *The Road to Democracy in South Africa*, 113–4.

36. For more on the history of the BCM in South Africa, see, for example, Gail M. Gerhart, *Black Power in South Africa: The Evolution of an Ideology* (Los Angeles: University of California Press, 1978); Millard Arnold, ed., *Steve Biko: Black Consciousness in South Africa* (New York: Random House, 1978); Baruch Hirson, *Year of Fire, Year of Ash: The Soweto Revolt: Roots of a Revolution?* (London: Zed Press, 1979); Lodge, *Black Politics in South Africa since 1945*; Robert Fatton, *Black Consciousness in South Africa* (Albany: State University of New York Press, 1986); Barney Pityana, Mamphela Ramphele, Malusi Mpumlwana and Lindy Wilson, eds, *Bounds of Possibility: The Legacy of Steve Biko and Black Consciousness* (Cape Town, London and Atlantic Highlands, NJ: David Philip and Zed Books, 1991); Badat, *Black Student Politics*; Daniel R. Magaziner, *The Law and the Prophets: Black Consciousness in South Africa, 1968–77* (Auckland Park: Jacana, 2010).

37. Wits CRO, Taffy Adler, 'University of Natal, Black Medical School', *Wits Student* 23, no. 9 (30 April 1971), 9.

38. Interview with Steve Reid, Hillcrest, 24 May 2003.

39. Badat, *Black Student Politics*, 153; and Mzamane, Maaba and Biko, 'The Black Consciousness Movement', 102.

40. Interview with Maila J. Matjila, Durban, 11 July 2003.

41. Mamphela Ramphele, *Across Boundaries: The Journey of a South African Woman Leader* (New York: Feminist Press, 1995), xi.

42. Badat, *Black Student Politics*, 62–5; and Mary A. Beale, 'Apartheid and university education, 1948–70' (PhD diss., University of the Witwatersrand, 1998), 4, 460.

43. Interview with Maila J. Matjila, Durban, 11 July 2003.
44. Interview with M.B. Kistnasamy, Durban, 26 August 2003.
45. Lindy Wilson, 'Bantu Stephen Biko: A Life', in *Bounds of Possibility: The Legacy of Steve Biko and Black Consciousness*, eds Barney Pityana, Mamphela Ramphele, Malusi Mpumlwana and Lindy Wilson (Cape Town, London and Atlantic Highlands, NJ: David Philip and Zed Books, 1991), 22.
46. Interview with Janet Giddy, Hillcrest, 24 May 2003. Also see UCT Faculty of Health Sciences, 'Truth and reconciliation: A process of transformation at UCT Health Sciences Faculty, (unpublished, obtained from Dr Gonda Perez, June 2002), 18; and Wits FHSR M3/40 Internal Reconciliation Commission, 1998, Jules Browde, Patrick Mokhoba and Essop Jassat, 'University of the Witwatersrand Faculty of Health Sciences Internal Reconciliation Commission Report' (November 1998), 30, 45.
47. Interview with Jerry Coovadia, Durban, 24 June 2003. A similar view is also evident in Interview with Mfanyana J. Ndlovu, Durban, 14 August 2003.
48. Sipho Buthelezi, 'The emergence of black consciousness: An historical appraisal', in *Bounds of Possibility: The Legacy of Steve Biko and Black Consciousness*, eds Barney Pityana, Mamphela Ramphele, Malusi Mpumlwana and Lindy Wilson (Cape Town, London and Atlantic Highlands, NJ: David Philip and Zed Books, 1991), 116.
49. Wits CRO, Taffy Adler, 'University of Natal, Black Medical School', *Wits Student* 23, no. 9 (30 April 1971), 9.
50. Karis and Gerhart, *From Protest to Challenge: A Documentary History of African Politics in South Africa*, 91.
51. Wits SAHA South African Political Materials, 1964–1990s, The Karis-Gerhart Collection, Part I: Interviews, Folder 41, Zuma, Nkosazana Dlamini (conducted by Gail Gerhart in London, 3 July 1988), 36.
52. Badat, *Black Student Politics*, 61–75; Majalefa Ralekhetho, 'The black university in South Africa: Ideological captive or transformative agent?' in *Knowledge and Power in South Africa: Critical Perspectives across the Disciplines*, ed. Jonathan D. Jansen (Johannesburg: Skotaville, 1991); and Hirson, *Year of Fire, Year of Ash*, 71.
53. Interview with TM, Pretoria, 21 August 2003.
54. Ina van der Linde, 'MEDUNSA at twenty', *South African Medical Journal* (December 1996), 1507–8.
55. Nimrod Mkele, 'Tragedy of the education system', *Star* (18 April 1983).
56. 'MEDUNSA closes after strike', *Sowetan* (10 June 1983); 'MEDUNSA is closed after row over SRC leaders', *Star* (10 June 1983).
57. 'Students at MEDUNSA hit police action', *Star* (1 October 1982); 'Baton charge', *Sowetan* (14 June 1983); Veleleni Mashumi, 'No peace at "ethnic" campus', *Pretoria News* (24 June 1983); 'Unrest: Fifty due for court', *Sowetan* (28 August 1984); 'MEDUNSA boycott erupts in violence', *Cape Argus* (15 April 1986); 'Students sent home after MEDUNSA riots', *Cape Times* (15 April 1986).
58. Interview with Maila J. Matjila, Durban, 11 July 2003.
59. Interview with Mfanyana J. Ndlovu, Durban, 14 August 2003.

60. Interview with Jerry Coovadia, Durban, 24 June 2003.
61. For more on Biko's biography, see Wilson, 'Bantu Stephen Biko: A Life', 15–77.
62. Interview with ZM, Durban, 6 October 2003.
63. Mbulelo Vizikhungo Mzamane and David R. Howarth, 'Representing blackness: Steve Biko and the Black Consciousness Movement', in *South Africa's Resistance Press: Alternative Voices in the Last Generation under Apartheid*, eds Les Switzer and Mohamed Adhikari (Athens, OH: Ohio University Centre for International Studies, 2000).
64. Interview with Maila J. Matjila, Durban, 11 July 2003.
65. M.W. Makgoba, *Mokoko: The Makgoba Affair: A Reflection on Transformation* (Florida Hills, RSA: Vivlia Publishers, 1997), 32–3.
66. Wilson, 'Bantu Stephen Biko: A life', 28; and Ramphele, *Across Boundaries*, 61.
67. Wits SAHA NAMDA – Uncatalogued, Core Newsclippings, Health Care, October 1991, Vasantha Angamuthu, 'Symbol of black struggle', *Daily News* (15 October 1991).
68. Interview with Breminand Maharaj, Durban, 10 June 2003.
69. Gerhart, *Black Power in South Africa*, chapter 8.
70. Wits SAHA South African Political Materials, 1964–1990s, The Karis-Gerhart Collection, Part I: Interviews, Folder 41, Zuma, Nkosazana Dlamini (conducted by Gail Gerhart in London, 3 July 1988), 35–6.
71. See chapters entitled 'Fear – An important determinant in South African politics', 'What is Black Consciousness?' and 'We Blacks', in Biko, *I Write What I Like*.
72. Mzamane, Maaba and Biko, 'The Black Consciousness Movement', 123.
73. *SASO Newsletter*, 'Who is Black' (September 1970), Aluka, http://www.aluka.org/action/showMetadata?doi=lo.5555/AL.SFF.DOCUMENT.1681.5777.000.000. Sep1970.
74. See, for example, 'Fragmentation of the black resistance', in Biko, *I Write What I Like*, 33–9. For more on the Bantustans, see Laurine Platzky and Cherryl Walker, *The Surplus People: Forced Removals in South Africa* (Johannesburg: Ravan Press, 1985).
75. Hirson, *Year of Fire, Year of Ash*, 86, 108. Hirson estimated that the total number of black students in universities across South Africa in 1972 was about 9 000 and that SASO claimed a student support base (based on *SASO Newsletter* sales) of between 4 000 and 6 000 students.
76. Interview with Y.K. Seedat, Durban, 14 July 2003. This view was supported by others: Interviews with S.B. Pitsoe, Durban, 17 July 2003; May Mashego, Durban, 14 October 2003; and Mfanyana J. Ndlovu, Durban, 14 August 2003.
77. UKZN Board of the Faculty of Medicine minutes, 29 May 1980, 17 August 1984 and 7 October 1985; UKZNA C10/9/1, 'Faculty of Medicine, Alan Taylor Residence', UN Council minutes, 21 September 1984; 'Alan Taylor Residence', 21 September 1984; 'Intimidation of students in the medical school', UN Council minutes, 16 November 1984; 'Inquiry into intimidation of students by the MSRC', UN Senate minutes, 21 November 1984; and 'Alleged intimidation of students in the Faculty of Medicine', UN Council minutes, 17 May 1985.

78. See Gerhart, *Black Power in South Africa*, 279–80.
79. Mosibudi Mangena, *On Your Own: Evolution of Black Consciousness in South Africa/ Azania* (Johannesburg: Skotaville, 1989), 13. Also see Donald Woods, *Biko* (New York: Henry Holt and Co., 1987), 157.
80. Interview with MM, Durban, 28 July 2003. This point was also discussed in an Interview with ZM, Durban, 11 September 2003.
81. Watts argues that by the late 1960s and early 1970s, two-thirds of Indians surveyed, many of whom originated from Natal, lived off-campus. H.L. Watts, 'Black Doctors. Part I: The students', 5, 24.
82. Shan Naidoo, Questionnaire, 2003 and Pooba Govender, Questionnaire, 2003.
83. B.T. Naidoo, 'The first twenty-five years', *Natal University News*, no. 2 (Autumn 1976), 9; Interviews with B.T. Naidoo, Durban, 10 November 2003, and May Mashego, Durban, 7 October 2003. Also see UKZNA C10/8/1, 'Natal medical students may lose bursaries', *Rand Daily Mail* (24 October 1977), and 'Boycott of lectures at medical school', UN Council minutes, 20 June 1980, 5.
84. Interview with Y.K. Seedat, Durban, 14 July 2003.
85. Interview with Jerry Coovadia, Durban, 24 June 2003.
86. Kogila Moodley, 'The continued impact of black consciousness', in *Bounds of Possibility: The Legacy of Steve Biko and Black Consciousness*, eds Barney Pityana, Mamphela Ramphele, Malusi Mpumlwana and Lindy Wilson (Cape Town, London and Atlantic Highlands NJ: David Philip and Zed Books, 1991), 145–6. For more on the in-between status that many Indian South African often found themselves in, see, for example, Bill Freund, *Insiders and Outsiders: The Indian Working Class of Durban, 1910–90* (Portsmouth, NH: Heinemann; Pietermaritzburg: University of Natal Press; and London: James Currey, 1995); and T.G. Ramamurthi, *Apartheid and Indian South Africans: A Study of the Role of Ethnic Indians in the Struggle against Apartheid in South Africa* (New Delhi: Reliance Publishing House, 1995).
87. Quoted in Mzamane, Maaba and Biko, 'The Black Consciousness Movement', 113.
88. Interview with Veronica Wilson, Durban, 6 November 2003.
89. Interview with Jerry Coovadia, Durban, 24 June 2003.
90. Interview with KM, Durban, 14 November 2003.
91. Themba Sono, *Reflections on the Origins of Black Consciousness in South Africa* (Pretoria: HSRC, 1993), 65; Badat, *Black Student Politics*, 86; Buthelezi, 'The emergence of black consciousness', 115–6, 124.
92. Ramphele, *Across Boundaries*, 55–6.
93. Interview with ZM, Durban, 11 September 2003.
94. Interview with Jerry Coovadia, Durban, 24 June 2003.
95. Buthelezi, 'The emergence of black consciousness', 116.
96. Mangena, *On Your Own*, 30.
97. In 1978 the Azanian Peoples' Organisation (AZAPO) was formed after black consciousness organisations were banned. AZAPO was established to carry forward black consciousness-inspired political ideologies, but became less popular in the 1980s as non-racial opposition politics emerged more strongly.

98. The UDF was formed in 1983 as a popular, non-racial and multi-class coalition of civic associations, churches, trade unions, student organisations, women's groups and sports bodies. It pursued a strategy of making South Africa 'ungovernable', promoting boycotts and protest actions like consumer and work stay-aways. Although the UDF did not formally affiliate itself to the banned ANC during the apartheid period, a strategy of survival in a repressive political environment, ANC leaders helped guide many of its policies and actions. See Tom Lodge and Bill Nasson, *All, Here, and Now: Black Politics in South Africa in the 1980s* (Cape Town: Ford Foundation and David Philip, 1991).

99. For more on the divisive nature and powerful impact of ethnicity and ethnic politics in South Africa, see Gerhard Maré, *Ethnicity and Politics in South Africa* (London and Atlantic Highlands, NJ: Zed Books, 1993); and Shula Marks, *The Ambiguities of Dependence in South Africa: Class, Nationalism, and the State in Twentieth-Century Natal* (Baltimore and London: Johns Hopkins University Press, 1986).

100. Interview with S.B. Pitsoe, Durban, 17 July 2003.

101. See, for example, 'Fragmentation of the black resistance' and 'Let's talk about Bantustans', in Biko, *I Write What I Like*; and Hirson, *Year of Fire, Year of Ash*, 113–7.

102. The first quotation comes from an African doctor who identified himself as Zulu.

103. UKZN Board of the Faculty of Medicine minutes, 13 January 1984, 1–2, and 25 March 1984, 1–2, and *Apartheid Medicine: Health and Human Rights in South Africa* (Washington, DC: American Association for the Advancement of Science, 1990), 29–30.

104. This interviewee did not want his name used. During the 1980s, many activists viewed doctors who worked in the homelands as sell-outs who propped up the homeland system. Of course, the situation was often more complicated than this. For example, married partners Janet Giddy and Steve Reid were forced to work in Bethesda, a KwaZulu-administered rural hospital during the late 1980s and early 1990s, as punishment for Reid's stance as a conscientious objector to military service. Both remember being labelled as political sell-outs at the time. Interviews with Janet Giddy, Hillcrest, 2 June 2003, and Steve Reid, Hillcrest, 24 May and 10 June 2003.

105. This Zulu interviewee's name has been omitted to protect his identity.

106. UWC MAC Medical Schools, 'We won't be silenced: SA pays Buthelezi, but he doesn't have to toe the line – students', *City Press* (22 January 1984).

107. On this issue, see Nkosinathi Gwala, 'State control, student politics and the crisis in black universities', in *Popular Struggles in South Africa*, eds William Cobbett and Robin Cohen (Trenton, NJ: Africa World Press, 1988), 179; Wits SAHA South African Political Materials 1964–1990s, The Karis-Gerhart Collection, Part III: Political Documents, NUSAS, Folder 583, Lawrence Boya, 'History of black student organisation', NUSAS July Festival Speeches, 1987, 48; and Debby Bonnin,

Georgina Hamilton, Robert Morrell and Ari Sitas, 'The struggle for Natal and KwaZulu: Workers, township dwellers and Inkatha, 1972–85', in *Political Economy and Identities in KwaZulu-Natal: Historical and Social Perspectives*, ed. Robert Morrell (Durban: Indicator Press, 1996), 161.

108. This interviewee's names has been omitted to protect his identity.

109. Fatima Meer, ed., *Resistance in the Townships* (Durban: Madiba Publications, 1989), 145.

110. Cedric de Beer, *The South African Disease: Apartheid Health and Health Services* (London: Catholic Institute for International Relations, 1986), 59.

111. UKZN MSA, 'Doctors turn tail on posts pledge: Controversy over oath of allegiance for hospital staff', *Sunday Tribune*, 31 August 1986; and Steve Reid and Janet Giddy, 'Rural health and human rights – Summary of a Submission to the Truth and Reconciliation Commission Health Sector Hearings, 17 June 1997', *South African Medical Journal* (August 1998), 980–1; Y.K. Seedat, 'The health crisis in Natal – A personal view', *South African Medical Journal* (7 July 1990), 3.

112. Interview with Breminand Maharaj, Durban, 10 June 2003; and Mamphela Ramphele, 'The dynamics of gender within black consciousness organisations: A personal view', in *Bounds of Possibility: The Legacy of Steve Biko and Black Consciousness*, eds Barney Pityana, Mamphela Ramphele, Malusi Mpumlwana and Lindy Wilson (Cape Town, London and Atlantic Highlands, NJ: David Philip and Zed Books, 1991), 214–5, 219. For more on the male-dominated nature of political organisations in South Africa more generally, see Cherryl Walker, *Women and Resistance in South Africa* (London: Onyx Press, 1982).

113. Ramphele, *Across Boundaries*, 110, 117; and Ramphele, 'The dynamics of gender within black consciousness organisations', 226.

114. Interview with May Mashego, Durban, 14 October 2003.

115. Wits SAHA South African Political Materials 1964–1990s, The Karis-Gerhart Collection, Part 1: Interviews, Folder 41, Zuma, Nkosazana Dlamini (conducted by Gail Gerhart in London, 3 July 1988), 14.

116. For more on this subject, see Daniel R. Magaziner, 'Pieces of a (wo)man: Feminism, gender and adulthood in black consciousness, 1968–77', *Journal of Southern African Studies* 37, no. 1 (March 2011).

117. Interview with Jerry Coovadia, Durban, 24 June 2003; Ramphele, 'The dynamics of gender within black consciousness organisations', 215; and Interview with Malusi Mpumlwana, conducted by Gail Gerhart in Tarrytown, 16 May 1978, 2.

118. For more on this, see Desiree Lewis, 'The politics of feminism in South Africa'. in *South African Feminisms: Writing, Theory, and Criticism 1990–94*, ed. Margaret J. Daymond (New York and London: Garland Publishing, 1996); and Gay W. Seidman, 'Gendered citizenship: South Africa's democratic transition and the construction of a gendered state', *Gender and Society* 13, no. 3 (June 1999).

119. Wits SAHA, South African Political Materials 1964–1990s, The Karis-Gerhart Collection, Part III: Political Documents, SASO, Folder 748, Maphiri Masekela, 'Black consciousness and the role of the black woman' (December 1971).

120. Wits SAHA South African Political Materials 1964–1990s, The Karis-Gerhart Collection, Karis-Gerhart Collection, Part I: Interviews, Folder 41, Nkosazana Zuma, 3 July 1988, 14.

121. Ramphele, 'The dynamics of gender within black consciousness organisations', 219–20.

122. 'We Blacks', 28–9. Emphasis added.

123. 'We Blacks' and 'What is Black Consciousness?', 29, 10–1.

124. For more on the history of the construction of 'struggle' masculinity amongst black South African men, see, for example, Thokozani Xaba, 'Masculinity and its malcontents: The confrontation between "struggle masculinity" and "post-struggle masculinity"' in *Changing Men in Southern Africa*, ed. Robert Morrell (Pietermaritzburg: University of Natal Press; and London and New York: Zed Books, 2001), 108–9; and Thembisa Waetjen, *Workers and Warriors: Masculinity and the Struggle for Nation in South Africa* (Cape Town: HSRC Press, 2004).

125. Interview with K.P. Naidoo, Durban, 4 June 2004.

126. Interview with Veronica Wilson, Durban, 6 November 2003. Similar points were raised in Interviews with B.T. Naidoo, Durban, 10 November 2003, and TM, Pretoria, 21 August 2003.

127. Interview with May Mashego, Durban, 7 October 2003.

128. Interview with Mfanyana J. Ndlovu, Durban, 14 August 2003.

129. Interview with Breminand Maharaj, Durban, 10 June 2003; and Interview with May Mashego, Durban, 14 October 2003.

130. Interview with Veronica Wilson, Durban, 6 November 2003.

131. Interview with Maila J. Matjila, Durban, 11 July 2003.

132. Interview with Breminand Maharaj, Durban, 10 June 2003.

133. Interview with Maila J. Matjila, Durban, 11 July 2003.

134. Michel-Rolph Trouillot, *Silencing the Past: Power and the Production of History* (Boston: Beacon Press, 1995), especially chapter 2, entitled 'The three faces of Sans Souci'.

135. *Students in the Barracks: Memories of Alan Taylor Residence* (University of Natal, Durban: Audio-Visual Alternatives, 1989). Also see UWC MAC Natal, 1988, Vasantha Angamuthu, 'Era ends as residence closes: Ex-military barracks gave Natal students a unique privacy', *City Press* (28 August 1988).

136. See, for example, *The University of Natal Durban Medical School: A Response to the Challenge of Africa* (Durban: Hayne and Gibson, 1954), 9; Interview with Soromini Kallichurum, Durban, 29 May 1999; B.T. Naidoo, 'A history of the Durban Medical School', *South African Medical Journal* (25 September 1976), 1625–6; *University of Natal Medical School Reconciliation Graduation Booklet 1995* (Durban: Indicator Press, December 1995), 3; and *University of Natal Nelson R. Mandela School of Medicine: 50 Years of Achievement*, 9.

137. David William Cohen, *The Combing of History* (Chicago and London: University of Chicago Press, 1994), 22.

138. Interview with Mfanyana J. Ndlovu, Durban, 14 August 2003.

CHAPTER 7

The 1970s and 1980s

Medical student political activism and its consequences

'Life was always like a state of emergency.'

— Breminand Maharaj

While it is clear that some medical students shied away from politics as a way to respond to the many hardships they endured, SASO, from the late 1960s and through the 1970s, stimulated a response from students at the other end of the spectrum too. Before it was banned by the state in 1977, SASO provided a confident and captivating anti-apartheid political message that helped to conscientise many medical students. However, it also politicised some students, who felt encouraged to stand up in defiant opposition to their oppressors. For activist students, this rebellious stance would continue after 1977 with the swing towards support for the United Democratic Alliance (UDF)/ANC-aligned politics in later years. During this period, Durban's medical campus became a vital seat of anti-apartheid political activity. Hugh Philpott recollected, whilst serving as dean of the medical school in the early 1980s, that P.W. Botha, who became the prime minister of South Africa from 1978 to 1984, and then the first state president from 1984 to 1989, said 'that he regarded the medical students' residence at Wentworth as the breeding ground for the ANC . . . as a breeding ground for young politicians'.[1] Often, their political activities made news headlines, providing a serious challenge to and something of an embarrassment for the state which had created this institution originally as the great showpiece of apartheid. It would also put the school in the firing line for police harassment.

This chapter will examine examples of specific issues and types of political activities that medical students got involved in during the 1970s and 1980s, as well as the diverse range of staff responses to their students' extracurricular political activities. Seeing student activism as an embarrassment, but also as a threat to their policies, the apartheid government often responded harshly to silence them. Some students paid a high price for their political activities. An analysis of the varied and sometimes serious consequences that involvement in extracurricular political activities had for these medical students will form the final part of this chapter.

Medical student opposition to apartheid: The 1970s
SASO community development work

> '[We] were at school but we were also very much concerned about what was happening in different communities . . . So we were not only students. We were also putting our ears [to the ground] and responding to other things outside the medical school.'
>
> — May Mashego

During the 1970s, SASO activists resisted the state's attempts to create a co-optable, black middle class supportive of its plans for separate development. It also opposed the production of an educated elite separated from the black working class which would prevent a commonality of interests. SASO activists worked hard to conscientise students about the significance of maintaining close links with, working within and providing services to their communities.[2] This message was particularly targeted at medical students, who had the most to gain in earning power and class privileges once they had graduated. An African medical graduate who studied in Durban during the latter half of the 1970s stated that SASO students were 'committed to community involvement' because their long training had a vital shaping role in students' perspectives:

> Remember . . . we got to campus as teens and medicine takes six years and by the time you're finished . . . you've sort of defined your outlook in terms of life. And if you're locked in there and you're doing [medicine] in that circumscribed environment and you don't interact with the community, you come out a stranger . . . [W]e were . . . cognisant of that very early [on] and we decided to interact with the community around us . . .[3]

For most students, SASO's community involvement message was not a difficult sell. However, while as students they were privileged because of their educational advantages, they did not feel isolated from events happening in their wider communities. In fact, they had been born and raised under the harsh realities of apartheid in such communities, as Steve Biko pointed out when he wrote: 'My friendships, my love, my education, my thinking and every other facet of my life have been carved and shaped within the context of separate development.'[4] Students could not easily disassociate themselves from what was happening outside the medical school's walls. Maila J. Matjila, who after graduating became a community health medicine specialist, made this point clear:

> ... you are part and parcel of the greater community ... you are also living in it so it affects you ... [A]ll the complaints and all the arrests [and other difficulties] that were taking place in the black communities ... [were affecting] our parents and our brothers and sisters. ... [Thus] we were affected [too]'.[5]

A popular slogan used by SASO activists in their speeches and writings was that they were '*Black* students and not Black *Students*', which placed the emphasis on their common black identity rather than on their educated and thus elite status as students.[6]

Mamphela Ramphele, who played a prominent leadership role in SASO during her student days in the early 1970s, helped open and run two community health clinics after she graduated. One was called Zanempilo Community Health Centre, which was opened near King William's Town in the Eastern Cape in 1975, while the other one was called Ithuseng Community Health Centre, which was opened a few years later in Lenyenye near Tzaneen in the north-eastern Transvaal. Of this work she wrote that she and other SASO activists were anxious to get involved in 'practical programmes to redress the inequalities of the past' and felt it was their duty to 'plough back their acquired skills into the community for the development of the poor'.[7]

Nkosazana Dlamini Zuma, another 1970s student activist, who later went on to become the minister of health in the first democratically elected government and worked to restructure the public health-care system to refocus on community-oriented primary health-care services, argued that 'there was a lot of emphasis on the fact that their own liberation would come from themselves'.[8] The idea was to 'popularise SASO and Black Consciousness not by just talking to people and . . . telling them, but by physically being there and being with them, sharing ideas with them . . . and help them to help themselves'. If local people were involved in improving themselves and conditions in their own communities, SASO leaders believed that the chances were much higher that these improvements would survive after the students left.

A key SASO initiative was the promotion of students' involvement in community development work. During the early 1970s, SASO activists started many different types of projects around the country which included, for example, improving literacy skills, helping communities to build durable homes, and providing clean water through water protection and sanitation schemes.[9] Malusi Mpumlwana, who was a medical student in Durban in 1971 until he failed his courses and then trained as a minister, remembered working in a rural Natal community that had a clean-water problem: 'We were working hard there to apply Paulo Freire's method [which entailed] gradually being accepted in [a] community, by going to beer drinks [occasions], then getting discussion going, having the villagers themselves initiate a solution of self-help for their problem.'[10]

Diliza Mji, who became the president of SASO in the mid-1970s, also recalled becoming involved in another of SASO's programmes, its literacy campaign, soon after starting his medical studies in 1972. In an interview conducted by Gail Gerhart in New York in June 1987, Mji discussed an example of this 'very important project' in the Natal region. He recalled how SASO medical students used to commute by 'kombi' (minibus) down to a rural village called Dududu on the south coast to a school where they spent their free time teaching illiterate members of this community to read and write.[11] For Mji, that was an attempt by SASO 'to forge links with non-students or community groups, and extend its influence beyond its constituency'.

In addition, community health projects formed an essential component of this work. For example, during the 1970s, SASO medical students worked closely with members of the Black Community Programmes (BCP). The BCP was a black consciousness organisation that generated local and international funds for black community development work in South Africa, including funds for the provision of health services for poverty-stricken black communities in and around Durban. Funds were also raised for this type of volunteer work from the University of Natal's Students' Representatuve Councils, particularly through its 'Rag Fund' and donations from the general public.[12]

On weekends, SASO medical students, in their clinical years, used a rotating volunteer roster system to provide free, primary health-care services, under the supervision of qualified volunteer doctors, to a number of low-income areas in Natal. These areas included the Happy Valley Clinic for the coloured community of Austerville/Wentworth near their Alan Taylor Residence (ATR), the African community in Inanda, and at the Mahatma Gandhi Clinic in New Farm, an impoverished Indian community near Phoenix.[13] Moreover, students who had not yet reached their clinical years, but wanted to get involved, could assist with the 'the administrative side' of running these clinics.[14] There are even examples of Durban SASO students giving up their university holidays to travel further inland to do volunteer development work, such as teaching literacy skills and providing basic health-care services at the Mabopane clinic for people living in Winterveld, an impoverished African settlement near Pretoria.[15]

At these clinic sites, students provided patients with basic curative services and preventive services, of which health education was a central concern.[16] Advice to address the causes and prevention of parasitic diseases, promotion of good hygiene methods, sanitation and nutrition were some of the main focus areas. In a report to the national executive committee of SASO in May 1974, it was noted that 'preventive and protective medicines is without any doubt the most important part of this field of our operation, even more than the healing and treatment of the patients'.[17] A bit later on, this report continued: 'Preventive medicine is in fact a must in clinics when one considers the fact that here you have a ready made model through which the basic elements and principles of Black [Consciousness] existence can be smoothly transmitted.'

For SASO activists, involvement in educational and preventive health-care work fitted in well with their black consciousness ideals. Primarily, this was concerned with providing their patients with the necessary knowledge and skills to encourage self-help as well as to empower black communities to take responsibility for their own health. This was viewed as a necessary prerequisite for black liberation from apartheid oppression.[18] Additionally, this type of work helped students to 'give back' to destitute black communities, and enabled them to spread their black consciousness message to a wider audience.

What is more, involvement in this type of extracurricular, health-care work extended the medical education acquired by students. The primary-level, community health work that SASO students got involved in provided a vital shift in perspective away from the expensive, curative medicine approaches taught at medical schools in South Africa at the time.[19] After Durban's innovative social and community health programme for undergraduates was abandoned in the early 1960s because of the state's refusal to fund what it considered a dangerous 'socialist' experiment, it took many years before there was a return to this focus in the formal curriculum. Indeed, it would take until the late 1970s and through the 1980s for a new community health department to once again plant solid roots on Durban's medical campus. Until then, primary-level community health care and preventive medicine were not priorities of this school's undergraduate curriculum; instead, like other schools around the country, the curriculum was geared towards encouraging specialisation and producing doctors highly trained in curative, hospital-based forms of medicine.[20]

At the time of MEDUNSA's launch in the 1970s, Durban's medical school was criticised for its 'conservative' curative and hospital-based curriculum that essentially tried to copy its white counterparts.[21] Between 1951, when the Durban school first opened its doors to students, to the early 1990s, a virtual explosion of academic departments and sub-departments had occurred from just a handful to over 30.[22] While high standards at the time were certainly equated with this type of medicine, these perspectives and approaches prevented a training of doctors that adequately met the primary health-care needs of the majority of the country's population. In contrast, when MEDUNSA was formed, one of the ways its ideologues distinguished their institution was to stress its foresight in focusing on primary-level care and community health services.

Therefore, if Durban medical students wanted to gain increased exposure to preventive and community health medicine after the Karks left and before the late 1970s, they either had to create their own reading groups on the subject or organise conferences around these themes themselves. Of course, they could also wait until after graduation to complete postgraduate diplomas on the subject, or get actively involved in community health work outside the formal curriculum.[23]

Unfortunately, despite their best intentions, SASO community health initiatives tended to be of limited scale and were often beset by problems.

Staff shortages, limited financial resources, lack of experience and transportation problems were some of the operational issues faced by these projects. The fact that students are by nature a transitory group, who move on to other things once they graduate, was also a notable factor. Expulsions from universities and the banning of SASO leaders (for instance, the large number of bannings that took place in 1973, including Steve Biko and Barney Pityana) did not help staffing matters either.

Furthermore, the compounded socio-economic problems faced by black communities in apartheid South Africa could not be easily solved by a few SASO students with limited training and resources. Mamphela Ramphele noted in a written piece on black consciousness and community development that whilst working in Winterveld, for example, SASO students were shocked by the level of poverty they encountered and 'the enormity of the problems people had to grapple with'. In addition, they had not prepared themselves for 'the bitter fruits of powerlessness' that plagued such poor areas, nor had they readied themselves for the huge problem of apathy and despair that enveloped people in these communities.[24]

Despite these problems, the provision of desperately needed health-care services and self-help health educational skills did nevertheless assist some patients over the years and provided medical students with experience in medicine practised outside the hospital's walls.[25] Moreover, for the 1970s' generation of students, involvement in SASO community health projects helped 'open . . . [their] eyes' to the inadequacies and inequalities of apartheid forms of medicine, and provided them with 'a much broader perspective' on health care, particularly some of the 'social, economic [and] political . . . factors which impinge[d] on it'.[26] Exposure to these situations had the effect of maturing the students in their social concerns and made them want 'to fight more', as it made them realise that apartheid health inequalities existed not only in their own communities but extended to affect all black communities in apartheid South Africa.[27]

Boycotts, commemorative events and mass marches
SASO medical students studying at the University of Natal also used a variety of tactics to voice their opposition and challenge the system of apartheid. Protest marches were sometimes organised down Umbilo or Sydney roads, the main arterial roads into and out of Durban that ran past the medical school. Academic boycotts, which entailed students abandoning lectures, thus undermining the functioning of university classes, were used

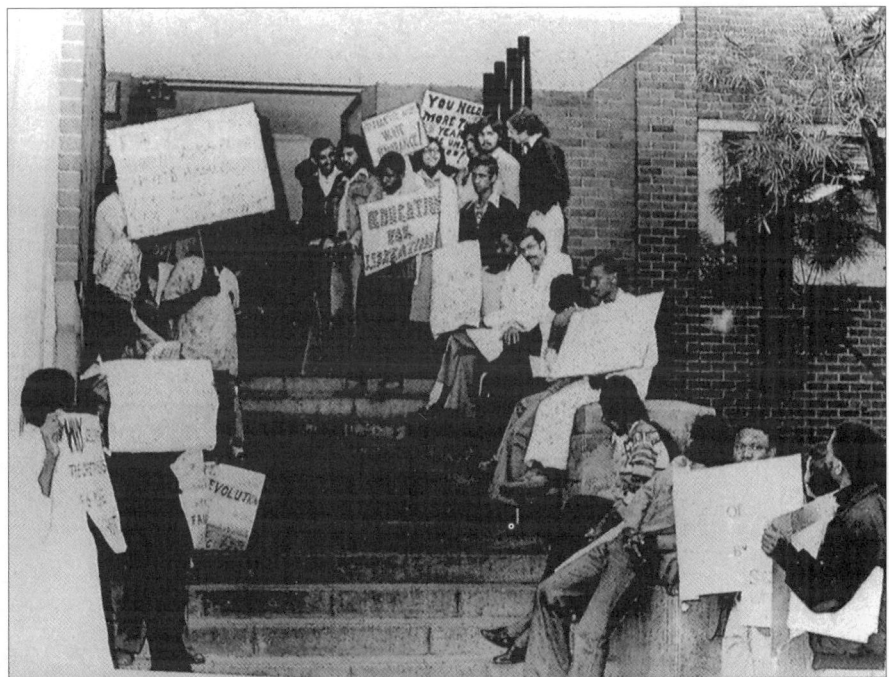

Photo 7.1   Student protest, August 1976. (*UKZN Medical School Archives*)

as an effective strategy. So too was the organisation of mass meetings or rallies. Additionally, commemorative services were often held for those who were killed by the apartheid police, providing another significant outlet for student opposition.

Specific examples of such tactics abound during the early 1970s. In 1970, a ten-year commemorative mass service was held at the medical school for the 69 people who were killed by police-fire on protesters who burned their pass books in Sharpeville. The organisation of such mass memorial services was a strategic mechanism that enabled student activists to remember the dead, but also to lambaste the apartheid system, often responsible for bringing about the deaths of activists. The untimely and shocking death of Steve Biko in detention in September 1977 provided another such occasion. It rallied medical students in Durban and indeed students across the country to critique the apartheid state and to mobilise support against its multiplicity of abuses.[28] Soromini Kallichurum, who lectured at the school at the time, remembered how after Biko was killed, '. . . afterwards when the facts started coming out about the way he was beaten up and all that, there was a lot of protest' on the campus and elsewhere.[29]

On some occasions, Durban medical students used the boycott tactic to show support for things going on in other parts of the country. For example, in 1972, Durban students joined other black university campuses and boycotted lectures for three days in protest against the expulsion of 1 146 African students from the University of the North. These students had been expelled because they had come out in support of their SRC president O.R. Tiro's attack on the discriminatory system of university education for black students.[30] The early 1970s were trying times for students. Reflecting on her time as a student, Nkosazana Dlamini Zuma noted in an interview that in 1973 'again there was quite a big confrontation at the University of Natal. There was a meeting there, it was [for the] March twenty-first celebration. While at the meeting, some Special Branch people were identified and they were beaten up' by the students.[31]

A couple of weeks later, it was reported that 300 students spent a number of days boycotting their lectures and attended another mass meeting organised by SASO on the medical school campus. This was to protest against the arrest and detention of several medical students who were suspected of beating up four security policemen who were caught spying at their Sharpeville commemoration meeting in March.[32] Student protests also broke out when it was heard in March 1973 that a number of SASO and BPC leaders, including Biko and Pityana, had been arrested and served with banning orders.[33]

Following these incidents, in September 1974, many SASO medical students participated in a mass pro-FRELIMO rally that took place in Durban and was organised by the BPC in support of Mozambique gaining independence from Portugal. This gathering was violently broken up by the security police, who arrested and detained a number of SASO and BPC leaders under the Terrorism Act. One of those detained was Aubrey Mokoape, who had been a medical student in Durban. Mokoape was tried and convicted under the Terrorism Act along with eight other people. After a seventeen-month trial, the SASO Nine, as they became known, were convicted and sent to Robben Island to serve prison sentences ranging between five and ten years.[34] These arrests sparked off further medical student protests, as well as wave after wave of campus unrest in other parts of the country.[35]

Anti-apartheid activities in the mid- to late-1970s brought continuous disruption to the medical school's curriculum. This was noted by Hugh Philpott, at the time a lecturer at the school and the head of the Department of Obstetrics and Gynaecology. Philpott remembered how students 'boycotted so many things' that he could not 'ever remember not being in the midst of a boycott'.[36] One incident that sparked heightened medical student protests was the 16 June 1976 Soweto Uprising. While there is much discussion in academic publications about what role SASO played in promoting this well-known uprising, which saw thousands of African school pupils abandon their classes to march in protest against the Bantu Education system, it has generally been accepted that the defiant and confident BC message that had filtered through to black township schools by this time period was key.[37] Several school pupils were injured or killed by the police who tried to stop their march.

Three days later, on 19 June, after the minister of justice had banned outdoor public gatherings in an attempt to curb the wave of country-wide civil disobedience and violence that followed the uprising, about 200 Durban medical students staged a demonstration and marched down Sydney Road towards the Durban city centre.[38] As they marched, they waved placards and distributed pamphlets to motorists and pedestrians, giving voice to their opposition to the state and support for the Soweto protesters. Although many of these students managed to flee when the police intervened to disperse them, 87 medical students were arrested and charged under the Riotous Assemblies Act, forcing the medical school to close early for its July holidays to accommodate the large number of students who were absent from classes.[39] University-appointed lawyers and the parents of arrested students managed, after several days of negotiations and the payment of fines, to get these students released from prison. A couple of months later, in August 1976, another student march was organised to protest the ensuing security police raids and harassment of students living at ATR, for suspected anti-apartheid political activities being organised there.[40]

The Soweto Uprising precipitated several months of widespread, national protests against apartheid. School pupils, university students, township residents and workers attacked and destroyed shops and properties belonging to the state. It took the deaths of over a thousand people, the detention of hundreds more and the banning of many key organisations (including SASO in October 1977) to restore 'law and order' to the country. One

African graduate, who recalled participating in these 1976 protest activities, said in an interview how 'we had really critical meetings trying to see whether we should actually abandon being at medical school or not, and then go and join the struggle . . . and going to take up arms' in the banned underground organisations like the ANC.[41]

The phase-out issue and MEDUNSA
The late 1970s was also an essential period for student protests against the state in other arenas. Towards the end of 1975, the University of Natal's Faculty of Medicine was notified of the state's decision that this campus should phase out Africans from its student body.[42] Basically, the faculty was instructed not to enrol any first-year African students from 1976; these students were from then onwards to receive their first year of training at one of the country's black universities, before continuing on at MEDUNSA, upon whose correlated opening this whole scheme depended.[43] In fact this plan had been on the cards since the mid-1960s, though it took the government time to work out the logistics of this idea and the funding for the scheme to put it into action.[44]

A growing shortage of African doctors, especially in the rural areas, was another reason this scheme materialised. In the fifteen year period between 1958 and 1973, when Durban was *the* primary medical-training site of black doctors in South Africa, only 167 African doctors had successfully graduated from this institution. This resulted in a total of about 350 African doctors to serve a population of about 16 million Africans at the time.[45] By 1984, the doctor-to-population ratio was 1:330 for whites; 1:750 for Indians; 1:12 000 for coloureds; and 1:91 000 for Africans.[46] MEDUNSA was built with the intention to train a variety of African health professionals, but especially physicians, to help ease the African doctor shortage in the country. Apartheid ideologues hoped that this institution would become a comprehensive, African, health sciences training school which would have an annual intake of about 200 aspiring African doctors, as well as 50 prospective individuals in each of its other disciplines.[47]

Moreover, in addition to giving notice of the phase-out of African students, the state made it clear that Indian and coloured medical students in Durban would start being phased out shortly after this process for Africans was completed. The aim was to force these black minority groups to attend their own ethnic universities too, such as the universities of Durban-Westville (UDW) for Indians and the Western Cape (UWC) for coloureds, where it was envisaged that separate medical schools would eventually be established to accommodate them.[48] Furthermore, in line with its separate-development plans, the state wanted to make way for the training of white medical students at the University of Natal.[49]

This phase-out decision was met with enormous resistance from students. In February 1976 a *Natal Mercury* reporter highlighted how more than 200 black medical students 'with raised fists symbolising Black Power' assembled outside their school in Durban to voice their opposition to the government's decision to phase out African students starting that year.[50] Robust efforts made by the university and particularly the managers of the Faculty of Medicine to argue against the proposal succeeded in securing a brief reprieve for the school in 1976. The state was made to see that the immediate implementation of this policy, before the actual completion and opening of MEDUNSA, would have actually worsened the country's African doctor shortage.[51] However, in 1977 the state made it clear that it would implement its phase-out policy from the start of the 1978 academic year, to correspond with the opening of MEDUNSA.

Joe Ndlovu, who was still in high school in 1977, remembered keenly following the events at the medical school as they unfolded in the media. This was the institution he hoped to attend once he had matriculated. During this year, numerous protest activities 'snowballed and kind of proliferated' into the declaration by student leaders, in September of that year, of an indefinite boycott of lectures by the entire medical student body to protest the state's decision to phase out African students from the University of Natal (UN) from 1978.[52] May Mashego, who participated in this boycott, discussed with passion how all students were stirred into action because this renewed focus on the phase-out policy would affect them all: 'We were told . . . they [the UN] were not going to take . . . [African students] next year . . . So this was when we kicked up a big fight . . . And for them to reverse that decision we had to fight, we had to go on a prolonged boycott.'[53] While on the boycott, students attended regular mass meetings at the school to keep informed about events. One alumnus, who was a senior student at the time, remembered how students also designed and printed pamphlets, and would 'drive around in the townships and give pamphlets asking for support', and inform the general public of the reasons for their boycott.[54]

Medical students gave two main reasons for their boycott actions. Firstly, they objected to the government's creation of yet another African-only facility in the Bantustans, rather than opening up existing medical-training facilities in the country for all students.[55] By 1977, these facilities included, in addition to Durban's medical school, two white English-medium medical schools at UCT and Wits, and three Afrikaans-medium schools at the universities of Pretoria, Stellenbosch and Bloemfontein. The state's aim was to build MEDUNSA at an exorbitant cost of about 30 million rand, when it was cheaper and easier to expand Durban's already tried and tested facilities.[56] For students, its creation was driven not by logic but by political considerations of separate development, which they actively opposed.

Secondly, students voiced opposition to what they regarded as the inferior educational standards of this apartheid institution. These concerns surfaced in the wake of many public discussions that raged during the 1970s about how best to alleviate the African doctor shortage. During this period, proposals as diverse as the creation of a shortened four-year medical-training scheme for Africans in the homelands, to the provision of supplementary training for African traditional healers working in the reserves, were suggested as possible ways forward.[57] The fact that MEDUNSA was prepared to accept students with lower entrance qualifications, including students who had failed in Durban, did not help matters either, despite assuring the public that its end degrees would meet the requirements set out by the South African Medical and Dental Council.

It was in this broader context, where general fears about the lowering of standards were being debated publicly, that medical students raised some of their strongest objections. As a result, in the years leading up to MEDUNSA's opening in 1978, this institution was tarred with a brush of negativity. Joe Ndlovu maintained that students' feelings were so strongly against the creation of MEDUNSA because they felt that 'it was being created as an inferior institution'. Indeed, in his opinion, the government had made it very clear that 'there were going to be no Indians and no coloureds. It was just going to be Africans only . . . And so it was viewed with suspicion immediately.'[58] When considering the issue, another African doctor, who trained in Durban between 1980 and 1986, concurred:

> We really didn't . . . believe that MEDUNSA was any good in the first place because, you know, the way that it came across, I was sort of like . . . this medical school [Durban] is too advanced for Africans and therefore

let's breed them something [else] at MEDUNSA.... And actually for quite some time ... lots of us who qualified from here, we had that mentality that whatever's coming out of MEDUNSA wasn't good quality.[59]

Many of the medical school's teaching staff were also opposed to MEDUNSA from the outset. One lecturer in the Department of Obstetrics and Gynaecology, S.B. Pitsoe, claimed that when MEDUNSA was opened, 'people looked down upon it' and it did not have a good name. It was 'an apartheid baby, so to speak', built in the Bantustan area of Ga-Rankuwa, and 'anybody who couldn't qualify here went up there'.[60] Andy Mogotlane, who was a senior lecturer in anatomy in Durban when MEDUNSA was established, recalled how '[i]t was a terribly unpopular idea' and he resisted it. 'Apart from the racial separation issues', he noted that he was concerned 'over rumours that "Bantu education medical training" would be confined to so-called African diseases that would have confined students to a limited area of medicine'.[61] Jerry Coovadia, who taught in the Department of Paediatrics, felt strongly about the issue too. 'The one thing they wanted to do was to take away African students from here and put them in MEDUNSA ... and I must say, a credit to the university and medical school faculty, it was rigorously opposed by everyone, from the bottom to the top. Everyone, everyone!'[62]

Reflecting on opinions such as these, one is struck by the uncannily similar arguments that were made against the Durban Medical School when it first opened nearly 30 years earlier. Funded by the state, it was also regarded by many as an apartheid-created institution, as well as an inferior 'tribal medical school' or 'bush college' that would not be able to compete with its white counterparts.[63] Having worked many long years to overcome these negative stereotypes, even by the 1970s the medical school's staff and students stood rigidly in defence of its high standards. And, MEDUNSA, the new 'apartheid baby' on the medical educational block, felt the brunt of this.

To ensure that negative comparisons were not made between MEDUNSA and the medical school, Durban students and staff worked hard to drive an ideological wedge between the two institutions. Since their own similar origins meant that they could not really push the argument that MEDUNSA was a creation of the apartheid government, they focused instead on what the medical profession feared most: that MEDUNSA was the creation of 'some indigenous healers' [school].[64] These negative comparisons were extended to the names students assigned MEDUNSA, as one alumnus remembered:

> The popular name of MEDUNSA became HERBUNSA – the Herbal University of South Africa. That's what we called it because . . . we felt that it was of lower standard, it was going to be herbal [or traditional] medicine, which is the way I think we were socialised that herbal medicine was inferior to western medicine. But that's how students expressed it.[65]

Like their lecturers, many students had internalised scientific medicine as the superior healing philosophy and approach, and anything that deviated from the standard medical school admissions and teaching norms was considered inferior.

Only in time would many come to see their earlier judgements of MEDUNSA as unduly harsh, and that this institution's more lenient admissions policies and supportive academic environment, which included carefully thought-out remedial and bridging programmes, ultimately did much to help graduate greater numbers of African doctors.[66] For Sam Fehrsen, a now retired family medicine professor who was at MEDUNSA from its inception, 'there was no intention of having a second-class doctor. This was attributed by the people furthest from us to us, that that was our aim.'[67] Fehrsen felt the Natal Medical School staff and students objected so strongly to MEDUNSA as they knew that the government wanted 'to close down Natal and it took some enormous amounts of pressure from their side to keep it open. And obviously they had to find every [means] that they could to shoot MEDUNSA down.'

To return to the 1977 phase-out protests, the medical students' prolonged boycott placed enormous pressure on students, but also on the state. On 19 October 1977, five weeks after the boycott had started, the state proved more receptive to another University of Natal delegation that had been sent to meet Piet Koornhof, the minister of national education in Pretoria, to negotiate on the medical school's behalf. This delegation consisted of the principal at the time, N.D. Clarence, the dean of the medical school, J.V.O. Reid, and a senior professor of medicine, E.B. Adams.[68] Their aim was to get the phase-out decision, due for implementation at the start of 1978, rescinded. By the time this delegation met the minister, the very public furore created by the student boycotts against the phase-out issue had drummed up national support for the medical school from other universities in the country, the South African Medical and Dental Council, as well as a number of international medical schools and other academic institutions.[69]

At this meeting, the state, already under considerable pressure to rectify its pariah status in the eyes of the international community, finally backed down. As had been the case in 1957 with sustained public opposition against the Separate University Education Bill, wide-scale public protests had served their purpose once again. In addition, the state was made to realise that if it continued with its plans, 623 medical students, the entire student body in Durban, would fail their end-of-year examinations. More importantly, this would include 94 final-year students scheduled to start their internship training in various black public hospitals around the country in 1978. In a situation where black doctors were in desperately short supply, and the new MEDUNSA facility would take years to start producing its first graduates, the state could not afford to lose black medical students already in training.[70] As a result of protracted and determined student protest actions, on 20 October 1977 the state retracted its decision to phase out African students from the Natal Medical School.[71]

To compensate for the prolonged boycotts, special arrangements were also made to help students catch up with their studies and write their final exams.[72] Breminand Maharaj, who was a final-year student at the time, captured the seriousness of this five-week boycott, and the uncertainty it held for students, in a recent interview:

> I was in my final year, we didn't actually write our final-year exams. We passed the date. This was a national issue. The minister of [education] . . . had to be involved and everybody because we said, 'No way' . . . And . . . we were not even sure we were going to graduate that year. Nineteen seventy-seven, I remember . . . we did our exams later . . . [when] the government actually backed down and African students were allowed to continue here.[73]

For the incoming class of 1978, the academic year started as it had done so many times before, with the school's admissions committee selecting a mixture of African, Indian and coloured candidates. However, this was achieved only after a drawn-out struggle waged largely on the backs of the school's black students. In the coming years, this would not be the end of the issue either. Although ultimately this institution's mixed-admissions policies would prevail through the 1980s and early 1990s, much uncertainty continued to shroud the future of the medical school, which also brought frustrating delays to building expansions and renovations.[74]

Medical student opposition to apartheid: The 1980s
The switch from black consciousness to UDF/ANC political alignment
In the same month that the prolonged phase-out boycott was called off, all black consciousness organisations – including SASO – were banned by the state as a way to suppress their opposition. This round of organisational bannings, however, did not dampen political activism in the way they had in the early 1960s. By the late 1970s, their bold anti-apartheid message had already laid the foundations for powerful defiance politics to emerge. This was particularly influential on the growing power of non-racial UDF/ANC-aligned organisations, whose defiant spirit mirrored earlier black consciousness organisations, but which stressed the inclusion of all population groups (including whites) in the struggle to overthrow apartheid.[75]

After the security police killed Steve Biko in detention on 12 September 1977, and SASO was banned in October 1977, a gradual shift occurred amongst student activists on the Durban Medical School campus in favour, as Barry Kistnasamy put it, 'of the ANC underground, and . . . the UDF as the front'. This political realignment, according to Joe Ndlovu, 'took beautifully at the medical school' through the 1980s.[76] Kistnasamy was a student in Durban between 1977 and 1982, while Ndlovu studied there between 1979 and 1984; thus both were witness to the shift.

Some activists spoke at length about why the transition of support from SASO to the UDF/ANC occurred relatively smoothly amongst medical students in Durban after SASO was banned. Speaking for herself, Nkosazana Dlamini Zuma told an interviewer that she did not see black consciousness as a contradiction to the ANC. Rather, she saw it as similar to what the ANC was like in 1912: 'If you look back at the ANC, they had a similar outlook at some stage and their outlook changed with experience of years and of changing international politics.'[77] In addition, Dlamini Zuma felt that students who made the transition to the UDF/ANC 'just saw Black Consciousness as a necessary stop during the development of political consciousness within the South African situation' in this later apartheid period.

While it is worth noting Dlamini Zuma's motives for making such a statement, including the effort by an ANC spokesperson to incorporate that political tradition under the broader ANC umbrella, the ANC did have a stronger presence in Natal than the PAC, and its non-racial policy line was more welcoming of diverse peoples.[78] These factors helped explain stronger support for it. Mamphela Ramphele concurred. 'When we started the Black Consciousness Movement in the late 'sixties,' she said,

> [w]e didn't see black solidarity as an end in itself. We saw the need for black people to . . . close ranks and just stop and reassert who they [were because] . . . black people had lost confidence in themselves and in their own human agency . . . The Black Consciousness Movement was a serious attempt to break away from the victim mentality that blacks had at the time, and to say to them that they are . . . active agents in history.[79]

By the late 1970s, the ideology had served its original purpose and the time had come, as it had done before, for a shift in political ideologies and strategies. By this time, after nearly a decade in existence, many black individuals and communities had been exposed to confidence-building ideologies, and 'people's entire attitude toward themselves had changed'.[80] According to Ramphele, black South Africans now demonstrated greater confidence in themselves. This enabled them to conceptualise the possibility of interacting with other people, including whites, 'as equal human beings'. Diliza Mji also asserted that 'when I was in SASO, I belonged to a School that said that SASO is purely filling in the gap'.[81] Once the older liberation movements, which had been 'battered into submission by the oppressive machinery of the state', had been unbanned, things would change. In the meantime, contact with older banned organisations like the ANC 'was done quietly'.

Reflecting on their student days, a number of ex-SASO activists have highlighted in more recent years that the move towards support for the exiled ANC was already in progress at the Durban Medical School from 1972/3. In the same interview mentioned above, Dlamini Zuma said how after the many political troubles during this period, including the banning of key SASO leaders, five medical students left the country and joined the exiled ANC, feeling that they needed to take their political consciousness further. SASO had nothing more to offer them. 'And so they felt that they had to leave the country to . . . see what form of higher political activity they could be involved in, you know, military activity or whatever.'[82]

In addition to the slow trickle of individuals who left because they felt they could make a contribution by joining the underground movement, Aubrey Mokoena felt that SASO experienced a serious split in the ranks by the mid-1970s. On the one side was SASO the exclusively black organisation, and on the other there was SASO, with 'the vision of a non-racial future and association with white liberals'. By the 1976 conference in Hammanskraal, he maintained, 'already SASO was tending to be pro-ANC'.[83] Keith Mokoape, a medical student who had in 1972 already called for the adoption in SASO of a policy supporting armed struggle as a strategy, as was being developed by the exiled ANC, agreed that this conference was key. He wrote:

> The 1976 General Student Council [of SASO] saw a sizeable shift in BC ranks to the ANC. This was particularly strong among University of Natal (Black Section) students, some of whom had recently visited Swaziland where contact was made with the ANC. Prior to this, in 1975, there had been an informal, clandestine meeting attended by some undelegated representatives from various organisations and areas. Steve Biko had felt that it was important at some level to brainstorm the issue of exile and the armed struggle.[84]

For Dlamini Zuma, who was SASO's vice-president at the time, this conference really tried to examine the BCM's successes and failures and 'to analyse the South African situation beyond Black Consciousness'. This included the need to 'bring in the broader issues of the country . . . and look at the real issues that were at stake rather than just . . . I mean, we are black and proud and all that'. This conference helped students see 'that SASO, the ideology of Black Consciousness as understood at the time, had reached a limit, and we had to look for something else'.[85]

After this conference and meeting with exiled ANC members, such as Thabo Mbeki in 1975 at the University of Swaziland, Dlamini Zuma highlighted how activist students in Durban like herself were then 'getting stuff from them [the ANC] in the mail, [and] having some duties to perform'. These students became avid readers of banned literature, such as the ANC's newsletter *Sechaba*, which helped spread understanding of the ANC's policies and strategies. Students also listened to 'Radio Freedom', an

ANC radio channel that was broadcast to South Africa from outside the country.[86] For Dlamini Zuma, the student movement had a central role to play in the fight against apartheid. While some students left to go into exile, 'some [also] remained behind and organised, [and] made it possible for the liberation movement to be able to put some of its ideas into action'.

During the 1980s, despite being banned, the ANC re-established itself as a powerful anti-apartheid organisation in South Africa and abroad. The exodus of hundreds of black activists into ANC military training camps, established in independent African states, such as Tanzania, and in the USSR after the 1976 Soweto Uprising and the 1977 banning of BC organisations, boosted the ANC's ranks and, according to Ramphele, 'breathed oxygen' into the ANC operations in exile.[87] A number of Durban medical students, such as Keith Mokoape and Nkosazana Dlamini Zuma, also went into exile as part of this exodus to escape being arrested or hounded by the security police. Many of these activists were young and prepared to return to South Africa to fight if necessary in guerrilla-type wars against the apartheid state after receiving their training.

Within South Africa's borders, the ANC used the formation in 1983 of the non-racial UDF – a national umbrella organisation eventually comprising over 500 affiliated civic, worker, student, religious, youth and women's organisations – as its above-ground organisational front. During the 1980s, many medical students in Durban joined the South African National Students' Congress (SANSCO), a non-racial student affiliate of the UDF.[88] Some were also involved as active members of the underground anti-apartheid movement. Returning to the example mentioned above, Keith Mokoape, once leaving South Africa, was sent for training in Egypt and then the USSR before he was infiltrated back into South Africa to work as part of the underground movement.[89]

Zweli Mkhize, who graduated in the early 1980s, was also a crucial ANC underground operative. May Mashego, who married Mkhize in the early 1980s after they both completed their medical degrees, spoke of the hardships she and her children had to endure, including going into exile in Swaziland and then Zimbabwe for the latter part of the 1980s, and spending much time apart from her husband, whilst he participated in ANC-coordinated activities that tried to bring down the apartheid state.[90] Some students and junior doctors participated in sabotage activities targeting particularly state buildings and installations. For example, in 1986 two junior doctors, who had completed their training in Durban, were charged under the Terrorism Act for involvement in over 22 counts against the state, including charges related to twelve bomb blasts and explosions in the Durban area between September 1983 and January 1986. According to a newspaper article at the time, other ATR students stood accused on various charges of what the apartheid state deemed 'terrorism' too.[91]

According to Barry Kistnasamy, student involvement in a variety of anti-apartheid activities during the 1980s made the Durban Medical School campus 'a hotbed of politics'.[92] This was reiterated by Janet Giddy, a white doctor who trained at UCT in the early 1980s and did her internship at King Edward in 1984. Many years after this period, she distinctly remembered how the Durban school was often in the news for the political activities some of the students were involved in. Her perception was that the school was 'always a thorn in the flesh' to the apartheid state and 'there was always this sense of simmering revolt'. In Durban, she told me,

> I think the medical students were far more politicised. I mean, when I was an intern . . . there was always some or other student unrest . . . going on . . . [And] the medical school was often closed down for a couple of days . . . [T]here was definitely far more political activity and I think . . . they were very challenging of the apartheid government . . . It was almost like every issue became politicised . . . [which led to] a protest march or let's refuse to go to lectures.[93]

Thinking back to the 1980s, Y.K. Seedat agreed. For this professor in the Department of Medicine, boycotts at the medical school 'became a way of life' during this period. In his opinion, student activists regarded education as less significant than liberation, and seemed to be continually responding to events that were negatively affecting their wider communities in apartheid South Africa.[94]

'Every little thing sparked off something with the students.'
— Soromini Kallichurum

There are many examples of students' protest activities in the 1980s. In April 1980, about 700 medical students went on another prolonged boycott of their classes in solidarity with the thousands of township school pupils in the Durban area, but also around the country, who abandoned their classes to protest against the unequal Bantu Education system.[95] One African doctor, who was studying at the time, recalled the occasion well: '[L]ots of schools in KwaMashu were on boycott and the medical school as well. In fact in 1980, when . . . [I was] doing first year, we were on boycott.' She recalled that the boycott went on for 'a long, long period' – 'something like . . . eight weeks'.[96] May Mashego, who completed her degree in 1982, recalled how during this 1980 boycott period, medical students used to go out and do volunteer work in communities like KwaMashu to provide education skills to pupils in makeshift classes, and 'we also assisted them in their struggles'.[97] This included helping them distribute pamphlets to conscientise surrounding communities about various political issues.

In fact, the potential value of students going out to work as volunteers in communities ignited during SASO's era did not disappear after SASO was banned in 1977. Indeed, they were actively taken up and promoted by UDF/ANC activists and groups in later decades too.[98] In the field of health, this was noticeable in the formation of a number of progressive organisations in the 1980s, which tried to counteract the rapidly deteriorating public health-care services provided for blacks by the apartheid state. For example, the National Medical and Dental Association (NAMDA), which was formed in 1982 in direct opposition to the largely white and apartheid-aligned Medical Association of South Africa (MASA), as well as other UDF-aligned health organisations,[99] promoted a community-oriented, primary health-care approach as the foundation of their policies.[100] These organisations publicly criticised the abusive and unethical practices of apartheid in medicine, demanded accountability for health professionals (especially those complicit in the deaths of political detainees such as Steve Biko) and campaigned at both national and international levels for health policy changes. In addition, they provided desperately needed primary-level, health-care services for many black communities around the country. This included trauma counselling for political prisoners, detainees and their families and emergency medical services for victims of state violence, such as civilians injured during clashes with the police that erupted in the townships during the 1980s.

Some Durban medical graduates and staff got involved in NAMDA, such as Diliza Mji and Jerry Coovadia, who both became executive members and played vital roles in its formation and operations. So did a number of medical student activists who keenly involved themselves in some of

NAMDA's above-mentioned community health-care projects. As well as providing them with hands-on experience, it gave students the opportunity to do something productive, where they could actively help people who needed health care in the townships. For many of these student activists, it was not enough merely to train as doctors to treat their patients' disease symptoms, many of which were preventable. They would just recur because of the socio-economic structural inequalities created by apartheid, as May Mashego highlighted:

> You admit this child today, he's got kwashiorkor, you give them good food, you send them home. But where are you sending them? They'll come back. So this was what was happening . . . [what] you were faced with as a black doctor . . . the type of diseases you were treating, the type of people you had to sit and look [at] suffering, and all you could do was just treat them . . . [T]his is why some of us couldn't shut up.[101]

This perspective was reinforced by another student – K.P. Naidoo, who started his medical studies in Durban in 1977, before dropping out in the early 1980s because of financial difficulties. In an interview conducted in 2004, Naidoo described as 'toxic' the situation he found himself in as a medical student in South Africa, which drove him to involvement in anti-apartheid politics:

> I was just feeling . . . [that] this place is not normal . . . I cannot function anymore in an abnormal situation. [So] . . . I became a political activist . . . I thought, you know, this place, it would stay the same; this country's going to stay the same. I'd be just helping to feed the system as an elite doctor to treat the masses and keep the status quo going . . . So . . . we cannot have a situation where the army [and] police . . . are bulleting people, detaining [and] jailing them, and when they bully them, they bring [them] to King Edward. Then we as students . . . must help the surgeons now remove [the] bullets.[102]

In addition to doing community activist work, many other examples of medical student anti-apartheid activities abound during the 1980s period. In 1981, students went on a three-day boycott of the twentieth-anniversary celebrations of South Africa's withdrawal from the British Commonwealth and the founding of the South African Republic in 1961. On this occasion, some medical students got involved in protest marches and even burnt a South African flag to show their resentment of this kind of celebration.[103] The following year, in July and August 1982, 800 Natal medical students undertook another prolonged boycott of classes in opposition to the suspension of 1 500 African students from the University of Fort Hare for their involvement in anti-apartheid protest activities.[104] As in the 1970s, they showed once again their ability to use the boycott strategy to support activities going on in other parts of the country.

One issue that caused much political ferment in the medical student body was the formation of the tricameral parliament in 1984. Developed as a crucial part of the state's 'divide-and-rule' strategy, it introduced limited representation in South Africa's parliamentary structure for Indian and coloured representatives, while African representation was excluded. Soromini Kallichurum, the first woman dean of the medical school at the time, vividly recalled the turmoil that this issue caused amongst the students: 'The students were angry, all students . . . I just found there was total non-acceptance of that and every little thing sparked off something with the students . . . The whole situation was volatile.'[105] These students saw the formation of the tricameral parliament as a further attempt by the government to divide Africans, Indians and coloureds, and an attempt to encourage Indian and coloured minority groups as collaborators who would work within the apartheid system to receive a few privileges, rather than against it.

As was discussed for the SASO period, anything promoting apartheid's separate-development policies and institutions was strongly opposed by many medical students, and this carried through to the 1980s too. This was captured by Maila J. Matjila, who described the medical school's student body as 'very much anti-apartheid in its outlook'.[106] For this doctor, the tricameral 'structures that were created by apartheid' were ones that the students 'couldn't really subscribe to' as they 'challenged exactly that very division of black people according to . . . [ethnic or] tribal political affiliation'. In Matjila's opinion, the students knew that this structure was 'a fabrication that we are [all] considered to be different . . . [this] was just a clear indication of divide and rule'.

A number of other issues sparked off protests amongst Durban students in the mid-1980s. During 1985 and 1986, the government declared numerous states of emergency in its attempt to suppress the growing tide of resistance to apartheid that had emerged amongst black communities across South Africa. During a state of emergency, the army was usually called in to support the police in their attempts to quell resistance in what were considered highly unstable black township areas.[107] During these periods of heightened state security, thousands of anti-apartheid activists were beaten up, arrested or detained, often for months at a time. Kallichurum remembered how during these explosive situations, when 'there was a lot of trouble all over the show', students in Durban often went on boycott as they worried about the safety of their loved ones:

> And the students came to me to say, 'A lot of us don't know what's happening to our parents, there's so much trouble. We feel that . . . because so many people will be absent, we'd rather just go on a boycott.' And I had to agree . . . because I know if you're worried about your family, how can you stay and study? And I said, 'Providing you return by Wednesday', and they did. [This went on] throughout my term of office . . . [B]ut I knew that it was either a few days or many weeks . . . and your whole university curriculum is disrupted.[108]

Natal medical students also boycotted and demonstrated for a number of other reasons. A glance through different newspapers in the mid-1980s provides evidence for many of these occasions. For example, students came out in support of striking workers who had been fired at King Edward VIII Hospital; students protested against the brutal killings of anti-apartheid protesters in other parts of the country; and students stood in solidarity with black school pupils and university students' protests against inferior education provisions. They also objected to police and army brutality and detentions; voiced opposition against international governments and businesses who profited from apartheid; and protested against their inferior working conditions in their clinical rotations.[109]

Asked to remember her mid-1980s internship training and work period at King Edward VIII Hospital, Janet Giddy, who came to the city of Durban from Cape Town, recalled the steep learning curve she experienced as a junior doctor. She vividly remembered the confusion and the fear the state of emergency caused in the city she had chosen to come to, the war-zone-like feel of the hospital's casualty wards and feeling that she was surrounded by many people secretly engaged in anti-apartheid political activities. The following quotation has been included at length as it does well to capture the nature of the environment that Durban medical students and doctors found themselves caught up in:

[During] the mid-1980s, there were all these bomb blasts going off in Durban. And so . . . the casualty [ward] was like a war zone and there were . . . lots of gunshot wounds and people who had been stabbed and whatever . . . [And wounded prisoners brought in under police guard]. And we got involved with this NAMDA group where we set up . . . a training course for township youth in first aid because sometimes things were so bad in the townships, and the troops were in the townships, that you couldn't, they couldn't get there or they were too scared to come to hospital . . . [As a member of NAMDA] Barry [Kistnasamy, who was completing his postgraduate degree at King Edward at the time] took me under his wing . . . [H]e was quite political and he used to take me to places. I remember one day . . . Alan Taylor Res. in Wentworth, he took me to some dances and things there and I was absolutely amazed at this Res. in the middle of all these oil refineries and it was like a barracks. And I remember being shocked that this is how . . . medical studentst . . . lived. And then one day he took me for a drive and there were lots of road blocks and policemen and they stopped us and they sort of wanted to search the car and then I suddenly thought, you know, maybe there's a whole lot more going on that we don't know about. And once he took me to meet a friend of his . . . He seemed quite quiet, didn't say very much . . . and this other chap . . . maybe 18 months later was arrested as being a mastermind behind a whole lot of the bomb blasts. And at that time [this man] he was a registrar in Surgery and he was one of these people who obviously was heavily involved but very quiet . . . [I] had the sense of being in a very, very political environment and then the state of emergency was declared . . . [in] '85. And there was a very tense feeling. The one department that I was in, one of the registrars . . . he was detained for months on end. The head of department, who was Jerry Coovadia, went off on an overseas trip and never came back also for about a year because he had had a tip-off that he was going to be picked up. And the other head of department went off to do a sabbatical in Saudi Arabia or somewhere and he didn't come back for months. So the [hospital] work was really affected by the politics . . . It felt

like a very steep learning curve and I learnt a lot about many, many things
. . . In retrospect, I could see how privileged and resourced [my training in
Cape Town had been] . . . Groote Schuur seemed more . . . [like] a fairy
tale . . . not really part of Africa . . . some other reality.[110]

Thus, during the 1980s, medical students in Durban were not isolated or
protected from the effects of apartheid in their wider communities. Many
were actively involved, if not actively affected. Some felt strongly the need
to respond politically to improve their lot. As a result, the 1980s period was
marked by intense and varied student protest actions. For Jerry Coovadia,
the 1980s period was one of numerous protests at the medical school: 'To
me it was just a continuous low-level opposition all the time, with the
occasional peaks of activity . . . It was just like a regular feature . . . I
mean, there were just numerous occasions . . . It just continued endlessly,
endlessly.'[111]

Protests against the University of Natal

'The Wentworth site, in short, is a very good one for breeding
malcontent revolutionaries.'[112]

While involvement in broader anti-apartheid protests took up much of
student activists' time, medical students in Durban also opposed
discriminations propagated by their alma mater. In a 2003 interview, Hugh
Philpott maintained that 'it wasn't just the government of the day that was
tough on them. It was the lack of care from the university [too]' which
stimulated students into action.[113] Once admitted, many Durban medical
students felt isolated from and even abandoned as a group by the main,
white, Howard College campus. Furthermore, this 'dichotomy', even though
technically they were all University of Natal students, made them feel like
'orphans' and 'not part of Natal', which could on occasion draw them
together as a more unified group of students.[114] As 'another sort of enemy'
over the years, students voiced much opposition to those running the
University of Natal.[115] There were many occurrences of this.

A major factor that ignited regular demonstrations was the high number
of students who failed, and the additional high rate of exclusion from the
medical school each year. One African graduate who attended the school

between 1980 and 1986 said that at the start of almost every academic year there would be boycotts because of exclusions. '[A] lot of African students would be excluded and . . . you know, the SRC, at the first meeting, we'd want to go through how many exclusions and why and then there would be a boycott and we would actually fight that.'[116] On one occasion, in February 1984, returning students found that 25 per cent of second-year students had failed and that 20 per cent were excluded from readmission. On this occasion, the high failure and exclusion rates provided the catalyst for a four-week boycott spearheaded by the black SRC.[117] Protests were also kindled by what students regarded as the 'unacceptable handling' of certain issues by the university, including the 'implementation of new and unfair rules'.[118] The decision to exclude students who had failed the notoriously difficult second year and the requirement that fourth-year students had to repeat the whole year, even if they failed only one clinical assessment, produced much opposition too.

In addition, during the 1970s and 1980s, students complained about the overcrowded, polluted and inferior accommodation facilities provided for those staying at ATR.[119] Unpopular authority figures, among them certain wardens, who were to students the front-line persons of the university's administration, were also not tolerated by students. During 1981, Hugh Philpott, who was dean at the time, remembered how the poor living conditions at ATR and the unpopular actions of a disliked warden, who imposed stricter residence rules on the students, provoked the students into action. 'Picture the scene,' he said. Black medical students were 'dumped' in 'atrociously' polluted and overcrowded conditions in ATR:

And one night I got a phone call from Pete Booysen . . . the vice-principal . . . and he said, 'Come down, we're in trouble. The students were going against the warden and they attacked the warden's house.' And we went down there at about half past eleven one night, and the students were swarming across the football field in the residence and throwing stones on the roof of the warden['s quarters]. And they were revolting against any authority at all there. And we eventually had to take the warden and his wife and his kids out of the back door and up onto the main campus into the transit accommodation.[120]

Students also staged demonstrations to protest against the lack of free university transport for students between the residence and the medical school campus on Umbilo Road.[121] Increases in tuition and residence fees also sparked opposition amongst students.[122] A good example of this is from the early 1980s, when a steep increase in students' tuition and residence fees formed part of a five-year programme imposed by the government to reduce its subsidy payment and bring the much-reduced medical school's fee structure into line with those at other South African medical schools. Numerous food boycotts against the inferior quality, rising costs and inadequate quantity and variety of food served in the medical school's canteen and at ATR were flashpoints of contention as well over the years.[123] Writing under the name of Adam Starz, a medical doctor who trained in Durban during the apartheid period provides an illustration of such a food strike in a book which draws on his personal experiences of the catering problems at ATR:

> The standard of catering deteriorated further and everyone became disgruntled. If you annoy the stomach, you provoke the brain; and if you provoke the brains you goad the person. That means only one thing: action. And that's exactly how the food strike began ... [T]he students would march into the dining hall, fill their plates, file out and dump the food in the bins outside the dining hall. They would also boycott the medical school canteen and sit on the lawn in front of it during lunch times ... The authorities finally acceded to most of the students' requests. The food improved.[124]

Furthermore, students demonstrated on occasion against what they regarded as unfair employment practices applied to African members of staff. During the 1970s and 1980s, a number of experienced African lecturers were bypassed for promotion to the level of professor or as heads of various departments in the medical school. Many senior lecturers, such as E.T. Mokgokong, M. Marivate and T. Mokoena, to mention but a few, left the medical school to take up appointments elsewhere, such as MEDUNSA after it was opened in 1978, where their work experience fast-tracked their promotions to professorial posts, and even to the office of vice-chancellor, in Mokgokong's case.[125]

Finally, as mentioned in chapter 5, annual graduation boycotts provided another outlet for student frustrations. From 1979 until 1995 (when a symbolic reconciliation graduation ceremony was held by the university to apologise to its medical graduates and the boycotts were stopped), the boycott of graduation ceremonies was adopted as the official stance of the whole medical student body.[126] During this time, these annual boycotts became an organised movement that saw whole graduating classes abstain from attendance at these ceremonies to demonstrate their opposition to the diverse discriminations they were forced to endure at the hands of their alma mater. These boycotts also reflected students' discomfort with the symbolism of the graduation ceremony, which served to separate them as professional elites from their wider communities. While students were prepared to attend these tertiary institutions 'under protest' as a way to acquire the education they desired, they were not prepared to accept the university's 'elaborate exit' ceremony, as one graduate was quoted saying: 'The pomp and ceremony, the paraphernalia . . . not to mention the Latin are meant to launch the graduate into a demi-God [status], different from your community. Can there be any doubt that this ceremony is meant to alienate us from our community?'[127]

Staff responses to medical student activism

Thinking back to her days as a medical student, and to her time later as a staff member at the medical school during the 1970s and 1980s, Soromini Kallichurum felt adamantly that many of her work colleagues, as well as people in management positions at the University of Natal, did not really understand the central importance of political issues in black students' lives. When Kallichurum became professor of anatomical pathology in the 1970s, she remembered that the medical students had a major boycott, angering the principal, N.D. Clarence. At a Faculty of Medicine board meeting, he asked the staff 'what this medical school stands for' and whether the students were there learning to be politicians or to receive a medical education:

And I thought, no, I had better stand up and tell him something. So I said, 'You know, there's one thing the university must understand. I was a student here and I know.' I said, 'My everyday life is politically determined. I study where I study for political reasons. I work where I work for political reasons. I drive through certain streets to reach home for political reasons. And I stay where I stay for political reasons. My whole life is determined by politics . . . You know, with the category of students we've got . . . here, we must understand every move they make is political. It's not that they have [a choice].' He said, 'Have they come here to study politics?' I said, 'Yes, life is political for us' . . . And I sat down and I think he was very angry . . . But it was a fact of life, which I felt the university never understood.[128]

But while academics and politics were often inseparable issues for medical students in Durban, many of their teachers and the administrative staff considered politics and academics as two separate issues. They had to remain separate to ensure the good academic reputation of the school and the continuance of its teaching programme.

Nevertheless, as with the student body, over the years there was a mixed bag of responses by the academic staff to their students' involvement in extracurricular political activities. Jerry Coovadia related how some of his colleagues were openly hostile and avidly opposed to student anti-apartheid activism and spoke out vehemently at faculty board meetings, coming down hard on students who boycotted their classes.[129] These lecturers worked to create not a supportive environment for their students, but a hostile one where some 'teachers were almost . . . [their] enemies, politically speaking'. Y.K. Seedat vividly remembered an example of this, where one time a dean, who also taught in his Department of Medicine,

> [p]ut out a notice: 'Will the following students come and see me'. And he put out their names on the board and when they went to see him, he handed the students over to the security branch. And that created a major problem within the medical school . . . That was in the . . . '70s . . . Those students were detained . . . You see, for the security branch to be effective they had to infiltrate every aspect of the medical school.[130]

Some of the academic staff displayed paternalistic attitudes: while they might have sympathised with their students' difficulties or understood why they became involved in anti-apartheid protest activities, they disagreed with the more radical means used by students to advance their cause. These individuals were usually concerned about the disruptions to the teaching programme and the issue of student failures, not to mention the dangers to students that participation in protracted boycott activities could cause. Liberals like J.V.O. Reid, who became the chairman of the Durban Coastal Branch of the Progressive Party and dean of the medical school in the 1970s, captured the slower, reformist attitude well. In an interview conducted with him in June 2002, Reid maintained that the students 'were people who were ahead . . . of us' and that most of his colleagues were being

> [f]orced into [doing things] . . . which we thought were too big for that moment. We were pushing slowly [for change]. They wanted to go quickly . . . [We had to] stop them from going too fast, from leading to the stopping of this medical school, it being closed down . . . And so sometimes we came into conflict with the students, although my heart was very much behind them. [But] there were some things that we couldn't agree with.[131]

Many were opposed to the medical school being used as a vehicle for protest by students, especially against issues over which the university had no control.[132]

A few individuals were remembered over the years as exceptions; for having 'a soft spot for blacks' and for striving to improve the learning and working experiences of black medical students and doctors.[133] Sidney Kark, Isidor Gordon, Hugh Philpott, Sam Ross and Theodore Sarkin were some of the lecturers who were mentioned by a number of graduates for the support they gave their students. Other than Kark (see chapter 2), who emigrated in 1958 after his far-sighted social, community and preventive medicine teaching experiment in Durban was shut down, all of the other lecturers were long-standing members of the Faculty of Medicine, and three of them even became deans of the medical school. Gordon was fondly remembered for a number of reasons. In 1998, Y.K. Seedat wrote in an obituary that 'Okkie', his friend, 'was a legend' in the South African medical arena. Seedat, who worked for many years with Gordon on the staff of the medical school, noted that, in his opinion, his biggest contributions were his 'struggle[s on the side] of underprivileged medical doctors', his 'strong stand against the injustices' of the apartheid years and his 'constant efforts to preserve the medical school' against outside attacks.[134] As dean, in 1957 he helped save the medical school from removal from the University of Natal, and 'in 1970 he played a very significant role in the struggle for equal pay for doctors of all races'.[135]

Philpott and Ross stood out in graduates' memories too for their many efforts to actively cross racial barriers through their involvement in Student Christian Fellowship (SCF) activities. A number of graduates argued that unlike many of their lecturers, Ross and Philpott took the time to discuss issues with their students and to try to understand the many problems facing them. May Mashego, who came to know these lecturers well through her involvement in the SCF, argued that they went the 'extra mile' in taking students into their homes, and treating them 'like family' during holiday breaks or during times of political controversy when the residence was closed.[136] They did this despite personal risks to themselves and their families for fraternising with black South Africans in their homes during the apartheid era.

Furthermore, Zweli Mkhize captured in a speech at the medical school's 50th-anniversary banquet in 2000 the essential supportive role Theodore Sarkin played as the chair of orthopaedic surgery and then dean of this medical school. For Mkhize, Sarkin even risked personal danger to protect his students. On one such occasion in 1981, when students were protesting on the campus against the Republic Day celebrations, which included their burning a South African flag to show their opposition, Mkhize vividly recalled the lone figure of the

> Dean of the School, Professor Sarkin, [who] stood at the gate, keeping the police outside until they could find a warrant of arrest. And on their return, of course, they found that the students had dispersed. When the police identified the culprits on the video on their return, the Dean had offered to replace the flag. No other campuses had that type of experience . . .[137]

The security police were regarded as an 'almighty force . . . [that] could get anywhere, anytime', so the bravery of some of the school's staff, who stood up against them to protect their students, stood out in the memories of many.[138] May Mashego, who also mentioned Sarkin's efforts in the early 1980s, firmly believed that 'he really didn't want the students to be prosecuted . . . because I think deep in his heart, he must have said, "I understand what is going on within them, I understand why they're being destructive"'.[139] In his obituary in 1998, Jerry Coovadia, his long-time colleague, wrote that his 'strength of character was best revealed in the courageous steps he took . . .

as a man to oppose and drive back apartheid. He never faltered in this mission to achieve the small victories . . . so that the larger battles could be won elsewhere.'[140]

By the 1980s, as larger numbers of black doctors trained in Durban were employed as part of the faculty of the medical school, some graduates felt that 'mindsets were changing . . . people like ourselves who had been on the other side had come in. So we could bring in a new perspective', which produced a more supportive environment for students.[141] The fact that the medical school also fell under the leadership of a more liberal vice-chancellor, Pete Booysen, in the latter half of the 1980s, was also mentioned by some. Joe Ndlovu noted that by this stage 'the governors of the university were . . . liberal white people who really, in a sense, you know, allowed or tolerated a lot of political activity. And sometimes they themselves actually got into trouble from the government . . . for allowing student protests . . . I think they tended to be more liberal and they tended more to want to listen . . .'[142]

During the late 1970s, and especially during the 1980s, when political disruptions to classes happened regularly, many staff members rearranged tests and exams and some lecturers tried to help students catch up on missed lecture time in the holidays.[143] Some supportive deans were also remembered for actively negotiating with the security police to have their students released from prison, for posting bail for students and for making special arrangements for students to write their exams in detention if they could not get them freed.[144]

However, many lecturers maintained their silence on political issues, and just wanted to carry on with their teaching. Another graduate of the school, B.T. Naidoo, highlighted how some of these lecturers 'didn't really fight for us as such. As far as they were concerned, this was government policy. "Don't rock [the boat]", and they carried on towing the line', which ensured the continuance of apartheid inequalities at the school.[145] Few were prepared to openly oppose apartheid policies because of the potential threats this posed to themselves, to their families and to their jobs. Some, such as Jerry Coovadia and Diliza Mji, who were active in NAMDA and the UDF, received numerous threats and even had to leave Durban on occasion to avoid arrest.[146] As demonstrated clearly in a 1998 report, which was prepared at the request of the South African Truth and Reconciliation Commission, NAMDA leaders were often 'harassed and sometimes arrested and detained without trial by security police. The homes of some NAMDA leaders were bombed, and many others received death threats. NAMDA offices were raided . . . by security police, and computer files and other documents were stolen.'[147] Additional hardships noted by the report include NAMDA members who were 'effectively barred' from getting jobs in the public health sector and being publicly and 'vehemently denounced' by MASA for their political activities. The risks were real for staff members who were politically active, which is why many preferred to remain, at least publicly, uninvolved. The consequences for student involvement in anti-apartheid politics, was just as severe.

Political involvement for students: the consequences

Participation in extracurricular political activities often brought harsh consequences for students. Despite the attempts made by some deans over the years to keep the security police off the campus to protect their students, they were not always successful. In fact, they were usually not. Many student activists suffered years of harassment by the security police, which deemed the medical school, by the early 1980s, 'a threat to national security'.[148] During the 1970s and 1980s, police raids at ATR, for example, became a common feature of student life.[149] Raids were conducted for a variety of reasons: to search and seize banned literature; to interrogate students for information; to disrupt anti-apartheid political activities that were being planned there; and to find and arrest activist leaders. And, because these raids often involved sealing off the entire residence as the police searched through students' rooms and questioned students, whether they were politically active or not, all students living there were implicated by association, and experienced their intimidating and often violent effects.

Many graduates experienced this terrifying experience. B.T. Naidoo remembered how they 'would drive down and just come into your residence, open your doors . . . bang into your rooms . . . and search'.[150] These raids were a stressful time for students, even for those who were not politically active, as they often had 'all sorts' of other contraband in their rooms, including sexual partners and liquor, which they would then have to explain to the warden on duty. Once the police arrived at ATR, Naidoo continued, 'they would just come and if they feel that they should take you in, they will take you in . . . harass your leaders, just to knock the daylights out of you . . . [We] were intimidated all the time.'

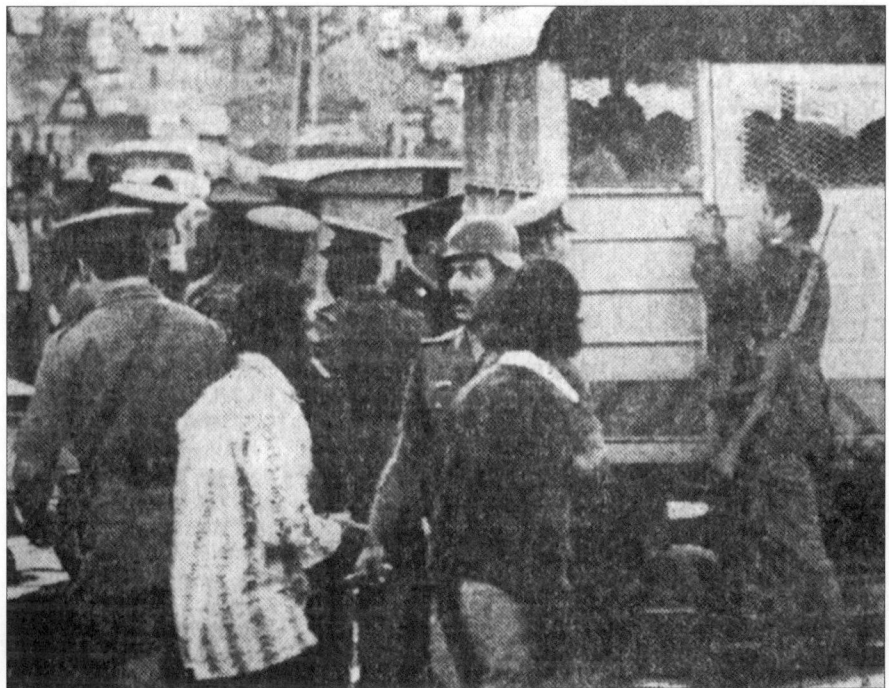

Photo 7.2   Police arresting students, newspaper unknown, 19 June 1976. (*UKZN Medical School Archives*)

Another African graduate, who completed his degree nearly twenty years after Naidoo, and preferred not to have his name mentioned, said that it was 'quite rough' as they used to have the police 'coming to raid us at night, wake us up, turn our rooms upside down looking for literature and so forth, threatening to shoot you if you don't open your door'. For him it was 'just constant' harassment.[151] As dean in the early 1980s, Hugh Philpott recalled having to drive down to ATR 'time and again', often at night, when a raid was in progress, to try to keep the students calm as these episodes 'could be violent':

> I mean, one night . . . I had to go down . . . the security police . . . were looking for some 'terrorists' . . . [I]t was two o'clock in the morning and they had everybody out on the football field . . . outside the Res. and some of them with no clothes on whatsoever, they just beat their doors down

and sjambokked [whipped] them out onto the football field and checked to find these terrorists. They never did find them and eventually the police disappeared.[152]

In addition to using overt measures to prop up apartheid policies and to punish student 'offenders', the police also used covert measures, which included the payment of informers within the student body, to get what they wanted.[153] This was highlighted by a number of graduates who studied in Durban during the 1970s and 1980s.[154] Breminand Maharaj asserted in an interview that the security police had 'a good informer system' at the medical school and were clearly 'paying people to study, who were informers inside'.[155] For him, 'there was no doubt about that because when . . . they would raid the residence . . . they knew exactly which rooms to go to . . . they were exceedingly well informed'.

But students could not usually tell who the informers were amongst them. Philpott declared with exasperation that the security police were sometimes more informed about student boycotts than he was as dean! During the early 1980s, he vividly recalled one such occasion when students had been on boycott for about a week and were in a student body meeting to discuss whether to return to classes. Whilst working in his office at the time of the meeting, he received a phone call from 'the notorious' Sergeant De Wet from C.R. Swart Square Police Station. In his own words, Philpott said:

> He phones me and says, 'I hear they've decided to go back [to classes].' And I said, 'Well, I don't know that. They're still in the meeting.' And he said, 'But you know they have decided.' He had planted in amongst them . . . informers, and he was sitting there in C.R. Swart monitoring the whole of that meeting. And before I, as the dean, knew anything, he just phoned to let me know that. I think he just did it because he wanted me to know where the power was . . . So all the time they had their own informers in and amongst the student body who kept them abreast of everything that was going to happen or had happened . . .[156]

The security police often approached students in dire financial straits to spy on their behalf in exchange for the payment of their fees or the provision of some other financial incentive. Threats to students' families were also used as a persuasive strategy. Recruitment of informers did not take place only once students reached the medical school, but often as early as high school. The aim of these undercover measures was to retrieve information for the police, but also to breed paranoia as well as fear and suspicion in the student body. It made students question the loyalties of those around them and kindled fear, as Veronica Wilson remembered:

> . . . you didn't know who was an informer and it was very stressful . . . I think especially emotionally and psychologically because . . . there were no structures in place to sort of assist you . . . like counselling and things like that. And even at the time also, I mean, who do you trust?[157]

Students knew 'informers were there . . . everywhere', and most 'just prayed that they would not talk to me next'.[158] Although it did not stop all students from participating in anti-apartheid political activities, it certainly made some students extremely wary of involvement.

The police sometimes clashed with students on campus grounds to break up mass gatherings. However, this type of violence inflicted upon students usually occurred on the streets, outside the protection of the medical school's grounds. In these public spaces, the police had more power to break up protest demonstrations, marches and mass meetings by using tear gas or rubber bullets, and by whipping or baton-charging students, all done ostensibly in the name of the public's general interest.[159] The restrictive apartheid laws passed to limit political activity resulted in much brutality, with many student leaders being harassed, arrested, banned, detained and assaulted, as Breminand Maharaj stressed in an interview:

> When the concept of black consciousness came in, it was regarded as a threat and so the security branch . . . would harass students at the time. And, I mean, they would raid us, detain people. In those days you could be detained for anything. It was first 90 day[s], then 180 day[s] and then . . . they were detained incommunicado [and] they were beaten up . . . To me life was always like a state of emergency . . . when, you know, the detentions and things were taking place, like casualties, and all would see.[160]

Other activist students had their studies cut short, either temporarily or permanently. For example, Dan Ncayiyana was arrested for his anti-apartheid activities in the 1960s, and after the judge granted him bail, he 'skipped' South Africa 'on a clandestine' journey, first to Lesotho for a few months, then 'from Lesotho to Botswana over several weeks on foot' because air traffic was being carefully monitored by the security police.[161] Then he stayed in Dar es Salaam and the Congo for a while, before making it to the Netherlands, where he completed his medical degree.

Several years after Ncayiyana's experiences, S.C. Moodley remembered 'the years 1975 and 1976 as indeed traumatic one[s]' too.[162] This was because one of his politically active, fifth-year colleagues at the medical school – Nkosazana Dlamini Zuma – who had joined the ANC underground movement whilst still a student, was forced to leave South Africa to escape being arrested by the security police. Some students were prepared to give up their professional degrees because they saw the anti-apartheid struggle as more important then getting an education. In an article published in the ANC newsletter *Sechaba* in 1977, shortly after she went into exile, Dlamini Zuma, reflecting on her decision to leave her medical studies in 1976, wrote:

> I just found myself getting on with my political work . . . [T]here was no point in leaving what I had started just for a degree. Even if I passed the degree I would still suffer the same oppression. It was a feeling; you know, that to make something of education – or anything else – there must be a complete political change. We all felt that we should rather concentrate on getting the people mobilised and politicised to bring political change, before we can enjoy education.[163]

Like Ncayiyana, Dlamini Zuma was one of the fortunate few. After making her way to Britain, she completed her degree at the University of Bristol in 1978, and managed to do a diploma in tropical child health at the School of Tropical Medicine at the University of Liverpool in 1986.[164] In Britain, she worked together with other health activists in exile until the ANC was unbanned in the early 1990s, as well as with a number of other colleagues in health organisations still operational in South Africa, to help create a national health plan in the lead-up to the 1994 democratic elections and in preparation for a new national health system for South Africa. Building on what Sidney and Emily Kark had pioneered during the 1940s and 1950s, on programmes that SASO medical activists had tried to reignite in the 1970s and on the work of progressive health-care organisations, such as

NAMDA and the National Progressive Primary Health Care Network (NPPHCN) in the 1980s, Dlamini Zuma, who became the new minister of health between 1994 and 1998, played a pivotal role leading the reconstruction of the national public health-care system. The new system aimed to draw the focus away from expensive tertiary-level services to community-oriented and more accessible and affordable primary health-care services.[165]

Some student activists were not lucky, however, with regards to completing their academic work. Loss of study time through boycott activities could have serious consequences for some students, especially those with weak educational backgrounds, and those trying to pass the notoriously difficult second-year subjects. For instance, May Mashego said she failed an already difficult second year of studies at the end of 1977 because of her involvement in the five-week boycott against the government's plans to phase out African students.[166] Fortunately, Mashego was allowed to repeat her second year in 1978, which she then managed to pass. Breminand Maharaj, who was doing his final year during 1977, recalled how he and his final-year colleagues all felt sure that they were going to fail that year as the date for writing their final exams passed them by during the boycott period. Unexpectedly, a last-minute decision by the university and frantic efforts by the staff to help them catch up lost study time enabled them to write their exams very late in the year, which he passed.[167]

Nevertheless, for many others, political involvement drew them away from their studies, which led to course failures that they did not recover from. Y.K. Seedat remembered the case of Steve Biko's failures and then his exclusion from the school in 1972:

> Biko wasn't attending classes . . . There was a whole write-up about Biko and that he was expelled from this medical school. But John Reid [the professor of physiology] wrote to *The Times* and corrected it, saying that he was not [just] expelled. It was in the second year that he kept failing the [physiology] exam . . . because he never used to attend classes. He had a vision. He said, you know, 'I'm not interested in medicine. I'm interested in politics in this country. That's more important to me.' So he didn't attend classes . . . Biko never came into the clinical years . . . because he was expelled from the second year because he never passed his exams.[168]

Between 1983 and 1985, when the failures were particularly high, between 25 and 27 students were excluded each year, usually for failing to pass the difficult second year. Indeed, the annual failure rate was often much higher. Depending on how badly a student had failed, some were given a second chance and allowed back to try again. In 1983, 45 per cent of the second-year class failed.[169] Other than failing, students also faced the worry of financial hardships and being forced to withdraw through loss of bursaries or loans if they participated in class boycotts or other political activities.[170]

Steve Biko provides a good example of the difficult choice that some medical students had to make between continuing with or abandoning their studies to fight for something bigger. These dilemmas were heavy burdens carried by students. If they completed their studies, they stood a good chance of improving their individual life chances, as well as those of their families, not to mention helping to improve the lives of their sick patients after graduating. If they abandoned their studies to join the anti-apartheid struggle, their immediate career aspirations could be shattered and patient care compromised with fewer doctors trained.[171] Anne Digby described the contradictions medical students and doctors often had to face 'between politics and medicine' and the 'ambiguity in reconciling collective and individual interests'. For her, these individuals had to make very difficult 'choices between legitimate – and often more profitable – professional aspirations and the urgent needs of disadvantaged black patients within an inequitable healthcare system'.[172]

For some, the only real choice to improve their lives, as well as the lives of their families, communities and patients, was to fight to replace the government oppressing them as black South Africans. This was the choice Biko made, as Lindy Wilson argues in her biographical chapter on Biko in the book *Bounds of Possibility*:

> In 1972, although reluctant to believe he could not manage both studying and political work, Biko chose the more difficult political road . . . [and was] dismiss[ed] from medical school . . . What was more painful was that he would also have to disappoint his family's ambitions for him and those of virtually the whole Ginsberg community. The choice he made was one that thousands of black students would come to face: the choice of either becoming a political activist or taking the time to gain some sort of qualification towards a professional life, whatever the compromise, under

apartheid. Biko thus sacrificed this chance of becoming a professional doctor. For the time being, his work lay elsewhere.[173]

Reflecting on his student days and the issue of politics, one African doctor, whose time in Durban overlapped with Biko's, argued that '[l]ots of people . . . focused their energies on things that they felt were bigger . . . they saw medical school as a privilege in which I think sometimes to conduct matters of the struggle'.[174] For some students like Biko, he continued, 'maybe medicine was the hobby rather than the thing that they were doing . . . It was *the* thing.' Unfortunately, for the liberation movement in South Africa that needed him, and for the many friends and family who loved him, Biko would pay the ultimate price for his choice. On 12 September 1977, his life was 'lost to the world' after receiving a fatal beating whilst being held in detention by the security police.[175]

In 1966, Edgar Brookes argued that the University of Natal's medical school developed in the wider socio-political context of apartheid South Africa and, as a result, continually found itself in the 'vortex' of apartheid politics.[176] Apartheid political issues were an inextricable part of students' lives, whether they chose to engage actively with it or not. While for some students, politics 'was just on the periphery of their vision',[177] which enabled them to remain less affected and thus able to continue with their medical studies, for others, such as Biko, active involvement in anti-apartheid political activities fundamentally affected their whole lives and would come at a great cost. The consequences varied enormously depending on the experiences and life choices of the individual student, as well as the historical time period in which they found themselves. While the 1950s and 1960s were a quieter time in the political activities of Durban medical students, the 1970s and 1980s brought a much louder oppositional voice that was not easily or quickly silenced.

While this book has done much to question simplistic portrayals of the medical school's history, celebratory 'struggle' narratives – which form the basis of this chapter – should not be dismissed either when trying to understand this institution's complex history. Indeed, there is much to learn from these narratives, so long as we also remain critically engaged. Undeniably, because of the extracurricular activities of some of its students in the 1970s and 1980s, the school proved almost a constant headache for the apartheid state. The school's anomalous set-up as a black faculty within a white liberal institution enabled the emergence of politically conscious and confident black activists, whose leaders challenged their alma mater and the apartheid government on many issues. And, despite the death in detention of Steve Biko and banning of black consciousness (BC) organisations towards the end of 1977, the spread of its defiant message through black communities in the years before ensured that students and other BC activists inspired a culture of fearlessness and pride which gave many black South Africans in the country and in exile renewed hope, as well as the strength to question and challenge their racial oppressors in the 1980s.

Taking a step back from appreciating the value of these alumni's memories for their content about the past, it is also useful to reflect on the usefulness of memories *as narratives* produced in the present. Building on earlier arguments that memories can silence as much as they reveal, memories are also narratives that do not just allude to the past, but do constructive 'work' in the present. As with all things, memories are social phenomena that are embedded in social environments. They serve to promote social cohesion and, ultimately, consensus. By producing common memories with a romanticised, harmonious and heroic 'struggle' lens, alumni were able to make sense of their individual experiences and assign a greater relevance to their hardships and achievements in line with broader ANC nation-building frameworks in the post-apartheid period. Whether done consciously or not, present-day social acceptance and public affirmation have been powerful motivators on the ways in which people have remembered. Thus, the past and present are closely intertwined in shaping how, when and why people remember their pasts, including their experiences at the Durban Medical School.

In the next chapter the focus turns to the present day and some of the key medical educational developments in the post-apartheid period. Educational and political struggles of the apartheid era bequeathed to the democratic era several notable contradictions and difficult legacies. An alteration in the political dispensation in 1994 did not bring automatic changes to many issues that had plagued the medical school during apartheid.

Notes

1. Interview with Hugh Philpott, Kloof, 14 July 2003.
2. Sipho Buthelezi, 'The emergence of black consciousness: An historical appraisal', in *Bounds of Possibility: The Legacy of Steve Biko and Black Consciousness*, eds Barney Pityana, Mamphela Ramphele, Malusi Mpumlwana and Lindy Wilson (Cape Town, London and Atlantic Highlands, NJ: David Philip and Zed Books, 1991), 112–3.
3. Interview with ZM, Durban, 6 October 2003.
4. See Biko quote in Wits SAHA South African Political Materials 1964–1990s, The Karis-Gerhart Collection, Part III: Political Documents, SASO, Folder 762, Sipho Buthelezi, 'The Black Consciousness Movement in South Africa in the late 1960s', *CEAPA Journal* 1, no. 2 (December 1987), 27.
5. Interview with Maila J. Matjila, Durban, 18 July 2003, and 22 September 2003.
6. Buthelezi, 'The emergence of black consciousness', 114; and Mosibudi Mangena, *On Your Own: Evolution of Black Consciousness in South Africa/Azania* (Johannesburg: Skotaville, 1989), 24.
7. Mamphela Ramphele, 'Empowerment and symbols of hope', in *Bounds of Possibility: The Legacy of Steve Biko and Black Consciousness*, eds Barney Pityana, Mamphela Ramphele, Malusi Mpumlwana and Lindy Wilson (Cape Town, London and Atlantic Highlands, NJ, David Philip and Zed Books, 1991), 156. Also see Mamphela Ramphele, *Across Boundaries: The Journey of a South African Woman Leader* (New York: Feminist Press, 1995), 94–9 and 138–42. For more on the Zanempilo Community Health Centre, see Leslie Hadfield, 'Biko, Black Consciousness, and "the system" eZinyoko: Oral history and Black Consciousness in practice in a rural Ciskei village', *South African Historical Journal* 62, no. 1 (2010).
8. Wits SAHA South African Political Materials, 1964–1990s, The Karis-Gerhart Collection, Part I: Interviews, Folder 41, Nkosazana Dlamini Zuma (conducted by Gail Gerhart in London, 3 July 1988), 5 and 13.
9. For more on these and other SASO projects, see Wits SAHA South African Political Materials 1964–1990s, The Karis-Gerhart Collection, Part III: Political Documents, Folder 750, SASO, 'Report of University of Natal (Black Section)', Reports presented at the third General Students' Council of the South African Students' Organisation, St Peter's Seminary, Hammanskraal, 2–9 July 1972; and SASO, Folder 753, 'Community Development', Commissions presented at the fourth General Students' Council of the South African Students' Organisation, St Peter's Seminary, Hammanskraal, 14–22 July 1973; and Ramphele, 'Empowerment and symbols of hope'.
10. Wits SAHA South African Political Materials, 1964–1990s, The Karis-Gerhart Collection, Part I: Interviews, Folder 26, Malusi Mpumlwana (conducted by Gail Gerhart in Tarrytown [?], 16 May 1987), 2.
11. Wits SAHA South African Political Materials, 1964–1990s, The Karis-Gerhart Collection, Part I: Interviews, Folder 23, Diliza Mji (conducted by Gail Gerhart in New York, 2 June 1987), 1–3.
12. Interviews with Breminand Maharaj, Durban, 10 June 2003; and May Mashego, Durban, 14 October 2003.

13. Interview with Maila J. Matjila, Durban, 18 July 2003; UKZN EGML, 'The caring kind: Medical students giving up their time to help the needy', *NU Focus* 10, no. 2 (1999), 33; Wits SAHA South African Political Materials 1964–1990s, The Karis-Gerhart Collection, Part III: Political Documents, SASO, Folder 755, 'Inanda', SASO Composite Executive Report to the sixth General Students' Council at the Wilgespruit Conference Centre, Roodepoort, Transvaal, 30 June – 7 July 1974; SASO, Folder 749, 'The "New Farm" project on preventive medicine, 1972'; and SASO, Folder 750, 'Community development', reports presented at the third General Students' Council of the South African Students' Organisation, St Peter's Seminary, Hammanskraal, 2–9 July 1972.
14. Interviews with B.T. Naidoo, Durban, 15 September 2003; and May Mashego, Durban, 14 October 2003.
15. Ramphele, 'Empowerment and symbols of hope', 159.
16. Interview with K.P. Naidoo, Durban, 4 June 2004.
17. Wits SAHA South African Political Materials 1964–1990s, The Karis-Gerhart Collection, Part III: Political Documents, SASO, Folder 755, 'UNB report to NEC', reports presented at the Federal Theological Seminary, Alice, 23–26 May 1974.
18. Ramphele, 'Empowerment and symbols of hope', 156–7.
19. Interviews with Maila J. Matjila, Durban, 18 July 2003; Jerry Coovadia, Durban, 27 June 2003; Janet Giddy, Hillcrest, 24 May 2003; and Steve Reid, Hillcrest, 24 May 2003. Anne Digby and Howard Phillips with Harriet Deacon and Kirsten Thomson, *At the Heart of Healing: Groote Schuur Hospital, 1938–2008* (Auckland Park: Jacana, 2008).
20. Aziza Seedat, *Crippling a Nation: Health in Apartheid South Africa* (London: International Defence and Aid Fund for Southern Africa, 1984); and Cedric de Beer, *The South African Disease: Apartheid Health and Health Services* (London: Catholic Institute for International Relations, 1986).
21. Interview with Sam Fehrsen, Pretoria, 22 August 2003.
22. UKZNA *UN Calendars*, Faculty of Medicine handbooks, 1950s–90s.
23. Interviews with Y.K. Seedat, Durban, 14 July 2003; and Maila J. Matjila, Durban, 22 September 2003; and Wits CRO 9847 Medicine, SMC Newsletters 'Natal Medical School conference', *Mednews* (21 July 1982).
24. Ramphele, 'Empowerment and symbols of hope', 159–60.
25. Saleem Badat, *Black Student Politics, Higher Education and Apartheid from SASO to SANSCO, 1968–1990* (New York and London: Routledge, 1999), 124–5; Ramphele, 'Empowerment and symbols of hope', 159, 170–2; and Ramphele, *Across Boundaries*, 63–5.
26. Interviews with ZM, Durban, 6 October 2003; and Jerry Coovadia, Durban, 27 June 2003.
27. Interviews with ZM, Durban, 11 September 2003; and Maila J. Matjila, Durban, 18 July 2003.
28. UKZNA C10/6/1-2, 'Death of Mr S. Biko: Student protest', UN Council minutes, 16 September 1977, 37.

29. Interview with Soromini Kallichurum, Durban, 29 May 1999.
30. See UKZNA Students, Societies, SASO, 'Student unrest spreads', *Natal Mercury,* 12 May 1972; Melville Herskovits Library of African Studies, Northwestern University, Chicago, EAA8618, SASO, Ongkopotse Ramothibi Tiro, 'Bantu Education', *South African Outlook* (June/July 1972); and Baruch Hirson, *Year of Fire, Year of Ash: The Soweto Revolt: Roots of a Revolution?* (London: Zed Press, 1979) 86–7.
31. Wits SAHA South African Political Materials, 1964–90, The Karis-Gerhart Collection, Part I: Interviews, Folder 41, Nkosazana Dlamini Zuma (conducted by Gail Gerhart in London, 3 July 1988), 10.
32. UKZN MSA, 'Six students detained', *Daily News,* 27 March 1973; 'Three on race charge', *Natal Mercury,* 23 May 1973; 'Student quizzed on revolution', *Daily News,* 23 May 1973; 'Students attacked me – policeman', *Natal Mercury,* 5 July 1973; and 'Medical students fined R375', *Daily News,* 20 April 1974.
33. Gail M. Gerhart, *Black Power in South Africa: The Evolution of an Ideology* (Los Angeles: University of California Press, 1978), 293.
34. Gerhart, *Black Power in South Africa,* 298–9. The nine SASO and BPC people convicted, in addition to Aubrey Mokoape, included Strini Moodley, Mosioua Lekota, Saths Cooper, Zithulele Cindi, Muntu Myeza, Pandelani Nefolovhodwe, Nkwenkwe Nkomo and Kaborane Sedibe.
35. Badat, *Black Student Politics,* 133–5, and Interview with TM, Pretoria, 21 August 2003.
36. Interview with Hugh Philpott, Kloof, 14 July 2003.
37. UFH, Centre for Cultural Studies, AZAPO/BCM Records, Publications C–F, Box 29, AZAPO, '1976–86: A decade of resistance. Make it a revolution', and Jonathan Hyslop, *The Classroom Struggle: Policy and Resistance in South Africa, 1940–90* (Pietermaritzburg: University of Natal Press, 1999).
38. Hirson, *Year of Fire, Year of Ash,* 187.
39. UKZN MSA, Pat Farley, 'There's more violence says race expert: Student march broken up', *Sunday Tribune,* 20 June 1976; 'Medical school closes early', *Natal Mercury,* 21 June 1976; and '87 students on Act charges', no paper, 24 June 1976.
40. UKZNA C10/6/1-2,. 'Alan Taylor Residence: Police raid', UN Council minutes, 20 August 1976, 15.
41. Interview with MM, Durban, 28 July 2003.
42. UKZN Board of the Faculty of Medicine, Minutes of a Special Meeting of the Board of the Faculty of Medicine held on 15 December 1975; and UWC MAC Medical Schools, 'Natal medical faculty is instructed to refuse blacks', *Cape Argus,* 17 December 1975.
43. UKZNA C205/1/1-3, Medical School Press Cuttings and Correspondence, 1970–1979.
44. NAR K296 E5/49 Medical Training, 1968–9, Vol. 2, Komittee: Mediese Opleiding Verslag. 'Govt plans to train more African doctors: Medical faculty for students at Pietersburg College', *Sunday Express* (30 June 1965).

45. For more on these statistics, see F.P. Retief, 'The Medical University of Southern Africa after five years', *South African Medical Journal* (27 November 1982), 841; and Phillip V. Tobias, 'Apartheid and medical education: The training of black doctors in South Africa', *The Leech* 60, no. 1 (March 1991), 85–6.

46. Wits, William Cullen Africana Library, Government Publications, 'Report and recommendations of the committee of enquiry on possible further facilities for medical and dental training – 1984' (The De Villiers Committee), 25.

47. UWC MAC MEDUNSA, 1984, 'MEDUNSA – Where medical history is in the making', *Citizen* (1 February 1978).

48. These schools never materialised. Instead, UWC established a dental school and UDW became a hub for allied health professionals. UKZN MSA, 'Black medical school plan', *Daily News* (29 May 1973); 'Mixed feelings on move to start separate Indian medical school', *Natal Mercury* (26 October 1974); G.C. Oosthuizen, A.A. Clifford-Vaughan, A.L. Behr and G.A. Rauche, *Challenge to a South African University: The University of Durban-Westville* (Cape Town: Oxford University Press, 1981), 110–4; and UWC MAC Medical Schools, 'Planning medical school for UWC', no paper, 29 November 1975; and 'UWC looks forward to training doctors', *Cape Times* (3 December 1975).

49. CC EGM File 463/7/3. KCM 56990 (88), 'Black medical school will go white', *Natal Mercury* (17 December 1975); UCT M&A, Rupert Gude, 'Apartheid and medical services', *The Pulse* 3, no. 1 (March 1977), 4–7; and Wits CRO, 'Natal medical school forced to toe the colour line', *Wits Student* 34, no. 18 (11 August 1982).

50. 'Black students in protest', *Natal Mercury* (28 February 1976).

51. UKZN MSA, 'University fights for its blacks', *Natal Mercury* (24 February 1976); UKZNA C205/1/1-3, Medical School Press Cuttings and Correspondence 1970–1979, 'A reprieve for black medical course', *Natal Mercury* (7 August 1976).

52. Interview with Mfanyana J. Ndlovu, Durban (14 August 2003). Also see UKZNA XS 10/1/1-2 Cuttings Medical School, 'State silent as medical students keep up boycott', *Daily News* (8 October 1977); 'Campaign goes on to save medical school', *Daily News* (12 October 1977).

53. Interview with May Mashego, Durban, 7 October 2003.

54. Interview with TM, Pretoria, 21 August 2003. Also see 'Black students in protest', *Natal Mercury* (28 February 1976) and 'Campaign goes on to save medical school', *Daily News* (12 October 1977).

55. Interviews with Maila J. Matjila, Durban, 18 July 2003; Mfanyana J. Ndlovu, Durban, 14 August 2003; Veronica Wilson, Durban, 6 November 2003.

56. Wits CRO Box No. Reg. 00886, File no. 3, B19/3, Training of Black Medical and Dental Students, June 1944 – July 1962, 'Memorandum from the University of Natal Vice Chancellor to Col. S.C. Smith on the need for the maintenance of training of Bantu medical students at the University of Natal', 17 February 1976, 2; and Retief, 'The Medical University of Southern Africa after five years'.

57. UKZN MSA, Education, Medical. '"Crash" medical course: Plan to beat African doctor shortage', *Daily News* (21 August 1971); '"Train more Africans": Doctor

shortage', *Daily News* (24 March 1973); C.J.H. Brink. 'Doctor shortage and health services', *South African Medical Journal* (14 August 1971); Charlotte Searle, 'The second-class doctor and medical assistant in South Africa', *South African Medical Journal* (31 March 1973); G.H. Roux, 'The medical profession and the witchdoctor', *South African Medical Journal* (8 October 1977); E.M. Mankazana, 'A case for the traditional healer in South Africa', *South African Medical Journal* (1 December 1979); and 'Motlana hits at "bush medical school"', *Star* (8 October 1980).

58. Interview with Mfanyana J. Ndlovu, Durban, 14 August 2003.

59. Interview with KM, Durban, 14 November 2003.

60. Interview with S.B. Pitsoe, Durban, 17 July 2003. Similar perspectives were mentioned by other doctors who were on the staff of the medical school at the time in Interviews with J.V.O. Reid, Plettenberg Bay, 16 June 2002; Y.K. Seedat, Durban, 14 July 2003; Dennis J. Pudifin, Durban, 2 July 2003; and Hugh Philpott, Kloof, 14 July 2003.

61. Ina van der Linde, 'MEDUNSA at twenty', *South African Medical Journal* (December 1996), 1508. This professor was vice-principal of MEDUNSA when he was interviewed for this article.

62. Interview with Jerry Coovadia, Durban, 24 June 2003.

63. UWC MAC MEDUNSA, 1989, 'Prof. rides the "white elephant" to glory', *Pace* (April 1988). This comment was made by Ephraim T. Mokgokong, who graduated from the Durban Medical School in 1961.

64. Interview with J.V.O. Reid, Plettenberg Bay, 16 June 2002.

65. Interview with MM, Durban, 28 July 2003.

66. Interviews with Hugh Philpott, Kloof, 14 July 2003; and ZM, Durban, 11 September 2003.

67. Interview with Sam Fehrsen, Pretoria, 22 August 2003.

68. MA, MEDUNSA Press Cuttings, 1977–1982, 'Varsity to tackle Koornhof on black students', *Pretoria News*, 17 October 1977; and 'Second time round . . .' *Cape Argus* (21 October 1977).

69. 'Second time round . . .' *Cape Argus* (21 October 1977).

70. MA, MEDUNSA Press Cuttings, 1977–1982, 'Doctor shortage if black students boycott exams', *Weekend World* (16 October 1977); and UWC MAC Medical Schools, 'Medical exams put off', *The World* (18 October 1977).

71. UKZNA, H6/1/1, Medical School – History, *NU Chronicle*, November 1977; UKZN MSA, 'Phasing-out', *MSRC Bulletin* (Special Edition), May 1982, and 'Report of the Faculty of Medicine: 1977' (20 June 1978).

72. UWC MAC Medical Schools, 'Koornhof backtracks on blacks', *Rand Daily Mail* (21 October 1977).

73. Interview with Breminand Maharaj, Durban, 10 June 2003.

74. UKZN Board of the Faculty of Medicine minutes, Mpala House, Minutes of the one hundred and fifty-seventh meeting of the Board of the Faculty of Medicine held on 8 May 1978; 'Multiracial medical school the aim of Natal', *Natal Mercury*, 24 August 1981; Wits, William Cullen Africana Library, Government Publications,

'Report and recommendations of the committee of enquiry on possible further facilities for medical and dental training – 1984' (The De Villiers Committee), 148–9.

75. As discussed in chapter 5, the number of people who supported more narrowly defined ethnic organisations, such as the South African Indian Congress and Inkatha, remained comparatively smaller than the broad-based organisations like the UDF/ANC in the 1980s. Formed in 1978, the Azanian People's Organisation (AZAPO), which adopted the BC philosophy for its programmes, also developed as only a small organisation. For more on the history of AZAPO, see 'Azanian People's Organisation', *South African History Online*, http://www.sahistory.org.za/topic/azanian-peoples-organization-azapo.

76. Interviews with M.B. Kistnasamy, Durban, 26 August 2003; and Mfanyana J. Ndlovu, Durban, 14 August 2003.

77. Wits SAHA South African Political Materials, 1964–1990s, The Karis-Gerhart Collection, Part I: Interviews, Folder 41, Nkosazana Dlamini Zuma (conducted by Gail Gerhart in London, 3 July 1988), 23.

78. See above, 8.

79. Wits SAHA South African Political Materials, 1964–1990s, The Karis-Gerhart Collection, Part I: Interviews, Folder 32, Mamphela Ramphele, Columbia University, New York, 26 October 1989. A short talk followed by questions and answers (notes by Gail Gerhart), 6–7.

80. Wits SAHA South African Political Materials, 1964–1990s, The Karis-Gerhart Collection, Part I: Interviews, Folder 26, Malusi Mpumlwana, Thoko Mbanjwa and Mamphela Ramphele (conducted by Gail Gerhart and TK in Cape Town), 3 November 1985, 1.

81. Wits SAHA South African Political Materials, 1964–1990s, The Karis-Gerhart Collection, Part I: Interviews, Folder 23, Diliza Mji (conducted by Gail Gerhart in New York, 2 June 1987), 7–9.

82. Wits SAHA South African Political Materials, 1964–1990s, The Karis-Gerhart Collection, Part I: Interviews, Folder 41, Nkosazana Dlamini Zuma (conducted by Gail Gerhart in London, 3 July 1988), 10–1.

83. Wits SAHA South African Political Materials, 1964–1990s, The Karis-Gerhart Collection, Part I: Interviews, Folder 23, Aubrey Mokoena (conducted by Gail Gerhart in Johannesburg, 8 July 1989), 1.

84. Keith Mokoape, Thenjiwe Mtintso and Welile Nhlapo, 'Towards the armed struggle', in *Bounds of Possibility: The Legacy of Steve Biko and Black Consciousness*, eds Barney Pityana, Mamphela Ramphele, Malusi Mpumlwana and Lindy Wilson (Cape Town, London and Atlantic Highlands, NJ: David Philip and Zed Books, 1991), 140. For more on links between BC organisations and the exiled ANC and PAC, see Mbulelo Vizikhungo Mzamane, Bavusile Maaba and Nkosinathi Biko, 'The Black Consciousness Movement', in South African Democracy Education Trust (SADET), *The Road to Democracy in South Africa: Volume 2, 1970–80* (Pretoria: UNISA Press, 2006), 152–7.

85. Wits SAHA South African Political Materials, 1964–1990s, The Karis-Gerhart Collection, Part I: Interviews, Folder 41, Nkosazana Dlamini Zuma (conducted by Gail Gerhart in London, 3 July 1988), 33–5.
86. See Interviews with M.B. Kistnasamy, Durban, 26 August 2003; and May Mashego, Ashburton, 18 October 2003.
87. Ramphele, *Across Boundaries*, 183–4. For more on the significance of youth politics in the 1980s, see Jeremy Seekings, *Heroes or Villains? Youth Politics in the 1980s* (Johannesburg: Ravan Press, 1993).
88. Interview with M.B. Kistnasamy, Durban, 26 August 2003. For more on the formation and operation of SANSCO, see Badat, *Black Student Politics.*
89. Stephen Ellis and Tsepo Sechaba, *Comrades against Apartheid: The ANC and the South African Communist Party in Exile* (London: James Currey; Bloomington: Indiana University Press, 1992), 72 and 75.
90. Interviews with May Mashego, Ashburton, 18 October 2003.
91. UKZN MSA, 'State links doctor to blasts', no paper, n/d [1986?]. For an earlier time period, also see UKZN MSA 'Durban Terror Bomber named', *Daily News* (17 March 1978).
92. Interview with M.B. Kistnasamy, Durban, 26 August 2003.
93. Interview with Janet Giddy, Hillcrest, 2 June 2003.
94. Interview with Y.K. Seedat, Durban, 7 and 14 July 2003.
95. UKZNA XS 10/1/1-2 Cuttings Medical School, 'Seven hundred at Durban Medical School decide to join in', *Daily News* (22 April 1980); 'Medical students to continue boycott', *Natal Mercury* (20 June 1980); 'Students end action', *Daily News* (30 June 1980). Also see UKZN Board of the Faculty of Medicine minutes, 6 June 1980, 2–3; and UKZNA C10/8/1, 'Boycott of lectures at medical school', UN Council minutes, 20 June 1980, 4.
96. Interview with KM, Durban, 14 November 2003.
97. Interview with May Mashego, Durban, 14 October 2003.
98. UKZN EGML C.C. 'Noddy' Jinabhai, 'The Other Struggle', *NU Focus* 11, no. 1 (2000), 12–3.
99. These included, for example, the Health Workers' Association (HWA), the National Emergence Services Group (NESG), the National Progressive Primary Health Care Network (NPPHCN) and the National Education, Health and Allied Workers' Union (NEHAWU). Other health professionals were included in these organisations too.
100. For more on this history, see the NAMDA collection at Wits, South African History Archive. Also see Laurel Baldwin-Ragaven, Jeanelle de Gruchy and Leslie London, eds, *An Ambulance of the Wrong Colour: Health Professionals, Human Rights and Ethics in South Africa* (Cape Town: University of Cape Town Press, 1999).
101. Interview with May Mashego, Ashburton, 18 October 2003. For a similar perspective, see UKZN MSA, 'The life and times of a medical student', *Embryo: A UNB Publication*, n/d [early 1980s?], 8–9. Kwashiorkor is a form of malnutrition that occurs especially in children when there is not enough protein in the diet. Its symptoms include fatigue, weight loss, diarrhoea, and a large, protruding stomach.

102. Interview with K.P. Naidoo, Durban, 4 June 2004.

103. Interview with May Mashego, Durban, 7 October 2003; and UKZN Board of the Faculty of Medicine minutes, Reports of two special meetings held on 25 May and 2 June 1981.

104. UKZNA XS 10/1/1-2 Cuttings Medical School, 'Parents upset by boycott', *Natal Mercury* (7 August 1982); 'Petition slams action at Fort Hare', *Daily News* (10 August 1982); 'Ripples from Fort Hare are lapping on Durban', *Daily News* (12 August 1982); and UKZNA C10/8/2, 'Boycott of lectures by medical students', UN Council minutes, 20 August 1982, 4.

105. Interview with Soromini Kallichurum, Durban, 29 May 1999.

106. Interview with Maila J. Matjila, Durban, 22 September 2003.

107. James Barber, *South Africa in the Twentieth Century: A Political History – In Search of a Nation State* (Oxford: Blackwell, 1999), 252; and Badat, *Black Student Politics*, 133–5.

108. Interview with Soromini Kallichurum, Durban, 29 May 1999. Also see UKZN MSA, Letter from P. Naidoo (MSRC president) to S. Kallichurum (dean), 26 July 1985; UKZNA C10/9/2, 'State of emergency', UN Council minutes, 15 August 1986, 260; and 'Shots at student demo', *Natal Mercury* (13 June 1986).

109. See UWC MAC H12 Doctors 1985, 'Medics decide to return to King Edward', *Natal Mercury* (14 February 1985); 'Three hundred demos hit Durban streets', *Natal Witness* (29 March 1985); H36 NAMDA 1986–1992, 'Treatment of Langa injured criticised by medics', *Eastern Province Herald* (20 May 1985); MEDUNSA, 1985, 'Protesting students dispersed in Durban', *Natal Witness* (31 May 1985); Natal, 1985, 'Medic students burn "symbol of apartheid"', *Natal Mercury* (1 August 1985); Natal, 1986, 'Shots at student demo', *Natal Mercury* (13 June 1986). Also see UKZNA C10/8/2, 'Faculty of Medicine', UN Council minutes, 18 March 1983, 186 and 'Student interns: Dissatisfaction', UKZN Board of the Faculty of Medicine minutes, 3 August 1987, 11.

110. Interviews with Janet Giddy, Hillcrest, 24 May and 2 June 2003.

111. Interview with Jerry Coovadia, Durban, 24 June 2003.

112. CC GP File 23, KCM 25915, University of Natal Medical School Miscellaneous, W.R.G. Branford and A.W. Rees, 'Pre-medical courses in arts and science and the non-European hostel', Addressed to all members of the Faculty of Arts, n/d [late 1950s?].

113. Interview with Hugh Philpott, Kloof, 14 July 2003.

114. Interviews with Maila J. Matjila, Durban, 11 July 2003, and B.T. Naidoo, Durban, 10 November 2003.

115. Interview with Breminand Maharaj, Durban, 10 June 2003.

116. Interview with KM, Durban, 14 November 2003.

117. Wits CRO, 'Natal med school closed', *Wits Student* 36, no. 2 (29 February 1984), 7; Wits SAHA S. Health, AL 2457, S.2.5 PPHC Committee, 'Crisis at University of Natal Medical School', SRC Academic Freedom Committee (February 1984); and UKZN Board of the Faculty of Medicine minutes, 4 June 1984, 2.

118. See, for example, UKZN MSA, 'Medical school students boycott lectures', *Post* (1 February 1984); UWC MAC Natal, 1984, 'Med school boycott', *Leader* (3 February 1984); 'Medical school shut down', *Natal Mercury* (4 February 1984); 'Students who "flunked" sparked off action: Backgrounder to medical school boycott and closure', *The Leader* (10 February 1984); UWC MAC Natal, 1986, 'Medical students out on boycott', *The Leader* (14 March 1986); UKZNA C10/9/2, 'Medical school boycott of lectures', UN Council minutes, 21 March 1986, 197.

119. UKZN Board of the Faculty of Medicine minutes, 'Memorandum on the need to increase the accommodation available for medical students at the Alan Taylor Residence', n/d [1972?]; UKZNA C10/6/1-2, 'Alan Taylor Residence', UN Council minutes, 18 March 1977, 215; and UKZNA C10/9/1, 'Residence accommodation', UN Council minutes, 20 December 1985, 177.

120. Interview with Hugh Philpott, Kloof, 14 July 2003. Also see UKZNA C205/1/3 Faculty of Medicine, Correspondence and Cuttings, 'Natal student boycott over residence warden', *Daily News* (13 February 1981); and UKZNA C10/8/1, 'Alan Taylor Residence: Resignation of warden', UN Council minutes, 20 March 1981, 151.

121. UKZNA C10/7/1, 'Transport for black students', UN Council minutes, 15 June 1979, 204.

122. UKZNA C10/8/1, 'Fees: Faculty of Medicine', UN Council minutes, 17 October 1980, 73; UWC MAC Natal, 1984, 'Natal medical students face 30 per cent fee hike', *Natal Mercury* (28 October 1983).

123. UKZN MSA, 'Student reply on food boycott', *Daily News* (13 August 1970); UKZNA C12/4/1-4, 'Alan Taylor Residence', UN Council minutes, 16 June 1972, 96, 114; UKZN Board of the Faculty of Medicine minutes, 13 February 1981, 1–2; and UKZNA, 'Boycott of Fedics Catering Services in the Faculty of Medicine and Alan Taylor Residence', UN Senate minutes, 21 May 1986, 204.

124. Adam Starz, *Between Laughter and Tears* (Ladysmith, RSA: Sinclair Publishing, 1986), 62–3.

125. See Thoko Mbanjwa ed., *Black Review, 1974/1975* (Black Community Programmes, 1975); Interview with Y.K. Seedat, Durban, 7 July 2003, and UKZN MSRC, Meeting of the Executive Committee, 28 July 1997, Committee Room, Mpala House, Medical School, 'University of Natal Medical School Submission to the Truth and Reconciliation Commission', 23 June 1997.

126. UWC MAC Natal, 1984, 'Students again in race boycott', *Natal Mercury* (16 April 1984); UKZN MSA, 'University of Natal reconciliation graduation ceremony to be held', *Daily News* (30 November 1995); and *University of Natal Medical School Reconciliation Graduation Booklet 1995* (Durban: Indicator Press, December 1995).

127. MA MEDUNSA Press Cuttings, 1977–1982, 'Natal graduation boycott', *Post* (20 April 1980). Also see Interview with Hugh Philpott, Kloof, 14 July 2003; and Kuper, *An African Bourgeoisie*, 159.

128. Interview with Soromini Kallichurum, Durban, 29 May 1999.

129. Interview with Jerry Coovadia, Durban, 24 and 27 June 2003. A similar view was discussed in Interview with Maila J. Matjila, Durban, 18 July 2003.

130. Interview with Y.K. Seedat, Durban, 14 July 2003.

131. Interview with J.V.O. Reid, Plettenberg Bay, 16 June 2002.

132. UKZN Board of the Faculty of Medicine minutes, 25 June 1980, 2.

133. Interview with B.T. Naidoo, Durban, 15 September 2003.

134. 'In memoriam: Isidor (Okkie) Gordon', *South African Medical Journal* 88, no. 6 (June 1998), 735.

135. Also see Interviews with Soromini Kallichurum, Durban, 29 May 1999; B.T. Naidoo, Durban, 15 September 2003; and Fatima Mayet, Durban, 4 June 1999; and UKZN MSA, '"Never" same pay for doctors: Professor called "agitator"', *Daily News* (23 April 1969).

136. Interview with May Mashego, Ashburton, 18 October 2003.

137. Speech given by Zweli Mkhize, *University of Natal, Nelson R. Mandela School of Medicine, Fiftieth Anniversary Banquet* (University of Natal, Durban: Audio-Visual Centre, 29 July 2000). A similar view of Sarkin was expressed in Interview with ZM, Durban, 6 October 2003.

138. Interviews with Maila J. Matjila, Durban, 18 July 2003, and Mfanyana J. Ndlovu, Durban, 14 August 2003.

139. Interview with May Mashego, Durban, 7 October 2003.

140. 'In memoriam: Theodore Leonard Sarkin', *South African Medical Journal* 88, no. 6 (June 1998), 734.

141. Interview with Breminand Maharaj, Durban, 10 June 2003.

142. Interview with Mfanyana J. Ndlovu, Durban, 14 August 2003. A similar view was discussed in Interview with Jerry Coovadia, Durban, 27 June 2003, and in a Speech given by Soromini Kallichurum. *Fiftieth Anniversary Banquet*. In contrast, Owen P.F. Horwood, who replaced E.G. Malherbe as principal and vice-chancellor from 1966 to 1969, was remembered as being pro-apartheid and afterwards became a National Party member of Parliament. Interviews with Fatima Mayet, Durban, 4 June 1999, and B.T. Naidoo, Durban, 15 September 2003.

143. UWC MAC Medical Schools, 'Medical exams put off', *The World* (18 October 1977). Interview with TM, Pretoria, 21 August 2003. Also see UKZNA C10/9/1, 'Faculty of Medicine: Boycott of lectures', UN Council minutes, 16 August 1984, 75; UKZN Board of the Faculty of Medicine minutes, 12 May 1980 and 29 July 1985; Deena Padayachee, 'Whites and Indians opposed apartheid of the medical school', *Natal Witness* (7 September 2000).

144. Interview with Maila J. Matjila, Durban, 18 July 2003. Also see UKZN Board of the Faculty of Medicine minutes, 11 November 1976, 2; UKZNA C10/6/1-2, 'Banning of medical students', UN Council minutes, 19 November 1978, 166; UKZNA C10/9/2, 'State of emergency', UN Council minutes, 15 August 1986, 260; and Maharaj, 'University of Natal Medical School submission to the Truth and Reconciliation Commission', 3.

145. Interview with B.T. Naidoo, Durban, 15 September 2003. A similar view was raised for discussion in Interview with Breminand Maharaj, Durban, 10 June 2003.

146. UWC MAC NAMDA, 1987, 'Mji's energy keeps fight alive', *Sunday Tribune* (26 July 1986); and UWC MAC Medical Schools, 1989, 'Police raid lecturer's home, office', *Natal Mercury* (23 August 1989).

147. The American Association for the Advancement of Science and Physicians for Human Rights, 'Human rights and health: The legacy of apartheid', 1998, http://shr.aaas.org/loa/sector.htm. Also see Interview with Jerry Coovadia, Durban, 27 June and 4 July 2003.

148. UKZNA C10/8/2, 'Faculty of Medicine', UN Council minutes, 18 March 1983, 186.

149. Interview with Barry Kistnasamy, Durban, 26 August 2003. Also see Wits SAHA South African Political Materials 1964–1990s, The Karis-Gerhart Collection, Part III: Political Documents, SASO, Folder 763, 'News in brief: Raids, detentions, protests', *SASO Bulletin – Extra-Ordinary* 1, no. 1 (November 1971), 2; UKZNA C10/6/1–2. 'Alan Taylor Residence', UN Council minutes, 20 August 1976, 110; UKZNA, 'State of emergency and unrest: Police raid at Alan Taylor Residence', UN Senate minutes, 11 September 1985, 155; and UKZNA C10/9/1, 'Police action at Alan Taylor Residence', UN Council minutes, 18 October 1985, 138.

150. Interview with B.T. Naidoo, Durban, 10 November 2003.

151. Interview with MM, Durban, 28 July 2003.

152. Interview with Hugh Philpott, Kloof, 14 July 2003.

153. During the apartheid years, spying on behalf of the police was noted on other liberal campuses like Wits and UCT too. See G.R. Bozzoli, *A Vice-Chancellor Remembers: The Memoirs of Professor G.R. Bozzoli* (RSA: Alphaprint Randburg, 1995), 179–81; Wits CRO, 'Spy story', *Wits Student* 36, no. 11 (July/August 1984); and Interview with Max Price, Johannesburg, 19 August 2003.

154. Interviews with Maila J. Matjila, Durban, 11 July 2003; Mfanyana J. Ndlovu, Durban, 14 August 2003; May Mashego, Durban, 14 October 2003; and Veronica Wilson, Durban, 6 November 2003.

155. Interview with Breminand Maharaj, Durban, 10 June 2003.

156. Interview with Hugh Philpott, Kloof, 14 July 2003.

157. Interview with Veronica Wilson, Durban, 6 November 2003.

158. Interview with MM, Durban, 28 July 2003.

159. See Wits SAHA South African Political Materials, 1964–90, The Karis-Gerhart Collection, Part I: Interviews, Folder 23, Diliza Mji (conducted by Gail Gerhart in New York, 2 June 1987) and Folder 41, Nkosazana Dlamini Zuma (conducted by Gail Gerhart in London, 3 July 1988); UKZN MSA, 'Six students detained', *Daily News* (27 March 1973); 'Students in detention', UKZN Board of the Faculty of Medicine minutes, 13 March 1978, 12; UWC MAC Natal, 1985, 'Two students held after demo', *Natal Witness* (30 July 1985) and NAMDA, 1987, 'Mji's energy keeps fight alive', *Sunday Tribune* (26 July 1986); and Speech by Zweli Mkhize, *Fiftieth Anniversary Banquet*.

160. Interview with Breminand Maharaj, Durban, 10 June 2003.
161. UKZNA MF3/1/18, *Mednews*. 'Homecoming for activist and scholar', *Mednews: Faculty of Medicine Newsletter* 3, no. 1 (January–December 2002).
162. S.C. Moodley, 'A personal perspective: 1973–95', *The University of Natal Medical School Reconciliation Graduation Booklet 1995* (Durban: Indicator Press, December 1995), 1.
163. Wits SAHA South African Political Materials 1964–1990s, The Karis-Gerhart Collection, Part III: Political Documents, SASO, Folder 761, (Nkosazana Dlamini, 'The ANC is the answer', *Sechaba* (Second quarter 1977), 25.
164. UKZNA BIO-S 842/1/1, Zuma, Nkosazana Dlamini.
165. Interview with Sidney and Emily Kark conducted by C.C. Jinabhai and Nkosazana Zuma, Durban, South Africa, 1992, 24–5; UKZNA BIO-S 1054/1/1 Coovadia, Hoosen 'Jerry'. Jerry Coovadia, 'Forsaking the revolution', *Focus* (Winter 1994), 9; UKZN EGML Rupini Vadyvaloo, 'Taking health care to the community', *NU Focus* 7, no. 2 (1996), 11; and C.C. 'Noddy' Jinabhai, 'The other struggle', *NU Focus* 11, no. 1 (2000), 12–3.
166. Interview with May Mashego, Durban, 7 October 2003.
167. Interview with Breminand Maharaj, Durban, 10 June 2003. Also see 'Students ask for more time', *Daily News*, 25 October 1977.
168. Interview with Y.K. Seedat, Durban, 7 July 2003; and Interview with J.V.O. Reid, Plettenberg Bay, 16 June 2002.
169. See UWC MAC Natal, 1984, 'Go back to class, dean tells students', *Natal Mercury* (2 February 1984), and 'Lecture boycott at NU Medical School', *Natal Witness* (4 February 1984); and UWC MAC Natal, 1986, 'Medical students out on boycott', *The Leader* (14 March 1986).
170. Interviews with May Mashego, 7 October 2003, and B.T. Naidoo, Durban, 10 November 2003. Also see UKZNA C10/8/1, 'Natal medical students may lose bursaries', *Rand Daily Mail* (24 October 1977) and 'Boycott of lectures at medical school', UN Council minutes, 20 June 1980, 5.
171. UKZNA XS 10/1/1-2 Cuttings Medical School, 'Doctors' dilemma: King Edward VIII Hospital faces severe staff shortage because of medical school boycott', *Natal Mercury* (12 June 1980).
172. Anne Digby, 'Early black doctors in South Africa', *Journal of African History*, 46, 3 (November 2005), 427–8.
173. Lindy Wilson, 'Bantu Stephen Biko: A Life', in *Bounds of Possibility: The Legacy of Steve Biko and Black Consciousness,* eds Barney Pityana, Mamphela Ramphele, Malusi Mpumlwana and Lindy Wilson (Cape Town, London and Atlantic Highlands, NJ: David Philip and Zed Books, 1991), 34.
174. Interview with MM, Durban, 28 July 2003.
175. Interview with Breminand Maharaj, Durban, 10 June 2003.
176. Edgar Brookes, *A History of the University of Natal* (Pietermaritzburg: University of Natal Press, 1966).
177. Interview with Hugh Philpott, Kloof, 14 July 2003.

CHAPTER 8

The legacies of medical-education struggles in post-apartheid South Africa

'A shining example of survival in spite of apartheid.'
— Soromini Kallichurum

In the early 2000s, a few students studying in Durban shared what they knew about their medical school's history. Ali Modiba, a fifth-year student at the time and an executive member of the Medical Students' Representative Council (MSRC), said:

> It was known for producing very good doctors but it was also known for its political education, considering that most of the people we knew in politics were from this medical school – Steve Biko, Mamphela Ramphele [etcetera] . . . So it was associated with the struggle but also very good doctors . . . It's a medical school that I think is rich in history . . . [T]he picture is that the students who came here . . . had actually seen the need to play a role in the struggle for this country.[1]

Yet, while Ali Modiba knew something about his medical school's complicated history, being a few years older than most of his classmates and having taken an interest in broader political and historical matters, he felt that most of his colleagues did not. Bandile Hadebe, another fifth-year student at the time, concurred. He became aware of the school's complex history because his early student years coincided with the school's much-publicised 50th anniversary celebrations in 2000, and later because of his position on the MSRC. Yet, he argued that he knew little if anything about the medical school's history when he first entered it, and felt sure that neither did most of his colleagues:

> I didn't know anything about its political history . . . It was just a matter of wanting to go and study somewhere and Natal was one of the options. I only found out about the historic background . . . [at] one of those talks, you know, when you come during orientation and the dean comes and addresses you . . . and that's one of the things they sort of reflected on. But it didn't stick . . . [It was only] subsequently, I think we were celebrating the 50th anniversary . . . [T]hat time it became very obvious, like I really understood the whole background.[2]

According to these individuals, most incoming generations of students were not interested in knowing about their institution's broader history.[3] For students like Modiba and Hadebe, the main reason for this was that this knowledge did not specifically help students to obtain their medical degrees. The MSRC leaders in this group felt that it was part of a larger problem of student apathy in political matters, a problem common at the medical school in the post-apartheid period. Students were more interested in getting on with their studies and leaving political matters to the politicians. As Modiba noted with frustration:

> [I]t's like everyone is focusing on their work. They've got no time for friends, no time for politics, no time for anything . . . You come here, you go to class, after class you go to the library or go to your room [to study]. And I think it's a disadvantage to this class . . . because they're missing out on a lot of things. They are not actually . . . well informed about what [went on] and is going on in South Africa.

In a separate interview, Bandile Hadebe's view coincided with Modiba's. He said that 'the level of apathy has gone too high'. For him, the intensity of the medical programmes created this apathy as, in his opinion, the students now 'just want to . . . [study] and get out in six years' time'.[4]

A number of doctors who had graduated during the apartheid era spoke of what they thought of medical students in the post-apartheid era. Jerry Coovadia maintained that 'an intense mercenary attitude to life' has now become the prime motivator of many students.[5] It was felt that the apartheid generation of students had a greater sense of social responsibility, while 'the values of dedication to science and service and people are just not there anymore'. Dennis J. Pudifin, a professor in the Department of Medicine at the time, opined ruefully during an interview: 'They're all too greedy. I have strong feelings about that. I mean, the immediate expectation of so many doctors is rapid wealth and opulence.'[6] However, despite supporting the need to train students with a greater sense of altruism, another professor felt that the political struggle in South Africa had been fought and won, and that present generations of medical students should be allowed to focus all their attention on their studies:

> I sometimes think that the students now have such wonderful opportunities. And when they grumble, I feel like saying to them there's something wrong with you guys . . . I just feel that they don't realise what they've got. They've got such marvellous opportunities that we had to struggle and struggle for, you know. And the doors were always closed, when now, doors are open . . . [But] I suppose each generation will look at it differently . . . [But then] why should you have to struggle? . . . [W]hat we need to teach them is to be good doctors. That's all they need to battle with. That should be the battle, not everything else.[7]

In the early 1990s, the African National Congress (ANC) and the National Party began the political negotiations that initiated the process of dismantling apartheid society.[8] This difficult process eventually led to the first democratic election in April 1994, when an ANC government came into power with a majority vote. President Nelson Mandela's government and those that succeeded him worked hard to undermine the decades of apartheid politics that divided South Africa's population by race. Nevertheless, the road to transformation has been a bumpy one, producing many positive changes but also problematic setbacks.

Many changes have occurred at the country's medical schools since the early 1990s. For this generation of students, the demands of studying and passing the difficult medical courses are still there. On the other hand, these students have the advantage of focusing exclusively on their studies. They do not feel the same compulsion to divide their study time between medical and political issues, as one African doctor, who studied in the 1970s, acknowledged:

> [T]hey don't have anything to fight for now. The enemy has disappeared, has become fuzzy . . . Politically they are dull but maybe that's necessary

for them academically . . . I mean, they now, I think, are living the lives of white kids, our contemporary white kids. So hopefully they will do better than us academically and they will be more directed towards the academic stream or the learning stream more than us who were trying to do both, you know.[9]

Admissions policies

In significant ways, the post-apartheid period has undermined white racial privileges. Although racial equality at all levels of society is still a long way off and the decades of compounded apartheid socio-economic and political discriminations will take time to dissipate, the democratic era has produced a more racially equitable political environment. This has provided greater opportunities for black South Africans generally, as well as for black students in the profession of medicine more particularly. For example, since 1994, most medical schools across the country have opened their doors to students of all races and have given them greater choice about where to apply to study medicine than ever before.[10]

Interestingly, admission transformation at the University of Natal's medical school in the early 1990s was delayed because of the fierce opposition raised by registered black students to the university's proposal to admit white students.[11] Protesting students felt that white students should be excluded from the medical campus until such time as greater numbers of black students were admitted to study in the country's historically white medical schools. They made a good case. By 1994, less than 1 500 out of a total of 35 000 doctors were African.[12] Also, in 1994, the overwhelming majority of students studying at the country's three Afrikaans medical schools – Stellenbosch, Pretoria and Bloemfontein – and about half of the students studying at the English-speaking medical schools – the Witwatersrand (Wits) and Cape Town (UCT) – were white, and thus did not yet reflect a demographic proportionality to the population numbers in the country, where Africans made up about a 70 per cent majority. Indeed, the situation had not improved that much even ten years later. By 2004, the three historically black medical institutions of Natal, MEDUNSA and the University of the Transkei (or UNITRA, which opened a third black medical school in 1985) remained predominantly black universities, while white students remained in the majority at Pretoria, Bloemfontein and Stellenbosch. Only on the Wits and UCT campuses did figures reflect how white students were now outnumbered by black students. Moreover, while by 2003, two-thirds (or 66 per cent) of total enrolments across the country's eight medical schools were made up of black students, African students formed only 41 per cent of these enrolments.[13]

Durban's medical school did eventually open its doors to students of all races in the 1995 academic year, though, in line with the apartheid era's skewed admissions system, its opening was conditional upon the identification of certain 'targets' or 'quotas' for student admissions.[14] With this system, the medical school favoured African applicants who met its admissions criteria, even if their overall marks were lower than candidates from other racial groups. This was done to try to align the school's admissions quotas with the country's demographic profile. Moreover, it aimed to encourage applications from promising students who came from disadvantaged schools, and to redress apartheid-era imbalances in the production of African doctors. Admission was based not only on academic achievement, but on a combination of matriculation results, students' extracurricular activities, in-depth personal interviews, as well as confidential reports completed by high school principals or teachers to determine students' leadership and personal qualities to adequately cope with the heavy workload.[15]

Since 1995, the medical school's admission committee has worked on achieving a selection target of 69 per cent Africans, 19 per cent Indians, 9 per cent coloureds, and 3 per cent whites. However, it has sometimes found it difficult to fill its African quota because the pool of qualified African applicants has remained low and in the post-apartheid period has also been divided amongst all the medical schools. A majority of at least 50 per cent of African students has been admitted to the school, however, with the remainder of spaces being divided up amongst Indian, coloured and white students.[16] From 1995 to the early 2000s, admission of white students was approximately 5 per cent per annum.

Furthermore, in terms of student dynamics, larger numbers of women were admitted to the medical school after 1994 in line with efforts made by South African universities to alter the predominantly male gender profile of their students. Nationally, women medical students' enrolments increased to roughly equal the number of male students in 1999 and have outnumbered their male colleagues since 2000, when about 51 per cent of total enrolments were women.[17] By 2005, women made up nearly 56 per cent of total student enrolments. This increase in women students occurred at the Natal Medical

School too. Interestingly, by the 2000s, women have made up the majority of students admitted to the school.[18] This was captured in a comment made by S.B. Pitsoe, a lecturer who worked over several decades in the Department of Obstetrics and Gynaecology, and was there to witness the gender transformations after 1994:

> What I've noticed now with the younger classes, more Africans that have come in. And what's more the [female] gender seems to be in the majority . . . that women are . . . now as medical students coming in . . . In my department now, there are days when I go into the labour ward [and] the whole team is just African females. This thing was unheard of in the past. So things have changed.[19]

In addition, although the profession of medicine still remains one dominated by men, the gender profile of the profession is changing, albeit more slowly. In the late 2000s, men still dominated the profession, comprising nearly three-quarters of all registered practitioners. Men have also continued to dominate certain specialities like surgery. However, between 2002 and 2006, statistics reveal that there was an increase of registered female doctors by 24 per cent, compared to an increase of only 6 per cent for male doctors and 11 per cent increase overall.[20]

During the 1990s, more determined efforts have also been made to address a wide range of structural inequalities experienced by women students and staff on their various campuses. The appointment at a number of universities of public commissions of inquiry has been one such attempt.[21] What is more, societal attitudes about women in the medical field have changed too. For instance, in 2003, May Mashego told me that in addition to demographic changes in student admissions and the number of women working as doctors, she felt that even 'the attitude of people' in terms of leadership has changed:

> The change has happened since after the elections. People have looked at women differently and women have been able to prove themselves . . . So I think there has been a change with the change of government generally . . . [and its] change of laws allowing women in . . . I think the outlook [on life] has changed . . . Women know that you don't have to sit at home and bring up your children . . . I think it's the change of attitude from the men

themselves, from the communities, and from the women themselves
. . . [There is more] support.[22]

Building expansions

During the 1990s and through the early 2000s, student numbers have
expanded at medical schools across the country. For example, the annual
intake of medical students increased at the University of Natal from about
120 in the early 1990s to about 190 in 1998 and to 200 by the year 2000.[23] In
fact, researchers Mignonne Breier and Angelique Wildschut argue that all
medical schools have felt the pressure to expand in recent years.[24] With
growing numbers of students matriculating each year and with the necessary
subject passes to enter medical school, some years have witnessed as many as
twenty times the number of applicants as places available at South Africa's
medical schools!

At various campuses, expansion has occurred to try to respond to the
greater overall student demand. It has also occurred to attempt to meet the
new admission quota requirements and to keep up with the growing
complexity of the medical field, which has seen an increase in the number of
academic specialities and sub-specialities that have needed to be accommod-
ated. At the University of Natal, the number of academic departments and
sub-departments reached 31 by 2001, a huge increase on the handful of
departments that existed when the medical school first opened in 1951.
There has also been a corresponding increase in the number of staff to run
these departments. An examination of the Faculty of Medicine's handbooks
between the early 1950s and 2000s highlight these dramatic changes.[25]

As a result, the 1990s have witnessed the erection of new buildings to
teach and accommodate expanding student and staff numbers. This has been
particularly noticeable on the Durban medical campus, when the University
of Natal entered negotiations with the Department of Health and the Natal
Provincial Administration to raise funds to build a new academic teaching
hospital. The aim was twofold. Firstly, it wanted to replace the rapidly
deteriorating and overcrowded King Edward VIII Hospital, which had been
repeatedly described from the 1970s through to the early 1990s as a
'nightmare', a 'social disgrace' and in 'crisis'.[26] Secondly, it wanted to build a
new and larger residence and medical school that could accommodate 200
students per annum in each year. By the 1980s, neither its teaching hospital
nor its medical school had been upgraded, nor, as a University of Natal

newsletter highlighted, had they been 'provided with the same facilities as their six counterparts elsewhere in the country, despite a massive increase in the service activities'.[27]

During the late 1980s, the first breakthrough came when a state subsidy was received to build a new medical residence.[28] This residence was opened in 1990 following the closure of the Alan Taylor Residence in Wentworth, which was taken over by Engen as part of its oil refinery plant. Its closure at the end of 1989 was the end of a bittersweet era, as one newspaper article highlighted, producing many conflicted emotions amongst graduates about their time spent at this residence.[29] Highlighting once again the politics of the present on the medical school's history, the new residence was named the Albert Luthuli Residence, in honour of Chief Albert Luthuli, the celebrated ex-president of the ANC and Nobel Peace Prize winner, and is located on Rick Turner Road, a residential area near the university's main Howard College campus. The university had received permission to build in this area in a reform era that saw the dismantling of Group Areas Act legislation. It was built to accommodate over 500 medical students studying in different years of their degree. It was also built in a more central location and, unlike ATR, was situated only about two kilometres away from the medical school's Umbilo Road campus.[30] With government relaxation of Group Areas legislation, the early 1990s saw the opening of the university's other residences to black students too.[31]

While the new residence building project was able to make progress by the late 1980s, largely because of relentless and heightening protests from students, the building of a new medical school and academic hospital complex experienced many complicated delays. Although discussions for a new medical school and a larger academic teaching-hospital complex in Cato Manor (an area close to the University of Natal) extended all the way back to the early 1980s, negotiations were stalled for a number of reasons.[32] The difficulty of finding suitable land close to the University of Natal was a key factor, as were the disruptions caused by the political transition in the early 1990s. Moreover, budgetary constraints and a temporary moratorium imposed by the transitional government on building new hospitals as it focused its attention on rolling out primary health-care services delayed progress.[33] In the interim, King Edward VIII Hospital was granted R30 million in 1990 to upgrade its facilities and to alleviate its critical patient overload, staff shortages and lack of essential equipment until a final decision could be made about building a new teaching hospital.[34]

In the early 1990s, the Natal Medical School's planners changed their tactics. The altered conceptualisation by the government of a future Cato Manor hospital required them to imagine something different. Originally, this hospital had been planned to become the new academic teaching hospital for the medical school, but as time passed and funding was raised for this building project, the government's view of this hospital's role broadened.[35] Instead, this hospital was envisaged – and eventually opened in 2002 – as a technologically sophisticated tertiary-level institution that would serve the educational needs of all institutions responsible for health training in the province of KwaZulu-Natal and nationally.[36] By the mid-1990s, Durban Medical School planners could estimate that, according to this revised plan, as little as 10 per cent of the school's teaching at the undergraduate level, and between 30 to 40 per cent at the postgraduate level, would take place at this hospital, making it illogical to build a new school adjacent to this Cato Manor hospital.[37] Growing financial restrictions in the post-apartheid era did not help their original plans to build a new school either, which would have cost, as a conservative estimate, in the region of about R115 million. This plan was therefore abandoned.

Managers in charge of these original plans decided to cut their losses and instead work on raising money to extend, renovate and refurbish the Umbilo Road medical school buildings. During negotiations, soon after implementing this change in strategy, the government quickly recognised the cost-effectiveness of this alternative plan, and granted the University of Natal additional subsidies for this purpose during the course of the 1990s.[38] An initial R3.2 million was allocated for extensions and renovations in 1991, and at the end of 1992, a further R6 million was granted for a second phase.

During the first phase, money was used to create additional space for various departments and to construct a 200-seat lecture theatre, additional seminar rooms, a new library and an improved student recreational area. Impala House, a former overnight residence for clinical students and residents, which was situated in the grounds of the medical school, was converted into an administrative centre, thus releasing further space inside the school for academic purposes. The second phase of expansion included the building of a six-storey tower block that enabled the expansion of office space in numerous departments. A further smaller amount of money was provided in the latter 1990s too, to fund Phase III, which entailed upgrading, decorating and executing minor changes to the medical school's old buildings, as well as the provision of 150 additional parking bays. During the 2000s, further substantial additions to the medical school's old building complex were made with the assistance of generous international sponsorships, such as the Doris Duke Medical Research Institute, which was opened in 2003, and the KwaZulu-Natal Research Institute for Tuberculosis and HIV (K-RITH), which was opened towards the end of 2012.[39]

Medical-educational challenges

One of the enormous challenges in health-sector services and medical school training in the post-apartheid era has been the devastating impact of HIV and AIDS, particularly in the province of KwaZulu-Natal, which in recent years has been much publicised as the epicentre of this pandemic. Studies of admissions to King Edward VIII Hospital, for instance, showed that the number of HIV-positive patients jumped from 19 per cent to 34 per cent between 1995 and 1997, and from 39 per cent to 53 per cent between 1997 and 1998, the vast majority being severely immunocompromised.[40] In 2001, between 55 per cent and 65 per cent of inpatients at King Edward VIII Hospital were HIV-positive. Another long-standing employee of the medical school and King Edward, Y.K. Seedat, said in 2003 that the 'public sector is getting worse in terms of the care of patients . . . Nobody predicted AIDS. In the medical wards 60 per cent are positive for HIV.'[41]

While some people interviewed felt that there were colleagues they knew who had been attracted to join the medical profession with the hopes of finding a cure for HIV/AIDS, much of this idealism was shattered once they started their clinical work in places like King Edward.[42] During the 1990s and through the early 2000s, despite their best efforts in a situation where a cure does not exist, and an environment where the post-apartheid government has been slow in its roll-out of free antiretroviral treatment, hospital employees, including attending academic teaching staff and medical students in clinical training, have been forced to watch many of their patients suffer and die.[43] The effects of the poor public health-care services and this HIV/AIDS health catastrophe have been overwhelming and devastating. In 2003, Jerry Coovadia spoke of the situation affecting him psychologically, as well as his colleagues who worked with him:

If you work in outpatients, when I was running Paediatrics, and you saw 80 patients – I mean, what is left of you? You are totally brutalised. You could be a saint, you know, but at the end of the day . . . [there is] no generosity or no humanity left in you . . . So it just weighs you down . . . And if that isn't bad enough, the AIDS epidemic comes in and just eliminates any trace of humanity that existed. Because now you see . . . all the problems magnify and then you can't do much for them . . . [and] you know that, for heaven's sake, if we had a programme which prevented this infection, and it's possible, this thing wouldn't be here . . . [T]here's treatment available and you can't give them this treatment, which is just terrible . . . So you got used to the idea . . . you develop the fatalistic approach . . . maybe you accepted death too easily because you couldn't help it. It was there every day.[44]

In 2004 Ali Modiba, who was doing his clinical training at the time, expressed his opinion of the effects of this disease on students' training. For him, the workload has increased under the impact of HIV/AIDS, as the health system's budget has not been sufficient to provide adequate staff to deal with the effects of this disease. In addition, he maintained:

It is making a very serious emotional trauma because . . . our graduates, even if they don't leave to go overseas, [some] will not practise medicine because of exactly what you see in the wards. You came to medical school thinking, you know, here I am going to train as a doctor and I'm going to help people. But when you see people die, day in [and] day out, and there isn't anything you can do about it . . . It's devastating emotionally . . . I don't think there are words to describe what we see in the hospital. It's all good and nice for people to talk about HIV . . . [and talk about] the numbers, [but when you see] the[ir] faces, [that's when] it really hits you . . .[45]

Ntuthuko Mahlaba, a student colleague of Modiba and the 2004 MSRC president, said he felt the virus has also completely shifted the focus of various departments at the medical school. Whether a student was studying in the departments of obstetrics and gynaeology, or in medicine, surgery, paediatrics or emergency medicine, students were now taught to 'always think of HIV/AIDS . . . and you find that every second patient you get to see . . . is HIV-positive'.[46] In a statement laced with strong emotion, Mahlaba said that students and staff were 'trying everything, doing [their] best, using a lot of resources, but the person, at the end of the day, is going to die'. Additionally, Mahlaba asserted that in terms of research, it seemed that almost 'everyone is doing HIV [work] . . . [in] this faculty' and that the school even has 'a big research centre' – the Doris Duke Medical Research Institute – to conduct this type of research.[47] For Mahlaba, HIV/AIDS had completely 'shifted . . . the focus of medicine' at the medical school in the post-apartheid period.

What is more, the dangers of working with patients with HIV/AIDS are real for students and doctors too, when clumsiness or exhaustion can lead to contamination with infected blood through needle-stick injuries, or contamination with other body fluids.[48] Some students just want to get their degrees as quickly as possible and plan to emigrate from South Africa to work in countries with lower HIV/AIDS rates. Veronica Wilson, a surgeon who has worked in the trauma section of King Edward for many years, highlighted this issue during an interview:

[W]ith the diseases, HIV/AIDS, the health-care workers are very, very exposed and TB also. And I don't think enough is being done because a lot of the health-care workers and doctors . . . are exposed. There are a number of doctors who've got TB and they've had severe forms, including TB meningitis and multi-resistant TB . . . So that I think is also going to be something . . . where people are not going to want to do medicine or they will do medicine and then they'll leave . . . So those are the hazards, it's needle-stick injuries, fluid contamination, and especially like working in an emergency department like mine, is that even if you practise universal precautions, you are at risk and especially if they bring in more than one resuscitation . . . and then somebody's got the needle with the injection and, you know, just blood and it pokes you and you know it's really [something].[49]

For the post-apartheid generation of student doctors-in-the-making, and especially those who plan to remain in South Africa and work as medical professionals, much of their present and future work will be focused on treating, preventing or researching HIV and AIDS in South Africa.

Adding to the stresses of older structural problems and dealing with new disease threats like HIV/AIDS, students and staff at the Durban Medical School and at medical schools in other parts of the country have also had to undergo significant curricula changes in the post-apartheid period in response to national health policy changes. During the 1990s the newly elected democratic government inherited a health-care system that was grossly fragmented and unequal, with many long-standing problems as a result of apartheid in health. Before the 1994 elections, for example, health provision was largely curative and hospital-based, as well as expensive, as public hospital facilities consumed close to 70 per cent of the nation's health budget.[50] The unequal distribution of medical personnel has also led to the concentration of doctors in urban areas, while private practice has remained the most attractive avenue for many doctors because of the lack of resources and poor working conditions in the public health service.[51]

The government's 1997 *White Paper for the Transformation of the Health System in South Africa*, which drew heavily on the experiences and writings of earlier primary health-care pioneers, such as Sidney and Emily Kark, as well as the Primary Health Care strategy that was promoted as the way forward at the 1978 international World Health Organization conference, provided a clear policy framework to develop a more equitable national health system in line with the realities and challenges of a developing country.[52] Governments in the post-apartheid era have committed themselves to improving health-care services for all. This has entailed shifting national health policy emphases and reallocating funds from an expensive hospital-centred approach to providing more appropriate, accessible and affordable community-level primary health-care services.[53] Recognition of the need to produce more doctors who understand the health needs of disadvantaged communities and who are motivated and trained 'to respond appropriately to the health needs of the people they serve' has also been a concern.[54] Finally, in an effort to provide doctors to help alleviate staff shortages in the public service and in underserved rural areas, at a policy level, the Health Professions Council of South Africa (the legislative body regulating medical standards that replaced the SAMDC) also introduced a community service requirement for doctors from 1998. This required that all new medical graduates who completed their internship do one year's paid community service in the public sector before being licensed to practise in South Africa.[55]

As a result of these broad health policy changes, medical schools across the country have undergone fundamental curricula changes in the 1990s and 2000s to accommodate the government's call for a community-based and primary-health-care-focused approach in the new South Africa.[56] Durban's medical school has been affected too. In fact, both the process and product of medical education had been under serious review at the school since the early 1990s to bring its curriculum into line with broader health-care trends occurring in the country.[57] Although experimental initiatives were introduced at the first-year level from 1996, under the guidance of a 'Curriculum Development Task Force', which aimed to make subjects taught more clinically relevant from the outset and saw a few lecturers take students out on clinic visits to help them appreciate better the wider social aspects of diseases, it was only in 2001 that a completely restructured curriculum was introduced.[58]

In a rapidly advancing medical world, the new curriculum, which continues to be taught today, aims to avoid training narrow specialists. Instead, it focuses on producing 'basic doctors' who can deal competently with a broad spectrum of common ailments at primary or general-practice level, though with sufficient academic background to allow students to pursue specialisation in postgraduate study if they so desire. In addition, the new curriculum seeks to shift the focus away from the older preclinical and then clinical 'layered curriculum' situation, where students only saw patients in the wards during their fourth year of medical school. In its place, it seeks to integrate the basic sciences and clinical subjects so that early clinical exposure stimulates experiential or 'hands-on' learning, which is more relevant and stimulating, and encourages better understanding of diseases from the outset.[59] Furthermore, more regular small-group learning situations, which are problem-based and student-centred, have replaced the large didactic lecture-theatre format. This approach requires students to take more responsibility for their own learning through self-directed research and study, while it also promotes the development of 'continuous life-long learning skills'.[60]

Moreover, this new curriculum focuses on producing doctors, as Sidney Kark and his team in the Department of Social, Preventive and Family Medicine and at the Institute of Family and Community Health tried to do in the 1940s and 1950s, taking a holistic approach to their patients' health as individuals, but also as integral members of families and communities. This means focusing on a patient's physical or clinical dimensions of care, but also on the social, emotional and psychological dimensions too.[61] What is more, this has opened the school to exploration of academic collaborations with people engaged in a diverse range of alternative and holistic healing approaches, such as Indian Ayurvedic healing, Traditional Chinese Medicine and African indigenous healing approaches. This has led to important research and the ability of interested individuals to complete postgraduate diplomas in diverse alternative and complementary therapies.[62]

Provision of a comprehensive training that is concerned with the promotion of good health as well as prevention and cure of diseases is viewed as essential too in this new curriculum. Students are encouraged to learn in multiple sites, such as hospitals, but also in community-level primary health-care facilities. This exposes students to the wider social causes of illnesses and gets them away from the clinical confines of the hospital into 'real-life' community-practice situations.[63] Furthermore, in the new curriculum, greater emphasis has been placed on moral and social ethics issues as well, including recognition of patients' rights, ethical research practices, and sensitivity and respect for the different cultural, racial and religious beliefs and practices of their patients.[64] Skills not commonly associated with a medical degree, such as basic Zulu language skills, are now also encouraged to enhance communication with and understanding of patients.[65]

Finally, in the post-apartheid period, the length of the school's curriculum has changed too. In 2001 the University of Natal's medical school was the second in the country to abandon the long-practised six-year Bachelor of Medicine and Bachelor of Surgery (MB ChB) degree programme in favour of a five-year degree. This was followed by the introduction of a two-year period of internship training to ensure the provision of adequate practical experience for graduates emerging from the shortened medical-training programme.[66] After a period of review, much discussion by medical-education experts and changes in health policies, this move was followed in the mid-2000s by all other medical schools in the country as the best way to train the country's future doctors. This school thus helped lead the way in the process of overall transformation in South African medical-education provisions, which now emphasise a five-year degree, followed by two years of internship and then one year of community service.[67]

Legacies of apartheid in the post-apartheid era

While some issues and problems are different for students and staff in the post-apartheid period, there are others that continue to haunt the Durban Medical School. In 2003 Dennis Pudifin, who had worked for decades at this institution, described the continued appalling conditions of work at the school's King Edward VIII teaching hospital, noting that 'conditions of work here are not good'. In his opinion, little had improved and 'it was better then than it is now'. In his view, conditions had deteriorated over the years, and 'in fact its deterioration has accelerated since 1994'. He added:

> It hasn't received [sufficient] funds. Attitudes to work, commitment, sense of responsibility, accountability, all seem to have been diluted . . . Staff is still too thin. We are quite severely understaffed compared to other teaching hospitals . . . It can be very depressing at times, particularly when the work pressures are really heavy as they can be. And you just struggle to manage with inadequate equipment, and equipment which is not working, inadequate support structures, help from the nurses, help from the porters, the communication system. There really [are] . . . many problems . . . [T]he effects are that very many people get out of the place as soon as they can. I mean, the commitments in the departments, particularly nowadays, [are] very heavy and retaining staff is very difficult.[68]

These numerous-public service-sector problems have resulted in the emigration of many doctors. Although emigration occurred during the apartheid years, since 1994 the rate of doctors leaving the country to settle elsewhere has grown substantially.[69] Statistics South Africa reported that there has been a steady increase in the number of doctors leaving since 1990, when 30 were recorded as having left, compared to a high in 2003 when 203 were recorded as having emigrated. The World Health Organization estimated that in 2006, when South Africa had 33 220 doctors on its medical register, there were as many as 12 136 South African qualified doctors practising in Australia, Canada, the United States, the UK, France, Germany, Portugal and Finland. Insecurity and crime, affirmative action policies, deteriorating conditions in the public service, the easy transferability of South African qualifications overseas and higher rates of pay abroad in part explain this increase. The emigration of doctors, as well as other health personnel, is one of the greatest concerns to the government. It has produced a large shortage of doctors in post-apartheid South Africa. In October 2002 the *Star* reported that there were at least 29 200 vacant health professional posts in public hospitals throughout the country![70]

The student body of the Durban Medical School has also remained fractured by race. This is evident in numerous ways. Firstly, in a situation where applications far exceed places available and a quota system continues to operate to redress educational imbalances, controversy around racially skewed admissions continues to beleaguer the school.[71] The favouring of African students, together with the acceptance of small numbers of white students after 1995, has reduced the number of places available for Indian students, despite their having obtained excellent matriculation passes. This has led to feelings of discrimination and accusations of reverse racism by some of the Indian applicants who had been denied admission.[72] Some of these cases have been highly publicised in the media, causing further tensions amongst the school's students.[73]

Secondly, many students' interactions at the medical school are still divided by race. This has been mentioned by a number of people who have worked either full-time or part-time at the medical school since 1994. B.T. Naidoo felt that while 'demographics' had 'changed remarkably' to now include 'a mixture of everyone' in the student body, 'polarised' racial groupings remained 'a disturbing feature' ensuring that medical students were not a cohesive group.[74] Reflecting on his many decades as a teacher at the medical school, Pudifin concurred. He expressed the view that 'one just had to walk past the cafeteria area during lunch breaks' to see apartheid racial categorisations still in operation in the student body: 'Generally you may find the odd white student mixing with one or other of the groups, but on the whole the Africans sit together, the Indians sit together and that's the way, it's always been the case.'[75] For May Mashego, separations between students would not simply disappear when apartheid had ended at the political level:

[T]he government of the day made . . . us grow up in terms of segregated groupings . . . And, I mean, it happens even now . . . you'll see these *klompies* [groups] . . . They don't have animosity towards each other but generally it's the way they are. And, I mean, we haven't [had] that much integrat[ion] that we don't see colour. We see a lot of colour, we are still very conscious of colour.[76]

These views were reiterated by medical students studying in Durban in the 2000s period. K.P. Naidoo felt adamantly that the impact of the previous apartheid governments' policies were great 'even today'. For this student, the 'vestiges of apartheid' separations were firmly ensconced amongst 'the psyche' of the students on his campus and would not change suddenly when they found themselves in a new, open, post-apartheid situation. People 'lived apart and they hated each other' for so long, and 'now for a few years to say, you know, shake hands and love each other . . . [that's] very artificial and unnatural . . . you just can't wish [the divisions] away over a few years'.[77] In 2004, Ntuthuko Mahlaba maintained that the MSRC was working hard, through educational initiatives and social events, to try to overcome the racial divisions amongst students. But, he said, 'we still have a lot to do as students' to bridge these separations, especially between African and Indian students:

> There is still a gap between us because you'll find that even if you go around outside, you'll find there's a group of Indian students sitting on that corner, and you'll find some . . . Africans sitting [over] there . . . And more tension is amongst blacks [Africans] and Indians. I must be honest. That is where the problem is . . . [The MSRC] want[s] to create a sense of community in the medical school, where we can [at least] all sit together.[78]

A third factor that has caused tensions in the student body was the unequal and discriminatory treatment African students felt they were continuing to receive at the hands of some of their lecturers who were of Indian descent. This was noted in a 2004 MSRC report, and included, for example, testimonies of being shouted at or belittled in front of their colleagues, being ignored in classes or during ward rounds, and claims of being unfairly victimised by being marked down in their clinical assessments.[79] African students also felt that their Indian colleagues received preferential treatment from their lecturers, and that the school provided a more supportive environment for them to advance.

These tensions and divisions extended to those studying at the postgraduate level and to those working at the medical school too. As mentioned in the introduction, accusations of racism and discrimination by African students and staff at the school that had bubbled just below the surface for many years erupted into the open at a glittering banquet held on 29 July 2000.[80] At this official banquet, which had been planned as a celebration of both the school's 50th anniversary and its renaming, the new Nelson R. Mandela School of Medicine was launched in the public domain not as a positive example of Mandela's rainbow nation in microcosm but, instead, as a school still deeply divided by race.

Kgotsi Letslape touched on some of the burning issues that came up for discussion in his impassioned speech on this occasion: 'At postgraduate level, we are accused of running to private practice and not really caring about post-grad. Nothing could be further from the truth. There's obstruction in terms of obtaining posts [and cases], there's harassment whilst in training, there's no support.'[81] Another African doctor reflecting on his postgraduate training experiences in Durban concurred: 'Many of us may have wanted to specialise but . . . the atmosphere under which you specialised . . . was hostile and people didn't want you there . . . because they felt that Africans belonged in private practice.'[82]

In addition to complaints about racism, the medical school was severely criticised at this occasion for its slow rate of transformation and for creating a hostile atmosphere for Africans to specialise, which, it was said, had driven most of them away. It was noted by African alumni that, comparatively, many Indian graduates had gone on to complete their specialist training at this institution, and filled key posts at the school and its teaching hospital.[83] A brief perusal through the school's faculty handbooks up until the 2000s shows how only a tiny number of Africans had been appointed as full professors and heads of departments at the school.[84]

When it came 'to fighting for turf, fighting for survival, fighting for positions', Maila J. Matjila argued in 2003 that in his opinion, Africans had been, and were continuing to be, 'sidelined' for jobs and promotions, which created much disharmony.[85] Disgruntled with their promotion prospects, especially into more senior academic positions, many Africans left to take up similar positions elsewhere. For Ntuthuko Mahlaba, the 'enemy' had changed. In an interview in 2004, he felt that in the post-apartheid period, 'the paradigm of sidelining or marginalising people has shifted. It's no longer that whites are sidelining blacks, but we, the people who are called blacks, now amongst ourselves, there is this struggle. There are certain people who want to monopolise things and [to] dominate.'[86]

As a consequence, the first decade of the twenty-first century has seen a number of UKZN-initiated committees of enquiry set up to deal with issues of racism and other discriminations in its medical school's 'institutional culture'. There have also been active attempts to recruit African employees into the institution, both at the teaching and management levels.[87] However, the process has been slow as it has been difficult to transform the institution at a structural level when positions were already filled. This has resulted in drastic measures and some ugly public mud-slinging. As the transformation process got under way in 2004, the dean at the time, Professor Barry Kistnasamy, was accused by some African students of what one newspaper reporter termed 'nepotistic' treatment of Indians and 'delaying transformation'.[88] Another journalist reported that he was 'physically frog-marched off the campus' by protesting MSRC students.[89] This was followed by the implementation of a controversial Deloitte and Touche audit as part of UKZN's transformation efforts, which led to the suspension and disciplinary hearings of several senior, mostly Indian, medical school academics in 2005.[90] They were accused of racism, discrimination, exam-paper leaks and unequal treatment of students.

At the eye of this storm was Kistnasamy, who was forced to relinquish his post as dean in December 2004. While taking his battle to the Durban High Court, he was publicly humiliated by being placed on forced leave, and then demoted to senior lecturer in the Department of Public Medicine in September 2006. Although eventually exonerated of racism and other charges in the Durban High Court in 2007,[91] the public denigration of Kistnasamy's character was serious and extreme. A journalist from *The New Age* – a newspaper often seen as sympathetic to the ANC government – labelled the treatment of Kistnasamy as a vicious 'ethnic cleansing' ritual by upper-level UKZN managers with the intent of removing powerful Indian academics who still 'roamed the corridors of this institution' in a new era.[92] These public attacks produced deep financial, emotional and psychological scars, which eventually saw Kistnasamy leave his alma mater to take up a position elsewhere.[93]

Although the other doctors charged with racial allegations in 2005 'were all later exonerated' too,[94] this 'culture of hostility' at UKZN, as two *Witness* reporters labelled it, and which extends beyond the bounds of the medical school, has produced much staff discontent and low morale at this institution.[95] It has also produced much criticism by academics and other concerned individuals for its 'misspending of taxpayers' money' on litigation and other processes against certain staff members.[96] What is more, these activities have produced a high turnover of academic staff in the medical school and in other departments of the university. In January 2012 *The New Age* reported that '[a] number of senior staff have been suspended or have resigned and this has long-term implications for the standard of education at the university. Numerous heads of department positions in the health sciences have been vacant for many years.'[97] Sadly, the tensions are not unique to the medical school or to UKZN, nor to the health sector. Accusations of 'racism' have also been made recently by doctors against their colleagues working at the Inkosi Albert Luthuli Central Hospital.[98]

At the time of the final editing of this book, racial tensions continued to simmer at the medical school as two further 'top UKZN academics' were suspended from their posts in April 2012. Professor Umesh Lalloo, a pulmonologist and former dean of the Nelson R. Mandela School of Medicine, and his wife, Professor Razia Bobat, a paediatrician, were suspended 'pending an internal disciplinary process' that was instituted by the university following allegations made on 'Tip-offs Anonymous', a fraud hotline that was designed purportedly 'to maintain academic integrity on campus'.[99] Although these charges were quietly dropped by June 2012,[100] a louder storm of controversy continues to wrack UKZN involving a dossier of allegations such as 'plagiarism, irregular staff appointments, the community's perception of racism, governance, unprofessional conduct of council members and the vice-chancellor, staff turnover and morale, favouritism, irregular procurement practices, perjury and financial irregularities' that was compiled by the Concerned Citizens Group of UKZN and sent to the public prosecutor for independent investigation.[101] UKZN's upper-level management will have much to answer for in coming months and years.

Future researchers will have the benefit of distance in time and perspective from which to describe and analyse these politically charged medical-educational controversies in the post-apartheid era. The telling and retelling of the story of the Durban Medical School has revealed, however, that ideological divisions around racial issues have had deep roots as well as very real consequences for particular individuals. Indeed, it would be naive to assume that they would have simply disappeared after the political settlements of the 1990s. As this book has shown, we can be assured that the medical school's staff and students will continue to exist in a world in which many aspects of the racially defined apartheid past will, unfortunately, remain obstinately in place.

Notes

1. Interview with Ali Modiba, Durban, 4 June 2004.
2. Interview with Bandile Hadebe, Durban, 7 June 2004.
3. Interviews with Ntuthuko Mahlaba, Durban, 7 June 2004, and K.P. Naidoo, Durban, 4 June 2004.
4. Interviews with Ali Modiba, Durban, 4 June 2004 and Bandile Hadebe, Durban, 7 June 2004.
5. Interview with Jerry Coovadia, Durban, 4 July 2003.
6. Interview with Dennis J. Pudifin, Durban, 2 July 2003.
7. Interview with MA, Durban, 6 November 2003.
8. For more on this subject, see, for example, James Barber, *South Africa in the Twentieth Century: A Political History – In Search of a Nation State* (Oxford: Blackwell, 1999); and Tom Lodge, *Politics in South Africa: From Mandela to Mbeki* (Cape Town: David Philip; Oxford: James Currey, 2002).
9. Interview with MM, Durban, 28 July 2003.
10. Dan Ncayiyana, 'Medical education challenges in South Africa', *Medical Education* 33, no. 10 (October 1999).
11. UKZN MSRC, Minutes of University Committees Executive Comm 02, Additional Documentation/Additional Item for a Meeting of the Executive Committee Scheduled for 28 July 1997, Committee Room, Mpala House, Medical School, 'University of Natal Medical School Submission to the Truth and Reconciliation Commission', 23 June 1997.
12. Ncayiyana, 'Medical education challenges in South Africa'.
13. Mignonne Breier with Angelique Wildschut, *Doctors in a Divided Society: The Profession and Education of Medical Practitioners in South Africa* (Cape Town: HSRC Press, 2006), 22, 24–7, 42.
14. UKZN Board of the Faculty of Medicine minutes, 25 July 1994, 24 October 1994, 2 May 1995 and 18 September 1995; Karen Jackman, Susan Miller and Praveen Naidoo, 'The quota quandary: Medical faculties are being forced to revise admission rules', *Daily News* (9 February 1995); UKZN EGML 'Med school to admit whites', *NU Info* 4, no. 11 (19 November 1994 – 14 February 1995); UKZN EGML Sarah Frost, 'Corrective action: The medical school's way', *NU Focus* 9, no. 2 (1998).
15. UKZN Board of the Faculty of Medicine minutes, 26 January 1996, 'Annexure 2: Admission criteria and procedures for first year MB ChB 1996'; UKZNA MF3/1/1-8, 'Focus on faculty's admissions policy', *Mednews: Faculty of Medicine Newsletter* (April–May 1999); and UKZN EGML Kathy Waddington, 'Redressing imbalances: Selection in search of caring doctors, *NU Focus*, 11, no. 2 (2000).
16. Breier with Wildschut, *Doctors in a Divided Society*, 101; UKZNA C10/12/1-6, 'Medical school: Legal case regarding non-selection of candidate', UN Council minutes, 30 April 1999; UKZNA C10/12/14-19, 'Admission policy: Faculty of Health Sciences', UN Council minutes, 22 June 2001.
17. Breier with Wildschut, *Doctors in a Divided Society*, 30. Also see Mignonne Breier and Angelique Wildschut, 'Changing gender profile of medical schools in South Africa', *South African Medical Journal* 98, no. 7 (July 2008), 557.

18. Sphumelele Mngoma, 'Education: Medical graduates from UKZN are mostly women', *Witness* (13 December) 2008.
19. Interview with S.B. Pitsoe, Durban, 17 July 2003.
20. Mignonne Breier and Angelique Wildschut, 'Changing gender profile of medical schools in South Africa', 557, 560; and Breier with Wildschut, *Doctors in a Divided Society*, 30.
21. See, for example, UCT M&A, 'Saunders sets up commission to investigate sexual harassment at UCT', *Varsity* 49, no. 3 (27 March 1990); L.R. Naidoo and D.R. Rajab, 'A survey of sexual harassment and related issues among students at the University of Natal Durban Campus' (Durban: UN Student Counselling Centre, December 1992); Wits CRO, 'Stamp out sexual harassment', *Wits Student* 45, no. 1 (February 1993), 3; and MA, 'What do you mean by sexual harassment?' *Student Voice* 4, no. 5 (June 1992), 3, 6.
22. Interview with May Mashego, Ashburton, 18 October 2003.
23. See UKZN EGML 'Forty years of excellence', *NU Focus* 2, no. 2 (Autumn 1991); UKZNA MF3/1/1-8, 'Extra room for new doctors', *MedNews: Faculty of Medicine Newsletter* (January–February 1998); and UKZN EGML Kathy Waddington, 'Redressing imbalances: Selection in search of caring doctors', *NU Focus* 11, no. 2 (2000).
24. Breier with Wildschut, *Doctors in a Divided Society*, 1, 22–5.
25. UKZN MSA, 'University of Natal Medical School: A centre of excellence in Africa' (UN Faculty of Medicine, 1998); Barry Kistnasamy, 'Ready to face the challenges of the twenty-first century', in Jack Moodley and Smita Maharaj, eds, *University of Natal Nelson R. Mandela School of Medicine: 50 Years of Achievement in Teaching, Service and Training* , (University of Natal Nelson R. Mandela School of Medicine: Communications Office, 2001); and UKZNA *UN Calendars*, Faculty of Medicine handbooks.
26. 'King Edward's daily nightmare', *Daily News* (25 June 1974); Isobel Shepherd Smith, 'This social disgrace: New-born babies, mothers and pregnant women are forced to sleep on the floor', *Sunday Tribune* (28 July 1985); and UKZN EGML, 'Crisis at King Edward', *NU Partners* 1, no. 2 (September 1990), 8.
27. UKZN EGML 'New hospital gets go-ahead', *NU Info* 3, no. 3 (15 April – 14 May 1993). Also see UKZN MSA, 'R620m city hospital project under way', *Daily News* (22 September 1993).
28. UKZNA C10/9/3 UN Council minutes, 30 June 1989.
29. UWC MAC Natal, 1988, Vasantha Angamuthu, 'Era ends as residence closes', *City Press* (28 August 1988). Also see *Students in the Barracks: Memories of Alan Taylor Residence* (University of Natal, Durban: Audio-Visual Alternatives, 1989); and UKZN Board of the Faculty of Medicine minutes, 12 May 2000.
30. UKZNA C10/9/2, UN Council minutes, 15 August 1986 and 21 November 1986; UKZNA Senate minutes, 28 September 1988; and UKZN EGML Pat Duminy, 'A day in the life: Medical student', *NU Focus* 2, no. 4 (Spring 1991).
31. UKZNA C10/9/3, UN Council minutes, 30 June 1989, and C10/10/7-15, UN Council minutes, 8 March 1990.

32. UKZNA XS 10/1/1-2, 'Plans for R2 500 000 medical residence at university on cards', *Natal Mercury* (6 March 1980); UKZNA C10/8/1, UN Council minutes, 16 April 1981 and 15 May 1981; UKZN Board of the Faculty of Medicine minutes, 9 August 1982, 14 March 1983, 21 March 1983, 9 May 1983, 8 August 1983 and 13 August 1984.

33. For more on these obstructions, see UKZNA C10/8/1, UN Council minutes, 20 November 1981; C10/8/2, UN Council minutes, 17 June 1983, 19 August 1983, 16 September 1983; C10/9/2, UN Council minutes, 21 November 1986, 20 February 1987; C10/10/1-6, UN Council minutes, 29 June 1990; C10/10/7-15; UN Council minutes, 25 October 1991; C10/11/1-17, UN Council minutes, 29 November 1993; UKZN Board of the Faculty of Medicine minutes, 13 August 1984, 11 April 1986, 30 March 1990, 30 July 1990, 19 March 1991, 18 September 1991, 19 September 1994, 2 May 1995, 24 July 1995.

34. UKZNA C10/10/1-6, UN Council minutes, 24 August 1990, 26 October 1990 and 14 December 1990.

35. UKZNA MF3/1/1-8, 'R600 million new Durban academic hospital gets green light', *MedNews: Faculty of Medicine Newsletter* (January–February 1996); UKZN EGML 'Academic hospital approved', *NU Info* 6, no. 2 (March 1996); and UKZN MSA, 'The new Cato Manor hospital', in *University of Natal Medical School: A Centre of Excellence in Africa* (UN Faculty of Medicine, 1998).

36. 'A first for health care', *Financial Mail*, 22 November 2002; and 'Inkosi Albert Luthuli Central Hospital' Special Feature, *Sunday Tribune* (17 December 2000), 25-8.

37. UKZN Board of the Faculty of Medicine minutes, 18 September 1995, 16 September 1996, and Minutes of a Joint Meeting of the Durban Academic Affairs Board and the Durban Executive Committee held on 25 November 1996.

38. See, for example, UKZN EGML 'New look for med school', *NU Info* 2, no. 1 (15 February – 14 March 1992); UKZN Board of the Faculty of Medicine minutes, 1 February 1993, 10 May 1993 and 20 September 1993; 'Medical school improvements', *Daily News* (6 October 1993); Minutes of a Joint Meeting of the Durban Academic Affairs Board and the Durban Executive Committee held on 25 November 1996 (Annexure 1 attached to the UKZN Board of the Faculty of Medicine minutes, 27 June 1997) and UKZNA C10/11/18-26, UN Council minutes, 6 December 1996.

39. See, for example, UKZNA MF3/1/1-8, Patrick Leeman, 'From humble beginnings to an institution of excellence', in *MedNews: Faculty of Medicine Newsletter*, (January–May 2000), 3; 'R40 Mln research facility opened at Durban Medical School', *Natal Witness* (20 July 2003); Lunga Memela, 'Groundbreaking ceremony of major tuberculosis and HIV research institute', *Mercury* (26 July 2011); and Leanne Jansen, 'R346m TB, HIV Research Centre', *Mercury* (10 October 2012), http://www.iol.co.za/mercury/r346m-tb-hiv-research-centre-1.1400411.

40. Chris Bateman, 'Can KwaZulu-Natal hospitals cope with the HIV/AIDS human tide?' *South African Medical Journal* 91, no. 5 (May 2001), 364; and Chris Bateman,

'Doctors overwhelmed at the AIDS coalface', *South African Medical Journal* 92, no. 6 (June 2002), 402.

41. Interview with Y.K. Seedat, Durban, 14 July 2003.

42. Interview with Bandile Hadebe, Durban, 7 June 2004. Also see Ronald Bayer and Gerald M. Oppenheimer, *AIDS Doctors: Voices from the Epidemic* (Oxford and New York: Oxford University Press, 2000); and Gerald M. Oppenheimer and Ronald Bayer, *Shattered Dreams? An Oral History of the South African AIDS Epidemic* (Oxford and New York: Oxford University Press, 2007).

43. 'KZN to roll out ARV treatment' (5 April 2004) www.polity.org.za/article/kzn-to-roll-out-arv-treatment-2004-04-05. For more on the history of the Treatment Action Campaign, the South African activist organisation formed in 1998 that eventually forced the South African government to start providing free antiretroviral drugs at public hospitals during the latter 2000s, see Mandisa Mbali, 'AIDS discourses and the South African state: Government denialism and post-apartheid AIDS policy-making', *Transformation* 54 (2004); and Mark Hunter, *Love in the Time of AIDS* (Pietermaritzburg: University of KwaZulu-Natal Press, 2010).

44. Interview with Jerry Coovadia, Durban, 27 June 2003.

45. Interview with Ali Modiba, Durban, 7 June 2004.

46. Interview with Ntuthuko Mahlaba, Durban, 7 June 2004.

47. Dasarath Chetty and Smita Maharaj, eds, *Doris Duke Medical Research Institute Brochure* (University of KwaZulu-Natal: Public Affairs and Corporate Communications, 2007).

48. Bateman, 'Can KwaZulu-Natal hospitals cope with the HIV/AIDS human tide?', 364; Interview with KM, Durban, 14 November 2003.

49. Interview with Veronica Wilson, Durban, 6 November 2003.

50. Ncayiyana, 'Medical education challenges in South Africa'. Also see Champak Jinabhai, 'High costs of poverty', *NU Focus* (Autumn 1994).

51. 'Bleak picture from the ministry of ill health', *Mail and Guardian* (3 March 1995); David Whittaker, 'Combating the disease', *Mail and Guardian* (20 October 1995); Ayanda Ntsaluba, 'The national health system: The way forward for health care in SA', *South African Medical Journal* 1 (1997), 18–19; Ann Eveleth, 'Cash is the only cure for ailing hospitals', *Mail and Guardian* (6 February 1998); Breier with Wildschut, *Doctors in a Divided Society*, 9 and chapter 2; Rural Doctors' Association of Southern Africa, Position Paper, 'Crisis in staffing of rural hospitals: South African Medical Association 2001', http://www.rudasa.org.za/download/crisis-staffing.doc; S.J. Reid, 'Crisis in rural South Africa', *South African Family Practitioners* 23 (2001), 17–8.

52. UKZN EGML Kathy Waddington, 'Doctors for Africa', *NU Focus* 11, no. 1 (2000).

53. UKZN EGML Hoosen Coovadia, 'Focus on primary health care: Crucial to resolve', *NU Focus* 2, no. 2 (Autumn 1991); Jim Day, 'Zuma's remarkable road to recovery', *Mail and Guardian* (23 May 1997); and UKZN EGML C.C. 'Noddy' Jinabhai, 'Medical school: The other struggle', *NU Focus* 11, no. 2 (2000).

54. Ncayiyana, 'Medical education challenges in South Africa'.

55. S.J. Reid, 'Compulsory community service for doctors in South Africa – An evaluation of the first year', *South African Medical Journal* 91 (2001), 329–36; UKZN EGML Greg Arde, 'Community service: The good and the bad', *NU Focus* 11, no. 2 (2000).

56. Breier with Wildschut, *Doctors in a Divided Society*, 22, 33–4, 98.

57. See, for example, UKZN EGML Derek Arbuckle, 'Looking ahead', *NU Focus* 2, no. 2 (Autumn 1991); UKZN Board of the Faculty of Medicine minutes, 26 July 1993, 'Strategic planning workshop: Undergraduate curriculum review'; UKZN EGML Champak Jinabhai, 'High costs of poverty', and Jerry Coovadia, 'Forsaking the revolution', both in *NU Focus* (Autumn 1994); and Stephen Reid, 'COPC experiences with medical students at the Valley Trust, South Africa', *COPaCetic* 5, no. 1 (Summer/Fall 1998).

58. UKZNA MF3/1/1-8, 'The coming together of Curriculum 2001', *MedNews: Faculty of Medicine Newsletter* (June–December 2001).

59. UKZN Board of the Faculty of Medicine minutes, 26 July 1993, 'Strategic planning workshop: Undergraduate curriculum review, Annexure 6: Educational philosophy underlying the medical curriculum'; Michelle McLean, 'Student perceptions of their first and second year experiences of medical studies at the University of Natal' (Masters in Education in the School of Education, University of Natal, 1999), 9, 11–3; UKZN EGML 'New dean at medical school', *NU Focus* 11, no. 2 (2000); and 'New approaches to learning', *University of Natal Nelson R. Mandela School of Medicine: 50 Years of Achievement in Teaching, Service and Training*.

60. UKZNA MF3/1/1-8, 'New deputy dean rises to the challenges of Curriculum 2001', *Mednews: Faculty of Medicine Newsletter* (January–May 2001).

61. UKZN Board of the Faculty of Medicine minutes, 8 July 2002, Appendix B: UN Faculty of Health Sciences, Nelson R. Mandela School of Medicine, School of Undergraduate Education Draft Constitution.

62. See, for example, UKZNA MF3/1/1-8, 'Ayurveda – The Science of Life', *Mednews: Faculty of Medicine Newsletter* (January-May 2001); 'The TCAM programme for traditional, complementary and alternative medicines', 'New plan to explore African traditional medicine', 'Medical school signs understanding with Chinese institution' and 'Academic programmes of the Ayurvedic initiative', all in *Mednews: Faculty of Medicine Newsletter* 3, no. 1 (January–December 2002); and Slindile Maluleka, 'Traditional healers and medical school fight HIV', *Daily News* (1 September 2009).

63. UKZNA MF3/1/1-8, 'Taking medicine to the people', *Mednews: Faculty of Medicine Newsletter* 3, no. 1 (January–December 2002).

64. UKZNA MF3/1/1-8, 'New deputy dean rises to the challenges of Curriculum 2001', *Mednews: Faculty of Medicine Newsletter* (January–May 2001); and UKZN MSRC, Minutes of University Committees Executive Comm 02, Additional Documentation/Item for a Meeting of the Executive Committee Scheduled for 28 July 1997, see attached: 'University of Natal Medical School Submission to the Truth and Reconciliation Commission', 23 June 1997.

65. 'New approaches to learning', *University of Natal Nelson R. Mandela School of Medicine: 50 Years of Achievement in Teaching, Service and Training.*

66. UKZNA MF3/1/1-8, 'Several major initiatives realised: The dean, Professor Barry Kistnasamy, reports on the faculty's major developments', *Mednews: Faculty of Medicine Newsletter* (January–May 2001).

67. See Breier with Wildschut, *Doctors in a Divided Society*, 19, 23, 33–4, 38, 98. For more on the reasons for the shift to two years of internship training, see Chris Bateman, 'Two-year internship a near certainty', *South African Medical Journal* 92, no. 5 (May 2002), 328; and Yvette Meintjes, 'The two-year internship training', *South African Medical Journal* 93, no. 5 (May 2003), 336–7.

68. Interview with Dennis J. Pudifin, Durban, 2 July 2003. Similar views were expressed in Interviews with Mfanyana J. Ndlovu, Durban, 14 August 2003, and Breminand Maharaj, Durban, 10 June 2003.

69. For more on this subject, see 'Training doctors who will stay in SA "is a dilemma"', *Business Day* (22 July 2008); 'Alarming lack of doctors', *Star* (8 July 2008); 'Salvaging the health system: Brain drain', *Citizen* (7 November 2008); Breier with Wildschut, *Doctors in a Divided Society*, 18.

70. N. Hlangani, 'Brain Drain: Health systems on life support', *Star* (22 October 2002).

71. In 1995, Durban's medical faculty received about 1 500 applications for 120 places available, while in 2007, it received more than 3 500 applications for roughly 210 places. See UKZN EGML, 'Med school to admit whites', *NU Info* 4, no. 11 (19 November 1994 – 14 February 1995); W.E.B. Edge, 'Student selection skewed', *Daily News* (15 March 2001); and Mbulelo Baloyi, 'Prof defends medical school entry system', *Independent on Saturday* (3 February 2007).

72. UKZNA C10/11/1-17, UN Council minutes, 17 February 1995; and C10/12/1–6 UN Council minutes, 30 April 1999.

73. See, for example, UKZN MSA, 'Matriculants threaten to sue medical school', *Daily News* (10 February 1995); UKZN EGML 'No entry for Ms Reddy: Racial quotas are operating at Natal University Medical School', *NU Focus* 14 (May 1999); Ishani Bechoo, 'Med school row goes on', *Daily News* (12 March 2001); 'Medical school criteria racially discriminating', *Daily News* (12 December 2001); and Barbara Cole, '"Not black enough" for medical school', *Daily News* (5 February 2004).

74. Interview with B.T. Naidoo, Durban, 10 November 2003.

75. Interview with Dennis J. Pudifin, Durban, 2 July 2003.

76. Interview with May Mashego, Durban, 7 October 2003. Similar perspectives were also raised in Interviews with Y.K. Seedat, Durban, 7 July 2003, and Steve Reid, Durban, 10 June 2003.

77. Interview with K.P. Naidoo, Durban, 4 June 2004.

78. Interview with Ntuthuko Mahlaba, Durban, 7 June 2004.

79. Ali Modiba, 'MSRC Racism Report presented to the faculty and students of the University of Natal, Nelson R. Mandela School of Medicine', 26 September 2004. Similar perspectives were raised in Interviews with KM, Durban, 14 November 2003; S.B. Pitsoe, Durban, 17 July 2003; and TM, Pretoria, 21 August 2003.

80. UKZN EGML 'Night of the Biko Affair: Criticising the medical school', *NU Focus* 11, no. 2 (2000); and UKZNA C10/12/713, 'Medical school fiftieth-year anniversary celebrations', UN Council minutes, 18 August 2000.

81. See *University of Natal, Nelson R. Mandela School of Medicine, Fiftieth Anniversary Banquet* (University of Natal, Durban: Audio-Visual Centre, 29 July 2000).

82. Interview with TM, Pretoria, 21 August 2003.

83. Interviews with TM, Pretoria, 21 August 2003; S.B. Pitsoe, Durban, 17 July 2003; and KM, Durban, 14 November 2003; and Mtutuzeli Nyoka, 'Day of shame for NU medical school: Selfishness has sullied the glorious history of a fabled institution', *Mercury* (11 August 2000).

84. See UKZNA *UN Calendars*, Faculty of Medicine handbooks.

85. Interview with Maila J. Matjila, Durban, 22 September 2003. Also see UKZN Board of the Faculty of Medicine minutes, 22 November 1996, 'Annexure 1: Response to recent protest action by nurses at KEH', and 28 November 1996, 'Special business: The recent demonstrations and subsequent events'; and Modiba, 'MSRC Racism Report', 26 September 2004.

86. Interview with Ntuthuko Mahlaba, Durban, 7 June 2004; and Interview with MM, Durban, 28 July 2003.

87. See Brenda Gourley, 'A symbolic platform', *University of Natal Nelson R. Mandela School of Medicine: 50 Years of Achievement in Teaching, Service and Training;* Interviews with M.B. Kistnasamy, Durban, 26 August 2003, and Maila J. Matjila, Durban, 22 September 2003.

88. 'Indo-African race row at South African university', *webindia123.com* (16 October 2005), http://h-net.msu.edu/cgi-bin/logbrowse.pl?trx=vx&list=h-sa-highereducation & month=0510&week=c&msg=YFCqlWqdLQOtL3Fqx6Rw9A&user=&pw=.

89. De Wet Potgieter, 'Talk of racism and hidden agendas', *The New Age* (6 March 2012), http://www.thenewage.co.za/mobi/Detail.aspx?NewsID=52580&CatID=1010.

90. Noloyiso Mchunu, 'Medical school row widens', *Witness* (8 October 2005), http://ccrri.ukzn.ac.za/archive/archive/files/pra20051008047057_ff87e3cf66.pdf; Angela Bolowana, 'Ex-students back racism report', *Mercury* (10 October 2005), http://ccrri.ukzn.ac.za/archive/archive/files/pra20051006047057_2ba7a66fe4.pdf; 'Suspension of lecturers welcomed', *Daily News* (17 October 2005), http://h-net.msu.edu/cgi-bin/logbrowse.pl?trx=vx&list=h-sa-higher-education&month=0510&week=c&msg=YFCqlWqdLQOtL3Fqx6Rw9A&user=&pw=; 'Indo-African race row at South African university', *webindia123.com* (16 October 2005); Santosh Beharie, 'UKZN Medical School hearings open in a veil of secrecy', *Sunday Tribune* (11 December 2005); Reena Budree and Pitika Ntuli, 'UKZN report change strategy workshops, Nelson R. Mandela School of Medicine', 12 April 2006; and 'Medical school students dissatisfied', *Daily News* (10 October 2006).

91. 'Top doc in legal battle', *Post*, (8 August 2007), http://www.highbeam.com/doc/1G1-167380171.html; and 'Academic goes to court over racism allegations', *Legalbrief* (13 August 2007), http://www.legalbrief.co.za/article.php?story=20070813080503581.

92. Potgieter, 'Talk of racism and hidden agendas', *The New Age* (6 March 2012). Also see De Wet Potgieter, 'University of dirty tricks', *The New Age* (6 January 2012), http://www.thenewage.co.za/52428-1007-53-University_of_dirty_tricks; and 'UKZN respond to rumble', *Post* (11 June 2008), http://lists.fahamu.org/pipermail/debate-list/2008-June/014169.html.

93. According to Potgieter, 'Talk of racism and hidden agendas', *The New Age* (6 March 2012), Kistnasamy is employed as the executive director of the National Institute for Occupational Health and National Cancer Registry based in Johannesburg. He was appointed to this position in 2009.

94. Potgieter, 'Talk of racism and hidden agendas', *The New Age* (6 March 2012).

95. Trish Beaver and Stephen Coan, 'Two UKZN professors suspended', *Witness* (26 April 2012), http://www.witness.co.za/index.php?showcontent&global%5B_id%5D=80257.

96. Stephen Coan, 'Doctors seek probe into UKZN', *Weekend Witness* (2 June 2012), http://www.witness.co.za/index.php?showcontent&global%5B_id%5D=82052.

97. Potgieter, 'University of dirty tricks', *The New Age* (6 January 2012).

98. 'Durban doctors take on professor over "racism"', *Daily News* (18 April 2012), http://www.iol.co.za/dailynews/news/durban-doctors-take-on-professor-over-racism-1.1278724.

99. Beaver and Coan, 'Two UKZN professors suspended', *Witness* (26 April 2012); and Laea Medley, 'Top UKZN academics suspended from posts', *Daily News* (27 April 2012), http://www.iol.co.za/dailynews/news/top-ukzn-academics-suspended-from-posts-1.1285369.

100. Taschica Pillay, 'Outcome of UKZN boss hearing due', *Sunday Times* (10 June 2012), http://www.timeslive.co.za/sundaytimes/2012/06/10/outcome-of-ukzn-boss-hearing-due.

101. Pillay, 'Outcome of UKZN boss hearing due', *Sunday Times* (10 June 2012). This Concerned Citizens Group of UKZN is made up of a coalition of UKZN academics, doctors and lawyers.

Reflections

This book has considered the complicated history of the production of black doctors in apartheid South Africa, the majority of whom received their training at the University of Natal Medical School. The school was established in 1951 after many decades of heated discussions, negotiations and failed earlier attempts by a variety of people to establish medical-training schemes for black students. For many years after 1959, when the Wits and UCT medical schools were forced to close their doors to black students (unless ministerial permission was received), and until MEDUNSA was opened for African students in 1978, Durban's medical school was the only place dedicated to the task of providing a full biomedical training for black doctors in South Africa. By the end of the apartheid period in 1994, the school had trained the largest number of black doctors in the country, most of whom would go on to provide much-needed professional medical services for their patients. In addition, the school had a profile beyond the national level. In fact, by the 1950s, it was one of only a handful of medical schools available to train black students as fully qualified medical practitioners in the whole of sub-Saharan Africa.

However, this book has also shown that the training of black doctors in South Africa has a history full of complex and often hurtful twists and turns. The history of Durban's medical school was closely interwoven with that of the apartheid state, which provided the school with the financial subsidies needed for its building and operation costs. With reliance on state funding, it was inevitable that apartheid policies would influence its operations in pivotal ways. From the outset, it was created as a black faculty separate from the University of Natal's main campus. The aim was to keep the university's black medical students strictly segregated from their white colleagues. Even the location of the medical campus, a few kilometres away from the main Howard College campus – which in itself was located on prime land on top of the Berea Ridge in Durban – flagged the school's status as different or 'other'. During the early 1950s, as construction of the new buildings progressed, this new school was celebrated by the state as an important showpiece of apartheid. It was an exciting moment for the Afrikaner-led Nationalist state. During these early years, the school was a good fit with the state's plans to create separate education facilities for black and white medical students, who, once they graduated, would go on to practise amongst their own communities in racially segregated health-care services.

On the other hand, the anomalous set-up of the medical school as a black faculty within the white University of Natal produced enormous contradictions and ambiguities, sometimes in line with, but at other times in opposition to, the state's desired policies and goals. This was evident in a number of ways. Despite being funded by an increasingly powerful apartheid state and developing in a racially segregated city in the 1950s, the school managed to attract a number of excellent academics as teachers and lecturers, some of whom were particularly forward-thinking and socially conscious for their time, and who worked to reorient the way modern medicine delivered health care to impoverished rural and urban communities. The 1950s, the school's more flexible 'teething years', gave some of these individuals, such as Sidney Kark and his team, the opportunity to pioneer an experimental teaching approach that was more humanistic in focus, and encouraged its students to consider prevention and health-promotion issues, not just curative approaches, to improve health-care services for the majority of black South Africans. Inviting their students to question the broader socio-economic structural inequalities producing ill health, Kark and his team also helped them examine health issues in community spaces beyond the walls of their teaching hospital.

Even though this educational experiment was short-lived, and was ultimately quashed in the early 1960s by the state and the conservative white medical profession for being too progressive for its time, it provides a telling commentary on the ironies of South Africa's history during the early apartheid period. It highlights how an innovative medical educational experiment could still be pioneered by progressive medical thinkers who were attracted to working with black medical students in Durban, and who exploited any gaps they could find to introduce innovative changes at a time of growing political conservatism and racial polarisation. This was not the last time academics in Durban worked to push the limits of, or challenge, apartheid policies. In fact, on at least two other occasions, not only individuals, but the school's whole academic staff, came out in strong, vocal opposition to the government's policies, such as its desire in 1957 to remove the medical school from the University of Natal, as well as its 1975–6 attempts to phase out black students from this school to coincide with the opening of MEDUNSA. From the late 1950s, the tertiary education sphere became a site of keen interest to the state, and with constant intervention the state worked to implement stricter racial segregation at the university level, which produced active responses from the academic staff.

Yet, while staff members played a significant role in opposing apartheid policies at particular moments over the years, from the late 1960s onwards it was really the school's students who were a thorn in the side of the apartheid state. In unexpected ways, the more liberal conditions at the Durban Medical School helped bring together students from culturally diverse backgrounds to live and study together, creating opportunities for interracial socialisation not available elsewhere in South Africa. On a black campus where the SRC and other student organisations were allowed to function, it provided opportunities for activist students to discuss, to organise and to mobilise in a highly repressive apartheid society. Involvement of many students in the formation and operation of the South African Students' Organisation, a black consciousness organisation at the school's Alan Taylor Residence in the late 1960s, and later in UDF and ANC activities, provided a broad political education that helped to conscientise its students and encouraged many to stand up in opposition to their apartheid oppressors. Led by charismatic student leaders such as Steve Biko, Mamphela Ramphele, Nkosazana Dlamini Zuma, Diliza Mji and Zweli Mkhize, the medical school's students in the 1970s and 1980s developed a strong anti-apartheid mindset and many engaged in both above-board and underground political activities. In opposition to the state's desired aims, this school thus became a fertile breeding ground for widespread anti-apartheid sentiment and action that helped reignite a defiant anti-apartheid nationalist politics that eventually contributed to the collapse of the apartheid state in the early 1990s.

Multifarious struggles

Looking back over the twentieth century, it is clear that segregated medical education developed as a result of many struggles by numerous people. This book traces the efforts over many decades of a handful of leading lights, especially medical missionaries, but also other medical pioneers, to win support within South Africa for the idea of providing a full biomedical education for black students. Various individuals struggled to raise funds to build, people and then run such an institution, as well as develop high-quality and innovative teaching approaches once the school was opened. For many of these pioneers, the goal was to ensure that its graduates were just as good as those trained at other white medical schools, even if this meant producing many failures, not to mention forcing students to deal with blatantly Eurocentric attitudes. However, while starting out with lofty intentions, compromises often had to be made by these managers and teachers along the way to ensure the school's survival.

Prospective students seeking enrolment at the medical school encountered many trying obstacles – financial, racial and those created by gender attitudes prevalent at the time. The odds were stacked heavily against them. And, for those lucky few who actually made it into the medical school each year, they soon realised that their hardships were set to continue. In addition to the very heavy workloads they had to contend with, the school's irregular formation as a black faculty within a white university forced its students to suffer many hurtful and humiliating racial inequalities and discriminations in their training and residential arrangements. For some, engagement in anti-apartheid struggle politics was a logical outcome, although this brought challenges serious enough to warrant constant surveillance and frequent police interventions.

The Durban Medical School's black students, though few in number and elite in their educational opportunities compared to other black South Africans of their time, are worth studying both for what they achieved during apartheid and what they have achieved since. For a few, hardships and struggle brought them to the highest political positions imaginable in the last decade of the twentieth century and some have gone on to play prominent roles in post-apartheid South Africa. Though small in overall number, some of these students went on to have impressive and influential careers in the country's various state formations, such as national and provincial governments, the tertiary education sector and state research bodies, and in key academic posts and organs of civil society. The collective political significance of these black doctors as a group in the longer term should not be overlooked.

Of course, it would be incorrect to assume that Durban Medical School students stood up every time in common unity in their struggle against apartheid adversity. While this book has tried to unpack a little-understood context underlying an essential site in the fight against apartheid, it has also developed views against the grain of a triumphant and romanticised, post-apartheid, national memory of the liberation struggle. It shows that during the apartheid years, as well as extending into the post-apartheid period, there were numerous struggles within both the student and staff bodies. While the training of doctors in Durban produced at certain key moments commonalities and political unity amongst African, Indian and coloured students who stood together in opposition to protest particular apartheid issues, it also ensured the production of deep divisions and tensions that muddied relationships over the years. This book has taken the reader into the fraught arena of student life, of the difficult and never-settled race, class and gender divisions among students, and the challenges of educational success in the context of extreme discrimination, unequal resources, segregated professions and uncertain futures.

The choices for those few black students entering the medical profession via Durban's medical school were complicated and diverse. For some, the hardships they endured produced a strong determination to focus on their studies and to pass their difficult medical courses. Although far from ideal, the medical school offered them the rare opportunity to improve their life chances and to attain elite status, respect, professional accolades and financial advantage once they graduated, particularly for those who entered private practice. While for some students, politics was on the periphery of their vision, for others, hardships were a powerful conscientising and mobilising force. Student doctors faced the challenges of an elite profession that grew out of an inferior social position in apartheid South Africa. Given the opportunity to overcome the barriers of class and achieve professional advancement, if they chose to work in South Africa, their careers were limited by the constraints of practising amongst 'their own communities' once they graduated. In this situation, the inequalities of race always trumped class advances, ensuring a subordinate position for black doctors in apartheid South Africa. Some could not accept this situation quietly. Instead they involved themselves in political struggles to try to address their grievances and to support their oppressed communities in a fight for something bigger. For these activist students, medicine and politics were not separate issues, and the Durban Medical School provided both a medical and political education for them.

Thus, while most black medical students saw themselves as future leaders of their communities, their choices became increasingly segmented. The first involved accepting the status quo and taking advantage of class opportunities created for elites in the separate-development structures of apartheid, as well as helping disadvantaged and impoverished black communities by graduating and working as doctors. The second entailed fighting to overthrow the larger apartheid system that oppressed them. Some students' lives were completely altered by their activism, resulting in their studies at times taking a back seat. This included the possibility of derailment of their professional careers, compounding an already acute shortage of doctors. Sometimes their choices shifted as the years progressed, as their work and family circumstances changed, but mostly as a result of changes in the wider political context. Whatever the circumstances, the difficulty of reconciling the interests of the group or collective and the private interests of the individual would have weighed heavily on the minds of these black medical students and doctors in apartheid South Africa.

In a similar approach to that advocated by Jacob Dlamini in his book *Native Nostalgia*, this book has considered the diverse stories of the people who studied and worked at Durban's medical school. It has tried to show that not everyone experienced their time at the medical school in the same manner, nor did they suffer or struggle against adversities in the same way. As Dlamini argued eloquently in his book, there were 'shades of grey, zones of ambiguity that individuals traversed daily as they went about their lives' and these 'were not experienced the same way'.[1] Furthermore, during the apartheid years, medical students' experiences in Durban were not all rosy and were certainly complicated by many things, despite being presented in recent years through a rosy lens that stressed a collective and unified entity in line with the harmonious nation-building narratives of those in government. A simple focus on the celebratory and heroic memories about this school, which dovetail well with the democratic government's triumphant struggle narratives of redemption and overcoming, hides the rich complexity of this school's messy history.

Taking seriously all sides of the complexity of this school's development during the apartheid years, not just the publicly celebrated accounts, is essential to understand more fully this school's fascinating history. This book is a celebration – not of an undifferentiated or indistinguishable group of medical heroes – but of the messiness of medical school life in Durban. It has focused on both the triumphs and tribulations, but also on the ambiguities, tensions and inconsistencies of those who helped build and run, teach at and study at this institution.

Over nearly half a century, segregated medical education in Durban developed as a site of great struggle against apartheid and a setting of deep contradictions. The provision of medical education in South Africa was always political in nature. During the 1950s to the early 1990s, this institution reproduced apartheid conditions, but at times its staff, and more importantly its students, also unlocked the essential failure of apartheid ideologies in their vociferous protest activities. This school thus fulfilled some of the objectives of policies of separate development, but also contributed to the apartheid state's eventual demise. Furthermore, a focus on the messiness of history sheds light on the construction of a racially divided medical profession in the country that has deep roots, and on the existence of a health-care system seriously compromised by decades of racial discrimination, whose unequal effects still haunt South Africa's post-apartheid health-care system today.

Note

1. Jacob Dlamini, *Native Nostalgia* (Auckland Park: Jacana, 2009), 30.

Appendices

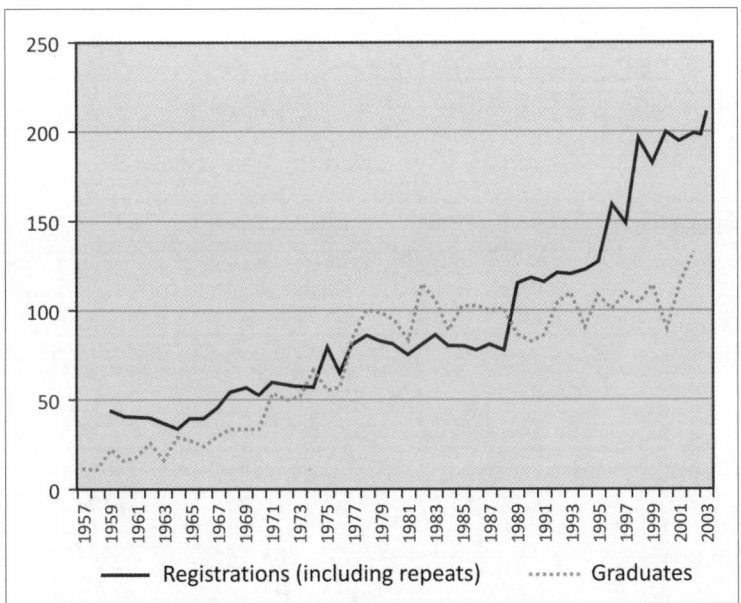

Appendix 1   Faculty of Medicine annual registrations (including repeats) and graduates. (*DMS Administration office*)

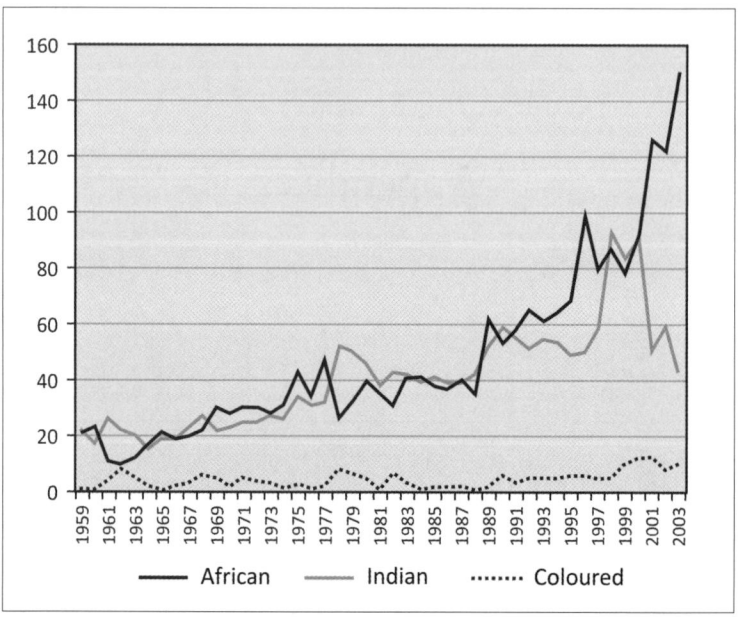

Appendix 2 First-year registrations (including repeats) by race. (*DMS Administration office*)

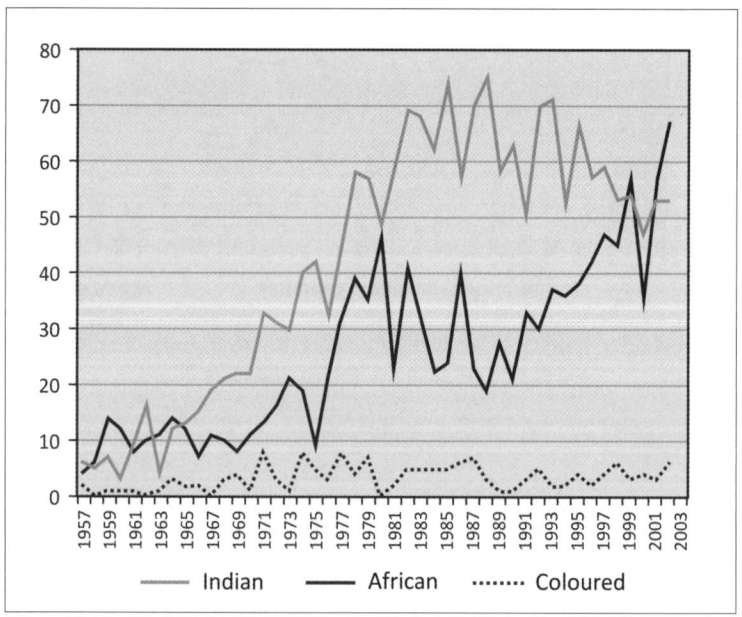

Appendix 3 Faculty of Medicine gratuates by race. (*DMS Administration office*)

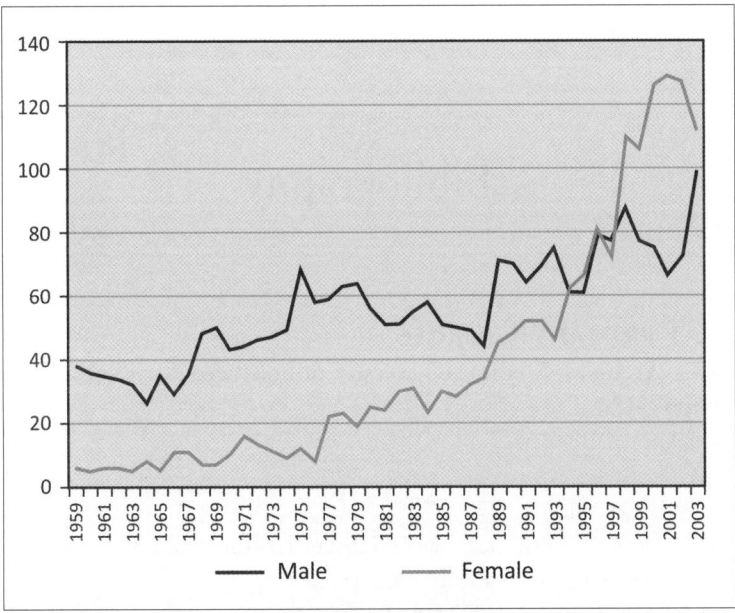

Appendix 4   Faculty of Medicine first-year registrations (including repeats) by gender. (*DMS Administration office*)

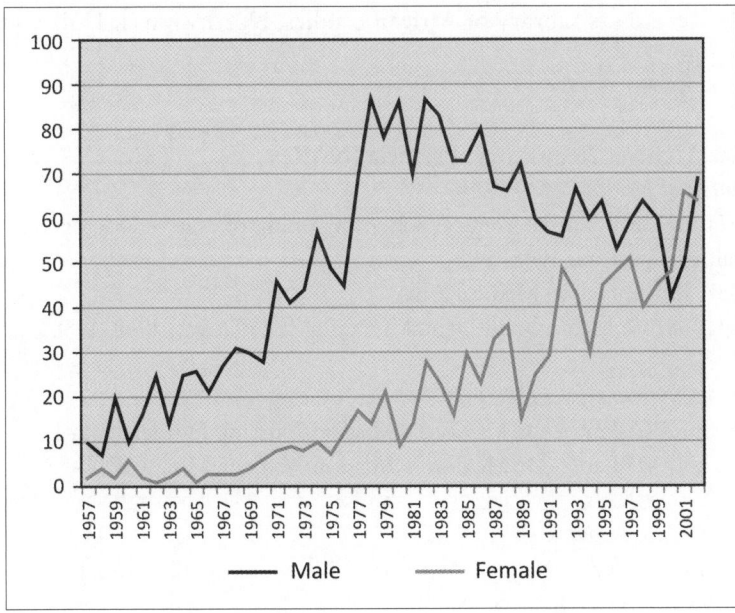

Appendix 5   Faculty of Medicine graduates by gender. (*DMS Administration office*)

Bibliography

ARCHIVAL PRIMARY SOURCES
MEDUNSA Archives, Medical University of Southern Africa, Garankuwa, Limpopo (MA)
Principal – Annual Reports.
MEDUNSA Brief.
MEDUNSA Yearbook.
MEDUNSA General. Periodicals with Substantial Information.
MEDUNSA General. Various Publications and Documents.
MEDUNSA Press Cuttings, 1977–1982.
Student Voice.

Melville Herskovits Library of African Studies, Northwestern University, Chicago
EAA8618, SASO.

National Archives Repository, Pretoria (NAR)
Department of Health (1900–1973)
GES 2271, 61/38B, Native Medical School Training of Native Doctors and Health Inspectors, 1933–39.
GES 2957, PN 5, Native Medical Aids.
GES 1831, 68/30, Medical and Dental Training for Natives, 1948–1958.

Secretary of Native Affairs (1880–1975)
NTS 2862, 7/303 Part 4 Dr McCord's Mission Nursing Home, 1942–45.
NTS 2862, 7/303 Part 5 Dr McCord's Mission Nursing Home 1944–49.

Secretary of Union Education (1911–68)
UOD 1546 U3/40/4, Natal University College for Establishment of Medical Schools for Natives, 1945–48.
UOD 56 U3/26/4/5, University of Natal Building Grants and Loans for Medical School Non-Europeans Durban 1949–53.

K87 Non-European Medical Schools, 1949.
K97 University Facilities for Non-Europeans, 1949.
K186 Non-European Medical Schools, 1965.
K296 E5/49 Medical Training, 1968–9. Komitee van Ondersoek oor Mediese Opleiding.

University of Cape Town, Cape Town (UCT)
Administrative Archives (AA):
Med/7 Medicine: General, 1953–8.
F2/1 Non Europeans, Vol. II.

Manuscripts and Archives (M&A):
Varsity.
UCT News.
The Pulse.

University of Fort Hare, Eastern Cape (UFH)
Centre for Cultural Studies, AZAPO/BCM Records.

University of KwaZulu-Natal (UKZN)
Nelson R. Mandela School of Medicine, Durban
Administration Office:
Board of the Faculty of Medicine Minutes, 1950s–2000s.

Medical School Archives (MSA):
Admissions information.
Correspondence.
Minutes of meetings.
Newspaper clippings.
Publicity materials.
Students' publications.

Medical Students' Representative Council Office (MSRC)
Minute books of the MSRC, 1970s–2000s.

Special Collection: Campbell Collections, Durban (CC):
E.G. Malherbe Collection (EGM):
File 463/4/1, KCM 56990 (15) b.
File 463/5/2, KCM 56990 (59) f.
File 463/7/2, KCM 57009 (12).

File 463/7/3, KCM 56990 (88).
File 464/2, KCM 56990 (130).
File 465/3, KCM 56990 (170).
File 465/5/1, KCM 56990 (194), (202), (206).
File 465/6, KCM 56990 (215).

Gordon Papers (GP):
File 1, KCM 25662.
File 6, KCM 25708.
File 8, KCM 22571.
File 13, KCM 25735, 25748, 25771.
File 17, KCM 25826, 25841.
File 18, KCM 25863.
File 21, KCM 25878.
File 23, KCM 25915, 25927 UN Medical School Miscellaneous.

Mabel Palmer Collection (MPC):
File 35, KCM 18254.

McCord Hospital (MH):
Aldyth Lasbery Papers, Box 8, Series II, *Isibuko.*
Box 7 Series II Medical Superintendents Reports 1956 to 1962.
McCord Hospital Board Minutes
Mouldy Box Scans.
Papers of the American Board of Commissioners for Foreign Missions, ABC 15
    Letters from Missionaries to Africa, 1834–1919, Southern Africa, Zulu Mission,
    1909–1929 from the Houghton Library, Boston.
Pretoria Disk 2 Doc 65, Annual Report of the Medical Superintendent of McCord
    Hospital, 1955.

Special Collection: E.G. Malherbe Library, Durban (EGML)
College of Health Sciences Newsletter.
Concept: Convocation of the University of Natal.
Dome.
Natal University News.
NU Chronicle.
NU Focus.
NU Info.
NU Partners.
University of Natal Gazette.

Bibliography

University Archives, Pietermaritzburg (UKZNA):
BIO P 3/2/5, SP 6/12/5 Cuttings, E.G. Malherbe 3/10/76–13/5/81.
BIO-S-506/1/1 Gordon, Isidor Prof.
BIO-S 842/1/1 Zuma, Nkosazana Dlamini.
BIO-S 1054/1/1 Coovadia, Hoosen 'Jerry'.
C10/1/1 through C10/12/14-19, Council Minutes, 1950s–2000s.
C205/1/1-3, Medical School Press Cuttings and Correspondence, 1970–1979.
C205/1/3 Faculty of Medicine, Correspondence and Cuttings (1981?).
CF 8/1/1- University of Natal Hippocratic Oath Ceremony, 1975.
H6/1/1, Medical School – History.
H6/2/1 Medical School.
H6/2/2 Medical School Advisory Committee Estimates and Expenditure, 1955.
UN Calendars, Faculty of Medicine handbooks.
H6/2/3 Correspondence concerning Establishment of the Department of Family
    Practice, 1953–55.
MF3/1/1-8 *MedNews: Faculty of Medicine Newsletter.*
MQ 1/1/1-5, *The Amoeba.*
Senate Minutes, 1950s–2000s.
Students, Societies, SASO.
XS 10/1/1-2 Cuttings Medical School.

University of the Western Cape (UWC)
Mayibuye Archives Centre (MAC):
H12 Doctors 1985.
H36 NAMDA 1986–1992.
Medical Schools.
Medical Schools, 1989.
MEDUNSA, 1984.
MEDUNSA, 1985.
MEDUNSA, 1989.
NAMDA, 1987.
Natal, 1984.
Natal, 1985.
Natal, 1986.
Natal, 1988.

University of the Witwatersrand, Johannesburg (Wits)
Central Records Office (CRO):
Box No. Reg. 00550, File no. 4, S6/5, Senate: Faculty of Medicine Documents,
    1984.

Box No. Reg. 00885, File no. 3, B19/2, Blacks – Training of Black Medical and
   Dental Students. June 1944 – July 1962.
Box No. Reg. 00886, File no. 3, B19/3, Training of Black Medical and Dental
   Students, June 1944 – July 1962.
Wits Student.
570 Medical School by Department.
9847 Medicine, SMC Newsletters – *Mednews.*

Faculty of Health Sciences Registry Archives (FHSR):
M3/40 Internal Reconciliation Commission, 1998.
M12/1/17/2 Black Students – Clinical Facilities, August 1980 – August 1984.

South African History Archive (SAHA):
S. Health, AL 2457.
NAMDA – *Critical Health* Publications, 1980–1992: *Critical Health.*
NAMDA – Uncatalogued, Core Newsclippings, Health Care.
South African Political Materials 1964–1990s, The Karis-Gerhart Collection:
Part I: Interviews.
Part III: Political Documents:
NUSAS, Folders 575, 583.
SASO, Folders 748, 749, 750, 753, 755, 761, 762, 763.

GOVERNMENT PAPERS
*Report and Recommendations of the Committee of Enquiry on Possible Further Facilities
   for Medical and Dental Training – 1984* (or the 'De Villiers Committee'). Pretoria:
   Government Printer, 1984.
*Report of the Committee Appointed to Inquire into the Training of Natives in Medicine
   and Public Health* (or the 'Loram Committee Report'). Pretoria: Government
   Printer, 1928.
Report of the Committee on Medical Training in South Africa, UG 25 of 1939. Pretoria:
   Government Printer, 1939.
*Report of the National Health Services Commission on the Provision of an Organised
   National Health Service for all Sections of the People of the Union of South Africa,
   1942–4.* Pretoria: Government Printer, 1944.

MEDICAL JOURNALS
American Journal of Public Health
COPaCetic
Journal of Medical Education
Journal of the Medical Association of South Africa
Journal of the National Medical Association

Leech
Medical Education
Medical Journal of South Africa
Medical Proceedings
South African Family Practitioners
South African Medical Journal
South African Medical Record

NEWSPAPERS
Business Day
Cape Argus/Argus
Cape Times
Citizen
City Press
Daily News
Eastern Province Herald
Financial Mail
Independent on Saturday
Leader
Mail and Guardian
Natal Mercury/Mercury
Natal Witness/Witness
Post
Pretoria News
Rand Daily Mail
Sowetan
Star
Sunday Express
Sunday Times
Sunday Tribune
The New Age
Weekend World
World

PUBLISHED SOURCES
Abramson, J.H. 'Natal medical students' attitudes to the social and preventive aspects of medicine', *South African Medical Journal* 35 (25 March 1961).
Apartheid Medicine: Health and Human Rights in South Africa. Washington, DC: American Association for the Advancement of Science, 1990.
Arnold, M. (ed.) *Steve Biko: Black Consciousness in South Africa*. New York: Random House, 1978.

Badat, S. *Black Student Politics, Higher Education and Apartheid from SASO to SANSCO, 1968–90*. Pretoria: HSRC; New York and London: Routledge, 1999.

Baines, G. 'The master narrative of South Africa's liberation struggle: Remembering and forgetting June 16, 1976', *International Journal of African Historical Studies* 40, no. 2 (2007).

Baldwin-Ragaven, L., De Gruchy, J. and London, L. (eds) *An Ambulance of the Wrong Colour: Health Professionals, Human Rights and Ethics in South Africa*. Cape Town: University of Cape Town Press, 1999.

Barber, J. *South Africa in the Twentieth Century: A Political History – In Search of a Nation State*. Oxford: Blackwell, 1999.

Bateman, C. 'Can KwaZulu-Natal hospitals cope with the HIV/AIDS human tide?' *South African Medical Journal* 91, no. 5 (May 2001).

Bateman, C. 'Doctors overwhelmed at the AIDS coalface', *South African Medical Journal* 92, no. 6 (June 2002).

Bateman, C. 'Two-year internship a near certainty', *South African Medical Journal* 92, no. 5 (May 2002).

Bayer, R. and Oppenheimer, G.M. *AIDS Doctors: Voices from the Epidemic*. Oxford and New York: Oxford University Press, 2000.

Becker, H.S., Geer, B., Hughes, E.C. and Strauss, A.L. *Boys in White: Student Culture in Medical School*. Chicago and London: University of Chicago Press, 1961.

Behr, A.L. *New Perspectives in South African Education*. Durban: Butterworth, 1978.

Beinart, W. *Twentieth-Century South Africa*. Oxford and New York: Oxford University Press, 1994.

Beinart, W. and Dubow, S. (eds) *Segregation and Apartheid in Twentieth-Century South Africa*. London and New York: Routledge, 1995.

Bhana, S. 'University Education'. In *South Africa's Indians: The Evolution of a Minority*, edited by B. Pachai. Washington, DC: University Press of America, 1979.

Biko, S. *I Write What I Like*. New York: HarperSanFrancisco, 1986.

Bonnin, D., Hamilton, G., Morrell, R. and Sitas, A. 'The struggle for Natal and KwaZulu: Workers, township dwellers and Inkatha, 1972–85'. In *Political Economy and Identities in KwaZulu-Natal: Historical and Social Perspectives*, edited by R. Morrell. Durban: Indicator Press, 1996.

Bozzoli, B. 'Marxism, feminism and South African studies', *Journal of South African Studies* 9, no. 2 (April 1983).

Bozzoli, G.R. *A Vice-Chancellor Remembers: The Memoirs of Professor G.R. Bozzoli*. RSA: Alphaprint Randburg, 1995.

Branford, W.R.G. 'Examination systems and selection: The experiences of the admissions committee of the Board of the Faculty of Medicine, University of

Natal'. In *Medical Education in South Africa: Proceedings of the Conference on Medical Education held at the University of Natal, Durban in July 1964*, edited by J.V.O. Reid and A.J. Wilcot. Pietermaritzburg: University of Natal Press, 1965.

Breier, M. and Wildschut, A. 'Changing gender profile of medical schools in South Africa', *South African Medical Journal* 98, no. 7 (July 2008).

Breier, M. with Wildschut, A. *Doctors in a Divided Society: The Profession and Education of Medical Practitioners in South Africa*. Cape Town: HSRC Press, 2006.

Brink, C.J.H. 'Doctor shortage and health services', *South African Medical Journal* (14 August 1971).

Brookes, E.H. *A History of the University of Natal*. Pietermaritzburg: University of Natal Press, 1966.

Burns, C. 'Louisa Mvemve: A woman's advice to the public on the cure of various disease', *Kronos: Journal of Cape History* 23 (November 1996).

Burns, C. 'A man is a clumsy thing who does not know how to handle a sick person: Aspects of the history of masculinity and race in the shaping of male nursing in South Africa, 1900–50', *Journal of Southern African Studies* 24, no. 4 (December 1998).

Burton, A. (ed.) *Archive Stories: Facts, Fictions, and the Writing of History*. Durham and London: Duke University Press, 2005.

Buthelezi, S. 'The Black Consciousness Movement in South Africa in the late 1960s', *CEAPA Journal* no. 2 (December 1987).

Buthelezi, S. 'The emergence of black consciousness: An historical appraisal'. In *Bounds of Possibility: The Legacy of Steve Biko and Black Consciousness*, edited by B. Pityana, M. Ramphele, M. Mpumlwana and L. Wilson. Cape Town: David Philip; London and Atlantic Highlands, NJ: Zed Books, 1991.

Candib, L.M. 'How medicine tried to make a man out of me'. In *Women in Medical Education: An Anthology of Experience*, edited by Delese Wear. Albany, NY: State University of New York Press, 1996.

Cartwright, A.P. *Doctors on the Mines: A History of the Mine Medical Doctors Association of South Africa*. Cape Town: Purnell, 1971.

Cassel, J. 'Cultural factors in the interpretation of illness: A case study'. In *A Practice of Social Medicine: A South African Team's Experiences in Different African Communities*, edited by S.L. Kark and G. Steuart. Edinburgh and London: E. and S. Livingstone, 1962.

Christie, P. and Collins, C. 'Bantu education: Apartheid ideology and labour reproduction'. In *Apartheid and Education: The Education of Black South Africa*, edited by P. Kallaway. Johannesburg: Ravan Press, 1984.

Cohen, D.W. *The Combing of History*. Chicago and London: University of Chicago Press, 1994.

Connerton, P. *How Societies Remember*. Cambridge: Cambridge University Press, 1989.

Conway, B. 'Active remembering, selective forgetting, and collective identity: The case of Bloody Sunday', *Identity: An International Journal of Theory and Research* 3, no. 4 (2003).

Coombes, A.E. *Visual Culture and Public Memory in a Democratic South Africa*. Durham and London: Duke University Press, 2003.

Cooper, F. 'Conflict and connection: Rethinking colonial African history', *American Historical Review* 99, no. 5 (December 1994).

Cooper, F. and Stoler, A.L. (eds) *Tensions of Empire: Colonial Cultures in a Bourgeois World*. Berkeley, Los Angeles and London: University of California Press, 1997.

Cooper, P. *The Need for Doctors in South Africa*. Cape Town: South African Medical Scholarships Trust, 1974.

Coser, L.A. (ed.) *Maurice Halbwachs: On Collective Memory*. Chicago and London: University of Chicago Press, 1992.

Crane, S.A. 'AHR Forum: Writing the individual back into collective memory', *American Historical Review* (December 1997).

Crichton, D. 'The clinical work of the Department of Gynaecology and Obstetrics of the University of Natal during 1957: A brief review', reprinted from *Medical Proceedings* 4, no. 19 (20 September 1958).

Davies, R., O'Meara, D. and Sipho Dlamini, S. (comps.) *The Struggle for South Africa: A Reference Guide to Movements, Organisations and Institutions*, Vol. 2. London and Atlantic Highlands, NJ: Zed Books, 1985.

De Beer, C. *The South African Disease: Apartheid Health and Health Services*. London: Catholic Institute for International Relations, 1986.

De Craemer, W. and Fox, R.C. *The Emerging Physician: A Sociological Approach to the Development of a Congolese Medical Profession*. Stanford, CA: The Hoover Institution, 1968.

'Department of Social, Preventive and Family Medicine, University of Natal: Appointment of Professor Sidney L. Kark', *South African Medical Journal* 10 (March 1956).

Digby, A. *Diversity and Division in Medicine: Health Care in South Africa from the 1800s*. Oxford: Peter Lang, 2006.

Digby, A. 'Early black doctors in South Africa', *Journal of African History* 46, no. 3 (November 2005).

Digby, A. 'From racial segregation towards transformation'. In *At the Heart of Healing: Groote Schuur Hospital, 1938–2008*, A. Digby and H. Phillips with H. Deacon and K. Thomson. Auckland Park: Jacana, 2008.

Digby, A. and Phillips, H. with Deacon, H. and Thomson, K. *At the Heart of Healing: Groote Schuur Hospital, 1938–2008*. Auckland Park: Jacana, 2008.

Bibliography

Digby, A. and Sweet, H. 'Nurses as culture brokers in twentieth-century South Africa'. In *Plural Medicine, Tradition and Modernity, 1800–2000*, edited by W. Ernst. London and New York: Routledge, 2001.

Dlamini, J. *Native Nostalgia*. Auckland Park: Jacana, 2009.

Dlamini Buthelezi, M.S.T. *African Nurse Pioneers in KwaZulu-Natal, 1920–2000*. Canada, USA, UK: Trafford Publishing, 2004.

Downs, L.L. *Writing Gender History*. London: Hodder Arnold; and New York: Oxford University Press, 2004.

Dreijmanis, J. *The Role of the South African Government in Tertiary Education*. Johannesburg: South African Institute of Race Relations, 1988.

Dubow, S. *Scientific Racism in Modern South Africa*. Cambridge: Cambridge University Press, 1995.

Dyer, C., Adams, E.B., Seedat, A.M. and Morfopoulos, J. 'Fifty years at King Edward VIII Hospital, Durban', *South African Medical Journal* (22 November 1986).

Editorial, 'The non-European medical school', *South African Medical Journal* (27 April 1957).

Elias, H.R. *Short Story Kaleidoscope*. Northmead, RSA: Prestige Publications, 1995.

Ellis, S. and Sechaba, T. *Comrades against Apartheid: The ANC and the South African Communist Party in Exile*. London: James Currey; Bloomington: Indiana University Press, 1992.

Fatton, R. *Black Consciousness in South Africa*. Albany: State University of New York Press, 1986.

Feierman, S. and Janzen, J.M. (eds) *The Social Basis of Health and Healing in Africa*. Berkeley and Los Angeles: University of California Press, 1992.

Field, S. 'Turning up the volume: Dialogues about memory create oral histories', *South African Historical Journal* 60, no. 2 (2008).

Flint, K. *Healing Traditions: African Medicine, Cultural Exchange, and Competition in South Africa, 1820–1948*. Athens, OH: Ohio University Press; Pietermaritzburg: University of KwaZulu-Natal Press, 2008).

Freund, B. *Insiders and Outsiders: The Indian Working Class of Durban 1910–90*. Portsmouth, NH: Heinemann; Pietermaritzburg: University of Natal Press; and London: James Currey, 1995.

Gale, G.W. 'The Durban Medical School: A progress report', *South African Medical Journal* (7 May 1955).

Gale, G.W. 'Medical schools in Africa: A short historical and contemporary survey', *Journal of Medical Education* 34, no. 8 (August 1959).

Gear, H.S. 'The South African Native Health and Medical Service', *South African Medical Journal* xvii, no. 11 (12 June 1943).

Geiger, J.H. 'Community-oriented primary care: The legacy of Sidney Kark', *American Journal of Public Health* 83, no. 7 (July 1993).

Gelfand, M. *Christian Doctor and Nurse: The History of Medical Missions in South Africa*. Sandton: Mariannhill Mission Press, 1984.

Gerhart, G.M. *Black Power in South Africa: The Evolution of an Ideology*. Los Angeles: University of California Press, 1978.

Gish, S. *Alfred B. Xuma: African, American, South African*. London: Macmillan Press, 2000.

Gluckman, H. *Abiding Values: Speeches and Addresses*. Johannesburg: Caxton, 1970.

Goonam, K. *Coolie Doctor: An Autobiography*. Durban: Madiba Publications, 1991.

Gordon, I. 'Experience in the establishment of a medical school for non-white undergraduate students in South Africa'. In *Medical Education in South Africa: Proceedings of the Conference on Medical Education held at the University of Natal, Durban in July 1964,* edited by J.V.O. Reid and A.J. Wilcot. Pietermaritzburg: University of Natal Press, 1965.

Gordon, I. *Further Report on the Government's Intention to Remove the Faculty of Medicine from the University of Natal*. Durban: Hayne and Gibson, 4 May 1957.

Gordon, I. 'King Edward VIII Hospital: The teaching hospital of the Durban Medical School', *South African Medical Journal* (2 December 1961).

Gordon, I. *Report on the Government's Intended Action to Remove the Faculty of Medicine from the University of Natal*. Durban: Hayne and Gibson, 4 March 1957.

Gordon, I. *Third Report on the Government's Intention to Remove the Faculty of Medicine from the University of Natal*. Durban: Process Printers, 25 February 1958.

Gwala, N. 'State control, student politics and the crisis in black universities'. In *Popular Struggles in South Africa*, edited by William Cobbett and Robin Cohen. Trenton, NJ: Africa World Press, 1988.

Hadfield, L. 'Biko, Black Consciousness and "the system" eZinyoka: Oral history and Black Consciousness in practice in a rural Ciskei village', *South African Historical Journal* 62, no. 1 (2010).

Hamilton, C., Harris, V., Taylor, J., Pickover, M., Reid, G., and Saleh, R. (eds) *Refiguring the Archive*. Cape Town: David Philip, 2002.

Harley, E.H. 'The forgotten history of defunct black medical schools in the nineteenth and twentieth centuries and the impact of the Flexner Report', *Journal of the National Medical Association* 98, no. 9 (September 2006).

Harrison, D. 'The National Health Services Commission, 1942–1944: Its Origins and Outcome', *South African Medical Journal* (September 1993).

Headrick, D. *The Tools of Empire: Technology and European Imperialism in the Nineteenth Century*. New York: Oxford University Press, 1981.

Healy-Clancy, M. *A World of their Own: A History of South African Women's Education*. Pietermaritzburg: University of KwaZulu-Natal Press, 2013.

Hirson, B. *Year of Fire, Year of Ash: The Soweto Revolt: Roots of a Revolution?* London: Zed Press, 1979.

Hofmeyr, I. *'We Spend our Years as a Tale that is Told': Oral Historical Narrative in a South African Chiefdom.* Portsmouth, NH: Heinemann; Johannesburg: Witwatersrand University Press; and London: James Currey, 1993.

Hooks, B. *Feminist Theory from Margin to Centre.* Boston: South End Press, 1984.

Horrell, M. *Bantu Education to 1968.* Johannesburg: South African Institute of Race Relations, 1968.

Horrell, M. *The African Homelands of South Africa.* Johannesburg: South African Institute of Race Relations, 1973.

'Hospital serves non-whites', *South African Panorama* (February 1962).

Hudson, C.P., Kane-Berman, J. and Hickman, R. 'Women in medicine: A literature review – 1985–1996', *South African Medical Journal* 87, no. 11 (November 1997).

Hunt, N.R. *A Colonial Lexicon: Of Birth Ritual, Medicalisation, and Mobility in the Congo.* Durham and London: Duke University Press, 1999.

Hunter, M. *Love in the Time of AIDS.* Pietermaritzburg: University of KwaZulu-Natal Press, 2010.

Hyslop, J. *The Classroom Struggle: Policy and Resistance in South Africa, 1940–90.* Pietermaritzburg: University of Natal Press, 1999.

Iliffe, J. *East African Doctors: A History of the Modern Profession.* Cambridge: Cambridge University Press, 1998.

'In memoriam: Theodore Leonard Sarkin', *South African Medical Journal* 88, no. 6 (June 1998).

'The Institute of Family and Community Health (Union Health Department): Summary of the report of the Medical Officer-in-Charge, for the year ending 30 June 1950', *South African Medical Journal* (24 November 1951).

'Institutional hearing: The Health Sector', in *Truth and Reconciliation Commission of South Africa Report,* Vol. 4. Cape Town: Juta, 1998.

'Interviews: South African women doctors speak', Special Issue on Women in Medicine, *South African Medical Journal* (November 1997).

Jeeves, A. 'Delivering primary care in impoverished urban and rural communities – South Africa's Institute of Family and Community Health in the 1940s'. In *South Africa's 1940s: Worlds of Possibilities,* edited by S. Dubow and A. Jeeves. Cape Town: Double Storey Books, 2005.

Kallaway, P. (ed.) *Apartheid and Education: The Education of Black South Africans.* Johannesburg: Ravan Press, 1984.

Karis, T.G. and Gerhart, G.M. *From Protest to Challenge: A Documentary History of African Politics in South Africa, 1882–1990,* Volume 5. Pretoria: UNISA Press, 1997.

Kark, S.L. 'Family and community practice in the medical curriculum: A clinical teaching program in social medicine', *Journal of Medical Education* 34, no. 9 (September 1959).

Kark, S.L. 'Health centre service: A South African experiment in family health and medical care'. In *Social Medicine*, edited by E.H. Cluver. Johannesburg: Central News Agency, 1951.

Kark, S. and Kark, E. *Promoting Community Health: From Pholela to Jerusalem*. Johannesburg: Witwatersrand University Press, 1999.

Kark, S.L. and Kark, E. 'A practice of social medicine'. In *A Practice of Social Medicine: A South African Team's Experiences in Different African Communities*, edited by S.L. Kark and G. Steuart. Edinburgh and London: E. and S. Livingstone, 1962.

Kauffman, K.D. and Lindauer, D.L. (eds) *Aids and South Africa: The Social Expression of a Pandemic*. New York: Palgrave Macmillan, 2004.

Kirsch, R. and Knox, C. (eds) *UCT Medical School at 75*. Cape Town: UCT Department of Medicine, 1987.

Kuper, H. 'Nurses'. In *An African Bourgeoisie: Race, Class, and Politics in South Africa*, by L. Kuper. New Haven, CT, and London: Yale University Press, 1965.

Kuper, L. *An African Bourgeoisie: Race, Class, and Politics in South Africa*. New Haven, CT, and London: Yale University Press, 1965.

Last, M. and Chavunduka, G.L. (eds) *The Professionalisation of African Medicine*. Manchester: Manchester University Press, 1986.

Lewis, D. 'The politics of feminism in South Africa'. In *South African Feminisms: Writing, Theory, and Criticism 1990–94*, edited by M.J. Daymond. New York and London: Garland Publishing, 1996.

Lewis, G. *Between the Wire and the Wall: A History of South African 'Coloured' Politics*. New York: St. Martin's Press, 1987.

Liebenberg, I., Lortan, F., Nel, B. and Van der Westhuizen, G. (eds) *The Long March: The Story of the Struggle for Liberation in South Africa*. Pretoria: HAUM, 1994.

Lodge, T. *Black Politics in South Africa since 1945*. London and New York: Longman, 1983.

Lodge, T. *Politics in South Africa: From Mandela to Mbeki*. Cape Town: David Philip; Oxford: James Currey, 2002.

Lodge, T. and Nasson, B. *All, Here, and Now: Black Politics in South Africa in the 1980s*. Cape Town: Ford Foundation and David Philip, 1991.

Louw, J.H. *In the Shadow of Table Mountain: A History of the University of Cape Town Medical School*. Cape Town: Struik, 1969.

Luedke, T.J. and West, H.G. (eds) *Borders and Healers: Brokering Therapeutic Resources in Southeast Africa*. Bloomington and Indianapolis: Indiana University Press, 2006.

Lyons, M. 'The Power to Heal: African Medical Auxiliaries in Colonial Belgian Congo and Uganda'. In *Contesting Colonial Hegemony: State and Society in*

Africa and India, edited by D. Engels and S. Marks. London and New York: British Academic Press, 1994.

Macquarrie, J.W. 'The Sociological Background of the African University Student'. In *Medical Education in South Africa: Proceedings of the Conference on Medical Education held at the University of Natal, Durban in July 1964,* edited by J.V.O. Reid and A.J. Wilcot. Pietermaritzburg: University of Natal Press, 1965.

Maforah, N. 'Black, married, professional and a woman: Role conflicts?' *Agenda* 18 (1993).

Magaziner, D.R. *The Law and the Prophets: Black Consciousness in South Africa, 1968–77.* Auckland Park: Jacana, 2010.

Magaziner, D.R. 'Pieces of a (wo)man: Feminism, gender and adulthood in black consciousness, 1968–77', *Journal of Southern African Studies* 37, no. 1 (March 2011).

Makgoba, M.W. *Mokoko: The Makgoba Affair: A Reflection on Transformation.* Florida Hills, RSA: Vivlia Publishers, 1997.

Malherbe, E.G. *Never a Dull Moment.* Southern and Eastern Africa and the UK: Timmins Publishers, 1981.

Mangena, M. *On Your Own: Evolution of Black Consciousness in South Africa/ Azania.* Johannesburg: Skotaville, 1989.

Mankazana, E.M. 'A case for the traditional healer in South Africa', *South African Medical Journal* (1 December 1979).

Maré, G. *Ethnicity and Politics in South Africa.* London and Atlantic Highlands, NJ: Zed Books, 1993.

Marks, S. *The Ambiguities of Dependence in South Africa: Class, Nationalism, and the State in Twentieth-Century Natal.* Baltimore and London: Johns Hopkins University Press, 1986.

Marks, S. *Divided Sisterhood: Race, Class and Gender in the South African Nursing Profession.* Johannesburg: Witwatersrand University Press, 1994.

Marks, S. 'Doctors and the state: George Gale and South Africa's experiment in social medicine'. In *Science and Society in Southern Africa,* edited by S. Dubow. Manchester and New York: Manchester University Press, 2000.

Marks, S. 'South Africa's early experiment in social medicine: Its pioneers and politics', *American Journal of Public Health* 87, no. 3 (March 1997).

Marks, S. and Andersson, N. 'Industrialisation, rural health and the 1944 National Health Services Commission in South Africa'. In *The Social Basis of Health and Healing in Africa,* edited by Steven Feierman and John M. Janzen. Berkeley and Los Angeles: University of California Press, 1992.

Martineau, R. 'Women and education in South Africa: Factors influencing women's educational progress and their entry into traditionally male-dominated fields', *The Journal of Negro Education* 66, no. 4 (Autumn 1997).

Marx, A.W. *Lessons of Struggle: South African Internal Opposition, 1960–90.* New York and Oxford: Oxford University Press, 1992.

Mashaba, T.G. *Rising to the Challenge of Change: A History of Black Nursing in South Africa.* Cape Town: Juta, 1995.

Maylam, P. and Edwards, I. (eds) *The People's City: African Life in Twentieth-Century Durban.* Pietermaritzburg: University of Natal Press, 1996.

Mbali, M. 'AIDS discourses and the South African state: Government denialism and post-apartheid AIDS policy-making', *Transformation* 54 (2004).

Mbanjwa, T. (ed.) *Black Review, 1974/1975.* Black Community Programmes, 1975.

McCord, J.B. *My Patients were Zulus.* New York and Toronto: Rinehart and Co., 1951.

McCord, J.B. 'A native medical service in South Africa', *Journal of the Medical Association of South Africa* 14 (September 1930).

McCord, J.B. 'The Zulu witch doctor and medicine man', *South African Medical Record* xvi, no. 4 (April 1918).

McCord, M. *The Calling of Katie Makanya.* Cape Town and Johannesburg: David Philip, 1995.

McCulloch, J. *Asbestos Blues: Labour, Capital, Physicians and the State in South Africa.* Oxford: James Currey; Bloomington and Indianapolis: Indiana University Press, 2002.

McEwan, C. 'Building a postcolonial archive? Gender, collective memory and citizenship in post-apartheid South Africa', *Journal of Southern African Studies* 29, no. 3 (September 2003).

Mdlalose, F.T. *My Life: The Autobiography of Dr Frank T. Mdlalose.* Wierda Park: Action Publishers, 2006.

Meer, F. (ed.) *Resistance in the Townships.* Durban: Madiba Publications, 1989.

Meintjes, Y. 'The two-year internship training', *South African Medical Journal* 93, no. 5 (May 2003).

Modisane, B. *Blame Me on History.* New York and London: Simon & Schuster, 1986.

Mokoape, K., Mtintso, T. and Nhlapo, W. 'Towards the armed struggle'. In *Bounds of Possibility: The Legacy of Steve Biko and Black Consciousness*, edited by B. Pityana, M. Ramphele, M. Mpumlwana and L. Wilson. Cape Town: David Philip; London and Atlantic Highlands, NJ: Zed Books, 1991.

Molteno, F. 'The historical foundations of the schooling of black South Africans'. In *Apartheid and Education: The Education of Black South Africans*, edited by P. Kallaway. Johannesburg: Ravan Press, 1984.

Moodie, G.C. 'The state and the liberal universities in South Africa: 1948–90', *Higher Education* 27 (1994).

Moodley, K. 'The continued impact of black consciousness'. In *Bounds of Possibility: The Legacy of Steve Biko and Black Consciousness*, edited by Barney Pityana,

Mamphela Ramphele, Malusi Mpumlwana and Lindy Wilson. Cape Town, London and Atlantic Highlands, NJ: David Philip and Zed Books, 1991.

Morantz-Sanchez, R. *Conduct Unbecoming a Woman: Medicine on Trial in Turn-of-the-Century Brooklyn*. New York and Oxford: Oxford University Press, 1999.

More, E.S. *Restoring the Balance: Women Physicians and the Profession of Medicine, 1850–1995*. Cambridge, MA, and London: Harvard University Press, 1999.

Morrell, R. 'Of boys and men: Masculinity and gender in southern African studies', *Journal of Southern African Studies*, no. 4 (December 1998).

Morrell, R., (ed.) *Political Economies and Identities in KwaZulu-Natal: Historical and Social Perspective*. Durban: Indicator Press, 1996.

Murray, B.K. 'Wits as an 'open' university 1939–59: Black admissions to the University of the Witwatersrand', *Journal of Southern African Studies* 16, no. 4 (December 1990).

Murray, B.K. *Wits the Early Years: A History of the University of the Witwatersrand Johannesburg and its Precursors, 1896–1939*. Johannesburg: Witwatersrand University Press, 1982.

Murray, B.K. *Wits the 'Open' Years: A History of the University of the Witwatersrand, Johannesburg, 1939–59*. Johannesburg: Witwatersrand University Press, 1997.

Mzamane, M.V. and Howarth, D.R. 'Representing blackness: Steve Biko and the Black Consciousness Movement'. In *South Africa's Resistance Press: Alternative Voices in the Last Generation under Apartheid*, edited by Les Switzer and Mohamed Adhikari. Athens, OH: Ohio University Centre for International Studies, 2000.

Mzamane, M.V., Maaba, B. and Biko, N. 'The Black Consciousness Movement'. In *The Road to Democracy in South Africa: Volume 2, 1970–80*, by the South African Democracy Education Trust (SADET). Pretoria: UNISA Press, 2006.

Naidoo, B.T. 'A history of the Durban Medical School', *South African Medical Journal* 50, no. 41 (25 September 1976).

Naidoo, P. *Footprints in Grey Street*. Durban: Far Ocean Jetty Publishing, 2002.

'The Natal Medical School – twenty-five years', *South African Medical Journal* 50, no. 41 (25 September 1976).

'The national health service', *South African Medical Journal* 19, no. 2 (27 January 1945).

Ncayiyana, D. 'Medical education challenges in South Africa', *Medical Education* 33, no. 10 (October 1999).

Noble, V. 'Health is much too important a subject to be left to doctors: African assistant health workers in Natal during the early twentieth century', *Journal of Natal and Zulu History* 24 and 25 (2006–7).

Noble, V. 'A medical education with a difference: A history of the training of black student doctors in social, preventive and community-oriented primary health care at the University of Natal Medical School, 1940s–1960', *South African Historical Journal* 61, 3 (September 2009).

Ntsaluba, A. 'The national health system: The way forward for health care in SA', *South African Medical Journal* 1 (1997).

Nuttall, S. and Coetzee, C. (eds) *Negotiating the Past: The Making of Memory in South Africa*. Oxford and New York: Oxford University Press, 2002.

O'Meara, D. *Forty Lost Years: The Apartheid State and the Politics of the National Party, 1948–94*. Johannesburg: Ravan Press and Athens, OH: Ohio University Press, 1996

Oosthuizen, G.C., Clifford-Vaughan, A.A., Behr, A.L. and Rauche, G.A. *Challenge to a South African University: The University of Durban-Westville*. Cape Town: Oxford University Press, 1981.

Oosthuizen, S.F. 'The intern year'. In *Medical Education in South Africa: Proceedings of the Conference on Medical Education held at the University of Natal, Durban in July 1964*, edited by J.V.O. Reid and A.J. Wilcot. Pietermaritzburg: University of Natal Press, 1965.

Oppenheimer, G.M. and Bayer, R. *Shattered Dreams? An Oral History of the South African AIDS Epidemic*. Oxford and New York: Oxford University Press, 2007.

Packard, R.M. *White Plague, Black Labor: Tuberculosis and the Political Economy of Health and Disease in South Africa*. Berkeley and Los Angeles. University of California Press, 1989.

Padayachee, D. *What's Love Got to Do with It? And Other Stories*. Johannesburg: COSAW Publishing, 1992.

Parle, J. *States of Mind: Searching for Mental Health in Natal and Zululand, 1868–1918*. Pietermaritzburg: University of KwaZulu-Natal Press, 2007.

Patton, A. *Physicians, Colonial Racism, and Diaspora in West Africa*. Gainesville: University of Florida Press, 1996.

Pearson, M.G. 'History of government hospitals in Durban, 1858–1945', *South African Medical Journal* (3 June 1961).

Perks, R. and Thomson, A. (eds) *The Oral History Reader*. 2nd ed. London and New York: Routledge, 2006.

Perry, A. *A Study of the Employment Experiences and Attitudes to Employment among African Secondary School Leavers in Durban* (Johannesburg: South African Institute of Race Relations, September 1974).

Phillips, H. *The University of Cape Town 1918–48: The Formative Years*. Cape Town: University of Cape Town Press, 1993.

Phillips, H. 'White coats and stethoscopes: Doctors and medical students at GSH'. In *At the Heart of Healing: Groote Schuur Hospital, 1938–2008*, A. Digby and H. Phillips with H. Deacon and K. Thomson. Auckland Park: Jacana, 2008.

Pillay, V.K.G. 'Some thoughts on intern training', *South African Medical Journal* (2 December 1961).

Pityana, B. Ramphele, M., Mpumlwana, M. and Wilson, L. (eds) *Bounds of Possibility: The Legacy of Steve Biko and Black Consciousness*. Cape Town, London and Atlantic Highlands, NJ: David Philip and Zed Books.

Platzky, L. and Walker, C. *The Surplus People: Forced Removals in South Africa*. Johannesburg: Ravan Press, 1985.

Portelli, A. 'What makes oral history different'. In *The Oral History Reader*, 2nd ed, edited by R. Perks and A. Thomas. London and New York: Routledge, 2006.

Posel, D. *The Making of Apartheid 1948–61: Conflict and Compromise*. Oxford: Clarendon Press, 1991.

'The proposed transfer of the Durban Medical School', *South African Medical Journal* (23 March 1957).

Radstone, S. and Schwarz, B. 'Introduction: Mapping memory'. In *Memory: Histories, Theories, Debates*, edited by S. Radstone and B. Schwarz. New York: Fordham University Press, 2010.

Ralekhetho, M. 'The black university in South Africa: Ideological captive or transformative agent?' In *Knowledge and Power in South Africa: Critical Perspectives across the Disciplines*, edited by J.D. Jansen. Johannesburg: Skotaville, 1991.

Ramamurthi, T.G. *Apartheid and Indian South Africans: A Study of the Role of Ethnic Indians in the Struggle against Apartheid in South Africa*. New Delhi: Reliance Publishing House, 1995.

Ramphele, M. *Across Boundaries: The Journey of a South African Woman Leader*. New York: Feminist Press, 1995.

Ramphele, M. 'The dynamics of gender within black consciousness organisations: A personal view'. In *Bounds of Possibility: The Legacy of Steve Biko and Black Consciousness*, edited by B. Pityana, M. Ramphele, M. Mpumlwana and L. Wilson. Cape Town, London and Atlantic Highlands, NJ: David Philip and Zed Books, 1991.

Ramphele, M. 'Empowerment and symbols of hope'. In *Bounds of Possibility: The Legacy of Steve Biko and Black Consciousness*, edited by B. Pityana, M. Ramphele, M. Mpumlwana and L. Wilson. Cape Town, London and Atlantic Highlands, NJ: David Philip and Zed Books, 1991.

Reid, J.V.O. 'A study of second-year examinations'. In *Medical Education in South Africa: Proceedings of the Conference on Medical Education held at the University of Natal, Durban in July 1964*, edited by J.V.O. Reid and A.J. Wilcot. Pietermaritzburg: University of Natal Press, 1965.

Reid, J.V.O. and Wilcot, A.J. (eds) *Medical Education in South Africa: Proceedings of the Conference on Medical Education held at the University of Natal, Durban in July 1964*. Pietermaritzburg: University of Natal Press, 1965.

Reid, S. and Giddy, J. 'Rural health and human rights – Summary of a submission to the Truth and Reconciliation Commission Health Sector Hearings, 17 June 1997', *South African Medical Journal* (August 1998).

Reid, S.J. 'Compulsory community service for doctors in South Africa – An evaluation of the first year', *South African Medical Journal* 91 (2001).

Reid, S.J. 'COPC experiences with medical students at the Valley Trust, South Africa', *COPaCetic* 5, no. 1 (Summer/Fall 1998).

Reid, S.J. 'Crisis in rural South Africa', *South African Family Practitioners*, 23 (2001).

'Report of the Department of Public Health for year ending 30 June 1925', *Medical Journal of South Africa* 21, no. 9 (April 1926).

Retief, F.P. 'The Medical University of Southern Africa after five years', *South African Medical Journal* (27 November 1982).

Rich, P. *Hope and Despair: English-Speaking Intellectuals and South African Politics, 1896–1976*. London: British Academic Press, 1993.

Rich, P. *White Power and the Liberal Conscience: Racial Segregation and South African Liberalism, 1921–60*. Manchester: Manchester University Press, 1984.

Riska, E. and Weger, K. (eds) *Gender, Work and Medicine: Women and the Medical Division of Labour*. London: Sage Publications, 1993.

Ritchie, D.A. 'Introduction: The evolution of oral history'. In *The Oxford Handbook of Oral History*, edited by D.A. Ritchie. Oxford and New York: Oxford University Press, 2011.

Ritchie, D.A. (ed.) *The Oxford Handbook of Oral History*. Oxford and New York: Oxford University Press, 2011.

Roux, G.H. 'The medical profession and the witchdoctor', *South African Medical Journal* (8 October 1977).

Salber, E.J. *The Mind is Not the Heart: Recollections of a Woman Physician*. Durham and London: Duke University Press, 1989.

Savitt, T. 'Abraham Flexner and the black medical schools', *Journal of the National Medical Association* 98, no. 9 (September 2006).

Searle, C. 'The second-class doctor and medical assistant in South Africa', *South African Medical Journal* (31 March 1973).

Seedat, A. *Crippling a Nation: Health in Apartheid South Africa*. London: International Defence and Aid Fund for Southern Africa, 1984.

Seedat, Y.K. 'The health crisis in Natal – A personal view', *South African Medical Journal* (7 July 1990).

Seekings, J. *Heroes or Villains? Youth Politics in the 1980s*. Johannesburg: Ravan Press, 1993.

Seidman, G.W. 'Gendered citizenship: South Africa's democratic transition and the construction of a gendered state', *Gender and Society* 13, no. 3 (June 1999).

Bibliography

Shapiro, E.C. and Lowenstein, L.M. (eds) *Becoming a Physician: Development of Values and Attitudes in Medicine*. Cambridge, MA: Ballinger Publishing, 1979.

Shapiro, K.A. 'Doctors or Medical Aids – The debate over the training of black medical personnel for the rural black population in South Africa in the 1920s and 1930s', *Journal of Southern African Studies* 13, no. 2 (January 1987).

'Shattering the male monopoly: The history and struggle of female doctors', *The Leech* 62, no. 3 (November 1993).

Sono, T. *Reflections on the Origins of Black Consciousness in South Africa*. Pretoria: HSRC, 1993.

Spencer, I. *Hope Beyond the Shadows*. Kloof: Forest Publishers, 1992.

Starz, A. *Between Laughter and Tears*. Ladysmith, RSA: Sinclair Publishing, 1986.

Stubbs, A. 'Martyr of hope: A personal memoir'. In *I Write What I Like*, by Steve Biko. New York: HarperSanFrancisco, 1978.

Susser, M. 'A South African odyssey in community health: A memoir of the impact of the teachings of Sidney Kark', *American Journal of Public Health* 83, no. 7 (July 1993).

Sweet, H. and Digby, A. 'Race, identity and the nursing profession in South Africa, c. 1850–1958'. In *New Directions in the History of Nursing: International Perspectives*, edited by S. McGann and B. Mortimer. London: Routledge, 2004.

Taylor, A.B. 'Presidential address'. In *Medical Education in South Africa: Proceedings of the Conference on Medical Education held at the University of Natal, Durban in July 1964*, edited by J.V.O. Reid and A.J. Wilcot. Pietermaritzburg: University of Natal Press, 1965.

Thomson, A. 'Memory and remembering in oral history'. In *The Oxford Handbook of Oral History*, edited by D.A. Ritchie. Oxford and New York: Oxford University Press, 2011.

Thompson, L. *A History of South Africa*. New Haven, CT, and London: Yale University Press, 1990.

Thornton, E. 'A medical and nursing service for natives in South Africa', *Journal of the Medical Association of South Africa* 5 (13 September 1930).

Tobias, P.V. 'Apartheid and medical education: The training of black doctors in South Africa', *The Leech* 60, no. 1 (March 1991).

Tollman, S.M. 'The Pholela Health Centre – the origins of community-oriented primary health care: An appreciation of the work of Sidney and Emily Kark', *South African Medical Journal* 84, no. 10 (October 1994).

Tonkin, E. *Narrating our Pasts: The Social Construction of Oral History*. Cambridge: Cambridge University Press, 1992.

Trostle, J. 'Anthropology and epidemiology in the twentieth century: A selective history of collaborative projects and theoretical affinities, 1920–70'. In *Anthropology and Epidemiology*, edited by C.R. Janes et al. Dordrecht: Reidel Publishing, 1986.

Trouillot, M. *Silencing the Past: Power and the Production of History*. Boston: Beacon Press, 1995.

Truth and Reconciliation: A Process of Transformation at the UCT Health Sciences Faculty. Cape Town: UCT Faculty of Health Science, 2002.

Truth and Reconciliation Commission of South Africa Report. Vol. 4. Cape Town: Juta, 1998.

Tunmer, R. 'Vocational aspirations of African high-school pupils'. In *Student Perspectives on South Africa*, edited by H.W. van der Merwe and D. Welsh. Cape Town: David Philip, 1972.

Unterhalter, B. 'Discrimination against women in the South African medical profession', *Social Science and Medicine* 20 (1985).

Unterhalter, B. 'Shattering the male monopoly: The history and struggle of female doctors', *The Leech* 62 no.3 (November 1993).

Vahed, G. 'The making of 'Indianness': Indian politics in South Africa during the 1930s and 1940s', *Journal of Natal and Zulu History* 17 (1997).

Van der Linde, I. 'MEDUNSA at twenty', *South African Medical Journal* (December 1996).

Vaughan, M. *Curing their Ills: Colonial Power and African Illness*. Cambridge: Polity Press, 1991.

Vietzen, S. 'Beyond school: Some developments in higher education in Durban in the 1920s and the influence of Mabel Palmer', *Natalia* 14 (December 1984).

Vietzen, S. 'Mabel Palmer and black higher education in Natal, 1936–42', *Journal of Natal and Zulu History* vi (1983).

Waetjen, T. 'Kitchen publics: *Indian Delights*, gender and culinary diaspora', *South African Historical Journal* 61, no. 3 (2009).

Waetjen, T. *Workers and Warriors: Masculinity and the Struggle for Nation in South Africa*. Cape Town: HSRC Press, 2004.

Walker, C. (ed.) *Women and Gender in Southern Africa to 1945*. Cape Town: David Philip, 1990.

Walker, C. *Women and Resistance in South Africa*. London: Onyx Press, 1982.

Walker, L. 'The colour white: Racial and gendered closure in the South African medical profession', *Ethnic and Racial Studies* 28, no. 2 (March 2005).

Walker, L. '"Conservative pioneers": The formation of the South African Society of Medical Women', *Social History of Medicine* 14, no. 3 (2001).

Wallace, M. *Health, Power and Politics in Windhoek, Namibia, 1914–1945*. Basel: P. Schlettwein Publishing, 2002.

Watson, W.H. *Against the Odds: Blacks in the Profession of Medicine in the United States*. New Brunswick, NJ, and London: Transaction Publishers, 1999.

Wendland, C.L. *A Heart for the Work: Journeys through an African Medical School*. Chicago and London: University of Chicago Press, 2010.

Who's Who of Southern Africa, 1964. Johannesburg: Wootton and Gibson, 1965.

Wilson, L. 'Bantu Stephen Biko: A life'. In *Bounds of Possibility: The Legacy of Steve Biko and Black Consciousness*, edited by B. Pityana, M. Ramphele, M. Mpumlwana and L. Wilson. Cape Town, London and Atlantic Highlands, NJ: David Philip and Zed Books, 1991.

Witz, A. *Professions and Patriarchy*. London and New York: Routledge, 1992.

Woods, D. *Biko*. New York: Henry Holt and Company, 1978, 1987.

Xaba, T. 'Masculinity and its malcontents: The confrontation between "struggle masculinity" and "post-struggle masculinity"'. In *Changing Men in Southern Africa*, edited by R. Morrell. Pietermaritzburg: University of Natal Press; London and New York: Zed Books, 2001.

Xuma, A.B. 'The training of natives in medicine: Notes on a native medical service in rural areas', *Journal of the Medical Association of South Africa* (24 January 1931).

Yach, D. and Tollman, S.M. 'Public health initiatives in South Africa in the 1940s and 1950s: Lessons for a post-apartheid era', *American Journal of Public Health* 83, no. 7 (July 1993).

UNIVERSITY OF NATAL/KWAZULU-NATAL PUBLICATIONS

Chetty, D. and Maharaj, S. (Managing editors) *Doris Duke Medical Research Institute*. University of KwaZulu-Natal: Public Affairs and Corporate Communications, 2007.

Moodley, J. and Maharaj, S. (Managing editors) *University of Natal Nelson R. Mandela School of Medicine: 50 Years of Achievement in Teaching, Service and Research*. University of Natal Nelson R. Mandela School of Medicine: Communications Office, 2001.

1951–1976: 25 Years of the Faculty of Medicine at the University of Natal. University of Natal: Communication and Publicity, 1977.

The University of Natal Durban Medical School: A Response to the Challenge of Africa. Durban: Hayne and Gibson, 1954.

The University of Natal Medical School 1951–1991: Meeting the Challenge of Change. University of Natal: Communication and Publicity, 1991.

University of Natal Medical School Reconciliation Graduation Booklet 1995. Durban: Indicator Press, December 1995.

UNIVERSITY OF NATAL/KWAZULU-NATAL AUDIO-VISUAL PUBLICATIONS

Students in the Barracks: Memories of Alan Taylor Residence. University of Natal, Durban: Audio-Visual Alternatives, 1989.

University of Natal Medical School Promotion Video. University of Natal, Durban: Audio-Visual Centre, 2001.

University of Natal, Nelson R. Mandela School of Medicine, Fiftieth Anniversary Banquet.
University of Natal, Durban: Audio-Visual Centre, 29 July 2000.

University of Natal Reconciliation Graduation Ceremony. University of Natal, Durban:
Audio-Visual Centre, 1995.

UNPUBLISHED SOURCES

Beale, M.A. 'Apartheid and university education, 1948–70'. PhD diss., University of the Witwatersrand, 1998.

Budree, R. and Ntuli, P. 'UKZN report change strategy workshops, Nelson R. Mandela School of Medicine', 12 April 2006.

Cassimjee, A. '"A good training ground": The lives of four South African Indian doctors who graduated in the Republic of Ireland during the 1960s and 1970s'. Honours thesis, University of KwaZulu-Natal, 2011.

Devenish, A. 'Negotiating healing: The professionalisation of traditional healers in KwaZulu-Natal between 1985 and 2003'. Master's diss., University of Natal, 2003.

Esselaar, P.A. '"Idealism tempered by realism": Dr E.G. Malherbe and issues of segregation and apartheid at the University of Natal, 1945–65'. Master's diss., University of the Witwatersrand, 1998).

Horwitz, S.J. '"A phoenix rising": A social history of Baragwanath Hospital, Soweto, South Africa, 1942–90'. DPhil diss., Oxford University, 2006.

Maharaj, B. 'University of Natal Medical School submission to the Truth and Reconciliation Commission', 23 June 1997.

Marks, S. 'Social medicine in South Africa in the mid-twentieth century: The international context'. Seminar Paper, WISER, Johannesburg, 17 July 2006.

McLean, M. 'Student perceptions of their first and second year experiences of medical studies at the University of Natal'. Master's diss., University of Natal, 1999.

Mindel, M.N. 'The construction of medical education in an unequal society: A study of the University of Cape Town Medical School, 1904–97'. PhD diss., University of London, 2003.

Modiba, A. 'MSRC Racism Report presented to the faculty and students of the University of Natal, Nelson R. Mandela School of Medicine', 26 September 2004.

Monamodi, I.S. 'Medical doctors under segregation and apartheid: A sociological analysis of professionalization among doctors in South Africa, 1900–80'. PhD diss., Indiana University, 1996.

Naidoo, L.R. and Rajab, D.R. 'A survey of sexual harassment and related issues among students at the University of Natal Durban campus'. Durban: UN Student Counselling Centre, December 1992.

Noble, V. 'Doctors divided: Gender, race and class anomalies in the production of black medical doctors in apartheid South Africa, 1948 to 1994'. PhD diss., University of Michigan, 2005.

Noble, V. '"A laboratory of change": A critical study of the Durban Medical School and its community health experiment, 1930–60'. Master's diss., University of Natal, Durban, 1999.

Rural Doctors' Association of Southern Africa. Position Paper. 'Crisis in staffing of rural hospitals', 2001.

Scholtz, M. 'Mervyn Susser and Zena Stein: Pioneers in community health and their Jewish identity as an orienting factor in their contribution'. Honours thesis, University of Natal, 1999.

Shuenyane, E.N. 'Black medical students' perceptions of medical school and the medical course'. M Ed. diss., University of the Witwatersrand, 1991.

Twine, J.L. '"I'm just an ordinary nurse": A life history of Matron Bongiwe Bolani'. Honours thesis, University of Natal, 1997.

Vis, L. 'We sow the seed: Perspectives of health educators at the Institute of Family and Community Health in Durban in the 1940s and 1950s'. Master's diss., University of KwaZulu-Natal, 2004.

Walker, E. 'The South African Society of Medical Women, 1951–92: Its origins, nature and impact on white women doctors'. PhD diss., University of the Witwatersrand, 1999.

Watts, H.L. 'Black doctors: An investigation into aspects of the training and career of students and graduates from the medical school of the University of Natal. Part I: The students'. University of Natal, Durban: Institute for Social Research, 1975.

Watts, H.L. 'Black doctors: An investigation into aspects of the training and career of students and graduates from the medical school of the University of Natal. Part II: The graduates'. University of Natal, Durban: Institute for Social Research, 1976.

Watts, H.L. 'Black doctors: An investigation into aspects of the training and career of students and graduates from the medical school of the University of Natal. Part III: The attitudes and opinions of staff'. University of Natal, Durban: Institute for Social Research, 1976.

INTERVIEWS

Conducted by the author (some interviewees preferred not to have their names disclosed)
Bolani, Bongiwe. Durban, 1 May 1999.
Coovadia, Jerry. Durban, 24 June 2003, 27 June 2003, 4 July 2003.
Fehrsen, Sam. Pretoria, 22 August 2003.
Giddy, Janet. Hillcrest, 24 May 2003, 2 June 2003.

Goonam, K. Durban, 13 October 1997.

Hadebe, Bandile. Durban, 7 June 2004.

Kallichurum, Soromini. Durban, 29 May 1999.

Kistnasamy, M. Barry. Durban, 26 August 2003.

KM. Durban, 14 November 2003.

MA. Durban, 23 September 2003, 6 November 2003.

Maharaj, Breminand. Durban, 10 June 2003.

Mahlaba, Ntuthuko. Durban, 7 June 2004.

Mashego, May. Durban, 7 October 2003, 14 October 2003; Ashburton, 18 October 2003.

Matjila, Maila J. Durban, 11 July 2003, 18 July 2003, 22 September 2003.

Mayet, Fatima. Durban, 4 June 1999.

MM. Durban, 28 July 2003.

Modiba, Ali. Durban, 4 June 2004.

Naidoo, B.T. Durban, 15 September 2003, 10 November 2003.

Naidoo, K.P. Durban, 4 June 2004.

Ndlovu, Mfanyana J. Durban, 14 August 2003.

Philpott, Hugh. Kloof, 14 July 2003.

Pitsoe, S.B. Durban, 17 July 2003.

Price, Max. Johannesburg, 19 August 2003.

Pudifin, Dennis J. Durban, 2 July 2003.

Reid, John V.O. Plettenberg Bay, 16 June 2002.

Reid, Steve. Hillcrest, 24 May 2003; Durban, 10 June 2003.

Seedat, Y.K. Durban, 7 July 2003, 14 July 2003.

Susser, Mervyn and Stein, Zena. Durban, 4 June 1999.

TM. Pretoria, 21 August 2003.

Wilson, Veronica. Durban, 6 November 2003.

ZM. Durban, 11 September 2003, 6 October 2003.

Conducted by other researchers

Interview with Albertina Luthuli, 10 January 1993, conducted by Padraig O'Malley, http://www.nelsonmandela.org/omalley/index.php/site/q/03lv00017.htm

Interview with Nomsa Ngakane, 26 August 1992, conducted by Padraig O'Malley, http://www.nelsonmandela.org/omalley/index.php/site/q/03lv00017.htm

Interview with Sidney and Emily Kark, conducted by C.C. Jinabhai and Nkosazana Zuma, Durban, South Africa, 1992.

Interview with S. Kark and I. Gordon on the 'Facts and Aspects of our Medical School which are not Recorded', conducted by S. Cameron-Dow, December 1980.

University of the Witwatersrand, South African History Archive, South African Political Materials 1964–1990, The Karis-Gerhart Collection, Interviews. Part I:

Folder 8, Coovadia, Jerry, conducted by Gail Gerhart and Steve Mufson in New York, 2 June 1988.

Folder 22, Mdlalose, Frank, conducted by TK, 24 May 1977.

Folder 23, Mji, Diliza, conducted by Gail Gerhart in New York, 2 June 1987.

Folder 23, Mji, Sikose, conducted by Victoria Butler in Lusaka, February 1988.

Folder 23, Mokoena, Aubrey, conducted by Gail Gerhart in Johannesburg, 8 July 1989.

Folder 26, Mpumlwana, Malusi, conducted by Gail Gerhart in Tarrytown, 16 May 1987.

Folder 26, Mpumlwana, Malusi, Mbanjwa, Thoko and Ramphele, Mamphela, conducted by Gail Gerhart and TK in Cape Town, 3 November 1985.

Folder 32, Ramphele, Mamphela, conducted by Gail Gerhart at Columbia University, New York, 26 October 1989.

Folder 41, Zuma, Nkosazana Dlamini, conducted by Gail Gerhart in London, 3 July 1988.

QUESTIONNAIRES

Pooba Govender, 2003.

HA, 2003.

Shan Naidoo, 2003.

AAH, 2003.

C, 2003.

WEBSITES

'Academic goes to court over racism allegations', *Legalbrief*, 13 August 2007 http://www.legalbrief.co.za/article.php?story=20070813080503581

'Afrikaner Broederbond', *South African History Online*, http://www.sahistory.org.za/organisations/afrikaner-broederbond

Aluka, http://www.aluka.org/action/showMetadata?doi=10.5555/AL.SFF.DOCUMENT.1681.577.000.000.Sep1970

'Azanian People's Organisation', *South African History Online*, http://www.sahistory.org.za/topic/azanian-peoples-organization-azapo

Beaver, T. and Coan, S. 'Two UKZN professors suspended', *Witness*, 26 April 2012, http://www.witness.co.za/index.php?showcontent&global%5B_id%5D=80257

Bolowana, A. 'Ex-students back racism report', *Mercury*, 10 October 2005, http://ccrri.ukzn.ac.za/archive/archive/files/pra20051006047057_2ba7a66fe4.pdf

Coan, S. 'Doctors seek probe into UKZN', *Weekend Witness*, 2 June 2012, http://www/witness.co.za/index.php?showcontent&global%5B_id%5D=82052

'Curriculum Vitae Y.K. Seedat', http://www.hospice.co.za/site/files/5600/CURRICULUM%20VITAE%201%20pageProf%20Seedat.doc

'Durban doctors take on professor over "racism"', *Daily News*, 18 April 2012, http://www.iol.co.za/dailynews/news/durban-doctors-take-on-professor-over-racism-1.1278724

'Frank Mdlalose', *Who's Who Southern Africa*, http://www.whoswhosa.co.za/frank-mdlalose-4125

Gerhart, G.M. 'Edgar Brookes 1897 to 1979', in the *Dictionary of African Christian Biography*, http://www.dacb.org/stories/southafrica/brookes_edgar.html

'History of MEDUNSA', http://www.medunsa.ac.za/faculties/nsph/nsph_about/about_medunsa1.htm

'Human Rights and Health: The Legacy of Apartheid', *The American Association for the Advancement of Science*, http://shr.aaas.org/loa/sector.htm

'Indo-African race row at South African university', *webindia123.com*, 16 October 2005, http://h-net.msu.edu/cgi-bin/logbrowse.pl?trx=vx&list=h-sa-higher-education&month=0510&week=c&msg=YFCqlWqdLQOtL3Fqx6Rw9A&user=&pw=

'Jerry Coovadia', *Who's Who Southern Africa*, http://www.whoswhosa.co.za/jerry-coovadia-2890

Lloyd, S.M. 'A short history of Howard University College of Medicine', http://medicine.howard.edu/about/history/default.htm

Makhaye, K. Article on Albertina Luthuli, http://www.northcoastcourier.co.za/2009/sep25/luthuli.htm

'Malegapuru Makgoba', *Who's Who Southern Africa*, http://www.whoswhosa.co.za/malegapuru-makgoba-5255

'Mamphela Ramphele', *Who's Who Southern Africa*, http://www.whoswhosa.co.za/mamphela-ramphele-4739

Mchunu, N. 'Medical school row widens', *Witness*, 8 October 2005, http://ccrri.ukzn.ac.za/archive/archive/files/pra20051008047057_ff87e3cf66.pdf

Medley, L. 'Top UKZN academics suspended from posts', *Daily News*, 27 April 2012, http://www.iol.co.za/dailynews/news/top-ukzn-academics-suspended-from-posts-1.1285369

'Nkosazana Dlamini Zuma', *Who's Who Southern Africa*, http://www.whoswhosa.co.za/nkosazana-dlamini-zuma-919

Pillay, T. 'Outcome of UKZN boss hearing due', *Sunday Times*, 10 June 2012, http://www.timeslive.co.za/sundaytimes/2012/06/10/outcome-of-ukzn-boss-hearing-due

Potgieter, De Wet. 'University of dirty tricks', *The New Age*, 6 January 2012, http://www.thenewage.co.za/52428-1007-53-University_of_dirty_tricks

Potgieter, De Wet. 'Talk of racism and hidden agendas', *The New Age*, 6 March 2012, http://www.thenewage.co.za/mobi/Detail.aspx?NewsID=52580& CatID=1010

'A short history', *Howard University College of Medicine*, http://medicine.howard.edu/about/history/default.htm

'Suspension of lecturers welcomed', *Daily News*, 17 October 2005, webindia123, http://h-net.msu.edu/cgi-bin/logbrowse.pl?trx=vx&list=h-sa-higher-education &month=0510&week=c&msg=YFCqlWqdLQOtL3Fqx6Rw9A&user=& pw=

'Top doc in legal battle', *Post*, 8 August 2007 http://www.highbeam.com/doc/1G1-167380171.html

'UKZN respond to rumble', *The Post*, 11 June 2008, http://lists.fahamu.org/pipermail/debate-list/2008-June/014169.html

'Wilson's disease', *MedlinePlus*, http://www.nlm.nih.gov/medlineplus/ency/article/000785.htm

'Zulu Chief Cyprian Bhekuzulu', *South African History Online*, http://www.sahistory.org.za/dated-event/zulu-chief-cyprian-bhekuzulu-born

'Zweli Mkhize', *Who's Who Southern Africa*, http://www.whoswhosa.co.za/zweli-mkhize-2310

Images source list

Figures

Index